RSSDI Atlas of Dermatological Conditions in Diabetes

RSSDI Atlas of Dermatological Conditions in Diabetes

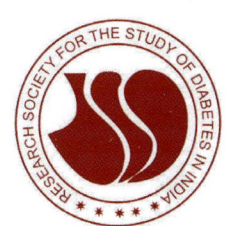

Editor-in-Chief

NK Singh MD FICP FACP F-RSSDI
Director
Department of Diabetology
Diabetes and Heart Research Centre
Dhanbad, Jharkhand, India
VICE President (Elect) 2026–2029, RSSDI
Founder CME INDIA

Assistant Editors

Akashkumar N Singh
MD(Medicine) MSc(Diabetes)
FRCP(Edinburgh and Glasgow) FACP
FICP FRSSDI Fellow Diabetes India
FIACM FISH FISC FCCDSI
Director
Department of Internal Medicine
and Diabetes
Manjalpur Hospital Private Limited
Vadodara, Gujarat, India

Anuradha Kapoor MD
PG diploma in Clinical Endocrinology
and Diabetes, Fellow ICCMD(CCDSI)
Preventive Diabetologist
Department of Diabetology
Lifeline Medicare Hospital
Mumbai, Maharashtra, India

Amit Kumar MD(Derm & STD)
Dermatologist
Department of Dermatology
CosmoDerma
Ranchi, Jharkhand, India

Foreword

Vijay Vishwanathan
Anuj Maheshwari
Sanjay Agarwal

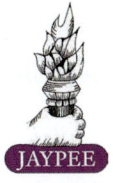

JAYPEE BROTHERS MEDICAL PUBLISHERS
The Health Sciences Publisher
New Delhi | London

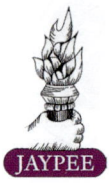

Jaypee Brothers Medical Publishers (P) Ltd

Headquarters
EMCA House, 23/23-B
Ansari Road, Daryaganj
New Delhi 110 002, India
Landline: +91-11-23272143, +91-11-23272703
+91-11-23282021, +91-11-23245672
e-mail: jaypee@jaypeebrothers.com

Corporate Office
4838/24, Ansari Road, Daryaganj
New Delhi 110 002, India
Phone: +91-11-43574357
Fax: +91-11-43574314
e-mail: jaypee@jaypeebrothers.com

Overseas Office
JP Medical Ltd.
83, Victoria Street, London
SW1H 0HW (UK)
Phone: +44-20 3170 8910
e-mail: info@jpmedpub.com

EU GPSR Authorised Representative
Logos Europe, 9 rue Nicolas Poussin
17000, La Rochelle, France
Phone: +33 (0) 6 67 93 73 78
e-mail: contact@logoseurope.eu

Website: www.jaypeebrothers.com
Website: www.jaypeedigital.com

© 2026, Research Society for the Study of Diabetes in India (RSSDI)

The views and opinions expressed in this book are solely those of the original contributor(s)/author(s) and do not necessarily represent those of editor(s) or publisher of the book.

All rights reserved. No part of this publication may be reproduced, stored or transmitted in any form or by any means, electronic, mechanical, photocopying, recording or otherwise, without the prior permission in writing of the publishers.

All brand names and product names used in this book are trade names, service marks, trademarks or registered trademarks of their respective owners. The publisher is not associated with any product or vendor mentioned in this book.

Medical knowledge and practice change constantly. This book is designed to provide accurate, authoritative information about the subject matter in question. However, readers are advised to check the most current information available on procedures included and check information from the manufacturer of each product to be administered, to verify the recommended dose, formula, method and duration of administration, adverse effects and contraindications. It is the responsibility of the practitioner to take all appropriate safety precautions. Neither the publisher nor the author(s)/editor(s) assume any liability for any injury and/or damage to persons or property arising from or related to use of material in this book.

This book is sold on the understanding that the publisher is not engaged in providing professional medical services. If such advice or services are required, the services of a competent medical professional should be sought.

Every effort has been made where necessary to contact holders of copyright to obtain permission to reproduce copyright material. If any have been inadvertently overlooked, the publisher will be pleased to make the necessary arrangements at the first opportunity.

Inquiries for bulk sales may be solicited at: jaypee@jaypeebrothers.com

RSSDI Atlas of Dermatological Conditions in Diabetes / *NK Singh*

First Edition: **2026**

ISBN: 978-93-7202-069-4

Printed at: Samrat Offset Pvt. Ltd.

RSSDI Executive Committe

President
Vijay Vishwanathan

President Elect
Anuj Maheshwari

Immediate Past President
Rakesh Sahay

Vice Presidents
Sujoy Ghosh
L Sreenivasa Murthy

Secretary General
Sanjay Agarwal

Joint Secretary
Pratap P Jethwani

Treasurer
JK Sharma

Executive Committee
Aravinda J
Manoj Chawla
NK Singh
M Shunmugavelu
Amit Gupta
Jothydev Kesavadev
Rakesh Parikh
Anil K Virmani

Co-opted
Neeta Deshpande
Sunil Gupta

Foreword

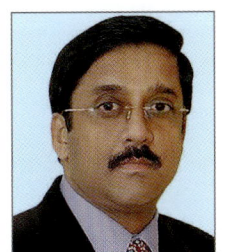
Vijay Vishwanathan
President RSSDI

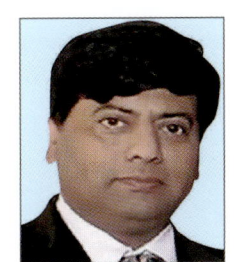
Anuj Maheshwari
President Elect RSSDI

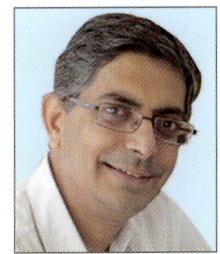
Sanjay Agarwal
Secretary

Diabetes mellitus is not merely a disorder of glucose metabolism—it is a systemic condition that touches virtually every tissue in the human body, and the skin is no exception. Yet, cutaneous manifestations of diabetes often remain overlooked, underdiagnosed, and underappreciated, despite being visible, accessible markers of underlying metabolic dysfunction.

This pioneering *RSSDI Atlas of Dermatological Conditions in Diabetes* represents a vital and timely contribution to clinical diabetology and dermatology alike. It bridges an important gap in our understanding by meticulously mapping the complex interplay between hyperglycemia, insulin resistance, microangiopathy, neuropathy, immune dysfunction, and the skin. The text reveals how the skin is not only a passive recipient of systemic insults but also an early marker of deeper metabolic imbalances, often preceding overt diabetic complications.

From the disruption of the stratum corneum barrier to the accumulation of advanced glycation end products (AGEs), from altered pH and hydration to impaired keratinocyte function and microvascular damage, this atlas navigates the intricate pathophysiology underlying diabetic dermatoses. It highlights classic entities such as acanthosis nigricans, diabetic dermopathy, and necrobiosis lipoidica while also shedding light on subtle yet clinically significant clues like xerosis, candidal intertrigo, and skin tags, which may serve as dermatological harbingers of insulin resistance and metabolic syndrome.

What distinguishes this atlas is its clarity, scientific rigor, and comprehensive scope. It decodes complex mechanisms such as epidermal dysfunction, immunologic compromise, and altered microbiota with lucidity, grounding them in current evidence and real-world relevance. Clinicians will especially appreciate the detailed correlations between skin changes and systemic diabetic complications, transforming skin into a window of opportunity for earlier diagnosis and intervention.

The RSSDI Skin Atlas of Diabetes is more than a reference—it is a call to action. It urges primary care physicians, diabetologists, dermatologists, and allied health professionals to recognize that effective diabetes care must extend beyond blood sugar control and encompass vigilant attention to skin health. Timely recognition and management of cutaneous clues may offer a crucial advantage in preventing disability, infections, and healthcare costs.

On behalf of the RSSDI, we commend the authors and contributors for this scholarly, clinically grounded, and visually enriching work. May it serve as a transformative resource, enhancing awareness, fostering interdisciplinary collaboration, and elevating the standard of care for people living with diabetes.

Preface

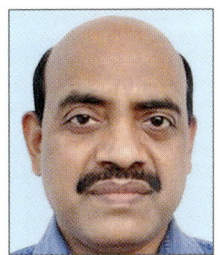 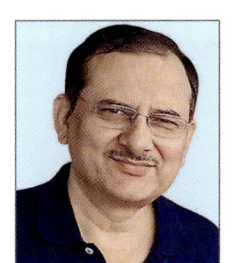 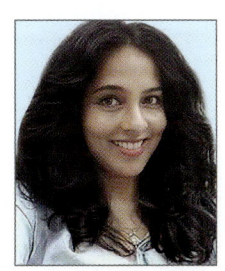 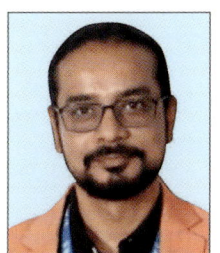

NK Singh
Editor-in-Chief

Akashkumar N Singh
Assistant Editor

Anuradha Kapoor
Assistant Editor

Amit Kumar
Assistant Editor

It gives us immense pleasure to present the *RSSDI Atlas of Dermatological Conditions in Diabetes*—a comprehensive, evidence-based compilation of the diverse cutaneous manifestations observed in people living with diabetes mellitus. This atlas is the result of a collaborative effort fueled by clinical observations, scientific inquiry, and a growing need to integrate dermatological insights into routine diabetes mellitus care.

Although the recognition of diabetes mellitus as a multisystem disorder has gained increasing attention, its dermatological manifestations often remain relegated to the background. Yet, as this book demonstrates, the skin can be both a mirror and a messenger—reflecting the internal metabolic milieu and signaling the onset of deeper systemic derangements. Subtle changes such as xerosis, altered pigmentation, recurrent infections, or acanthosis nigricans are often the first clinical indicators of insulin resistance, hyperglycemia, or microvascular complications.

This atlas brings together current research and clinical pearls to explain the underlying pathophysiology, from advanced glycation end products (AGEs) and stratum corneum dysfunction to immune compromise and microvascular damage. The chapters are organized to provide a logical and layered understanding of how diabetes influences skin biology at the cellular, structural, and functional levels.

Each section is enriched with:
- Detailed mechanistic explanations grounded in current evidence
- Clinical relevance for both type 1 and type 2 diabetes
- Visual aids to facilitate diagnosis and pattern recognition
- Practical insights for early detection, prevention, and management
- We aim to empower physicians, diabetologists, dermatologists, and postgraduate students with a deeper understanding of dermatological signs as potential diagnostic markers and prognostic indicators. We also hope this work stimulates interdisciplinary dialogue between skin and systemic medicine, fostering a more holistic and proactive approach to diabetes care.

We extend our heartfelt thanks to the esteemed contributors, researchers, and reviewers whose insights have shaped this volume. Special gratitude goes to the Research Society for the Study of Diabetes in India (RSSDI) for its unwavering support and visionary commitment to addressing this often-overlooked intersection of skin and systemic disease.

It is our sincere hope that this atlas not only enhances clinical acumen but also promotes a culture of vigilance toward diabetic skin changes, because in diabetes, the skin often speaks first.

Preface

Ankur Kumar
Assistant Editor

Samreen Ahmad
Assistant Editor

Alagarsamy M Shaik
Assistant Editor

BN Singh
Editor-in-Chief

- Case studies...
- Lesions more often emphasized, grounded in clinical evidence
- Clinical relevance for both type 1 and type 2 diabetes
- Visual aids to facilitate diagnostic and pattern recognition
- Practical insights for early detection, prevention, and management

We aim to empower physicians, diabetologists, dermatologists, and postgraduate students with a deeper understanding of dermatological signs as early and prognostic indicators. We also hope this work stimulates interdisciplinary dialogue between skin and systemic medicine, fostering a more holistic and proactive approach to diabetes care.

We extend our heartfelt thanks to the esteemed contributors, researchers, and reviewers whose insights have shaped this volume. Special gratitude goes to the Research Society for the Study of Diabetes in India (RSSDI) for its unwavering support and visionary commitment to addressing this often-overlooked interface of skin and systemic disease.

It is our sincere hope that this atlas not only enhances clinical acumen but also promotes a culture of vigilance toward diabetic skin changes, because in diabetes, the skin often speaks first.

Contributors

Aarathy Kannan MD Dip(Diabetology) FDI MBA(HM)
Consultant Physician and Diabetologist
Governing Council Member of TN RSSDI (2025–2028)
Assistant DNB Coordinator
Co-opted EC Member
RSSDI Tamil Nadu

Abhinav Jain MBBS MD DVD
Senior Resident 3rd Year
Department of Dermatology
DY Patil Medical College
Navi Mumbai, Maharashtra, India

Akashkumar N Singh MD(Medicine) MSc(Diabetes) FRCP(Edinburgh and Glasgow) FACP FICP FRSSDI Fellow (Diabetes India) FIACM FISH FISC FCCDSI
Director
Department of Internal Medicine and Diabetes
Manjalpur Hospital Private Limited
Vadodara, Gujarat, India

Amalkumar Bhattacharya MD(Medicine)
Professor
Department of Medicine
SBKS Medical College and Research Centre
Vadodara, Gujarat, India

Amit Kumar MD(Derm and STD)
Dermatologist
Department of Dermatology
CosmoDerma
Ranchi, Jharkhand, India

Anil Patki MD(Skin and VD) MNAMS
Dermatologist
Department of Dermatology
Akshay Hospital
Pune, Maharashtra, Inida

Ankur Kothari MS(Surgery)
Associate Professor of Surgery
Department of Surgery
SSG Hospital and Medical College
Vadodara, Gujarat, India

Anuradha Kapoor MD PG diploma in Clinical Endocrinology and diabetes, Fellow ICCMD(CCDSI)
Preventive Diabetologist
Department of Diabetology
Lifeline Medicare Hospital
Mumbai, Maharashtra, India

Arijit Singha MD DM
Assistant Professor
Department of Endocrinology and Metabolism
Institute of Post Graduate Medical Education and Research
Kolkata, West Bengal, India

Arjun Khadse MBBS
3rd Year Resident
Department of Medicine
Vedantaa Institute of Medical Sciences
Palghar, Maharashtra, India

Armaan Mishra MBBS
Junior Resident
Department of General Medicine
RSDKS Government Medical College
Ambikapur, Chhattisgarh, India

Arti Muley MD(Medicine)
Professor and Head
Department of General Medicine
Parul Sevashram Hospital
PIMSR, Parul University
Vadodara, Gujarat, India

Ashma Surani MD DNB
Assistant Professor
Department of Dermatology
BJ Medical College and Civil Hospital
Ahmedabad, Gujarat, India

Avina Jain MBBS MD(Dermatology)
Consultant Dermatologist
Founder and Chief Dermatologist
Auro Skin Clinic
Mumbai, Maharashtra, India

Bela J Shah MD
Professor and Head
Department of Dermatology, Venereology and Leprology
BJ Medical College and Civil Hospital
Ahmedabad, Gujarat, India

Bharat Bhushan Kukreja MBBS MD(Medicine)
Consultant Physician
Department of Medicine
Marwari Hospitals
Guwahati, Assam, India

Chaitanya Bhandekar MBBS
2nd Year Resident
Department of Medicine
Vedantaa Institute of Medical Sciences
Palghar, Maharashtra, India

Chinmayee Anand N MBBS
Junior Resident
Department of Dermatology
KIMS Hospital and Research Centre
Bangalore, Karnataka, India

Deepak Das MD
Associate Professor and Diabetologist
Department of Physiology
SRMS Institute of Medical Sciences
Bareilly, Uttar Pradesh, India

Dhaivat Joshi MBBS 3rd Year MD DVL
3rd Year Resident
Department of Dermatology,
Venereology and Leprosy
BJ Medical College and Civil Hospital
Ahmedabad, Gujarat, India

Dipali Rahirkar MBBS
3rd Year Resident
Department of Medicine
Vedantaa Institute of Medical Sciences
Palghar, Maharashtra, India

Firdous Shaikh MBBS Dip DIAB (RCP UK)
Dip DIAB(Emory School of Medicine USA)
CPS. DIAB(Mumbai) Fellow ISCM Fellow DI
Consultant Diabetologist and
Metabolic Physician
Department of Diabetology
Dr Firdous Rasheeda Shaikh's
Diabetes and Obesity Management
Research Centre
Mumbai, Maharashtra, India

Gaurav Gupta MBBS
Junior Resident
Department of Medicine
Sarojini Naidu Medical College
Agra, Uttar Pradesh, India

Gururaj B Sattur MD(Medicine)
Senior Physician and Diabetologist
Department of Diabetology
Sattur Medical Care
Hubli, Karnataka, India

Hiral Shah MD(Skin and VD)
Associate Professor
Department of Skin and VD
SSG Hospital and Baroda Medical College
Vadodara, Gujarat, India

J Thadeus MD(DVL)
Professor
Department of Dermatology
GTKM College
Thoothukudi, Tamil Nadu, India

Leena Singh MBBS DCP(Path)
Managing Director
Department of Diabetology
Diabetes and Heart Research Centre
Dhanbad, Jharkhand, India

Namrata C Manjunath MBBS
MD(Dermatology) FRGUHS(Dermatology)
Associate Professor
Department of Dermatology
KIMS Hospital and Research Centre,
Bangalore, Karnataka, India

Nipul Vara MD(Dermatology)
Associate Professor
Department of Skin and Venereal
Diseases
SSG Hospital and Medical College
Baroda, Gujarat, India

Niraj MD
Associate Professor
Department of Skin and Venereal
Diseases
Varun Arjun Medical College and
Rohilkhand Hospital
Banthara, Uttar Pradesh, India

NK Singh MD FICP FACP FRSSDI
Director
Department of Diabetology
Diabetes and Heart Research Centre
Dhanbad, Jharkhand, India
VICE President, (Elect) 2026–2029, RSSDI
Founder CME INDIA

Prabhat Kumar Agrawal MBBS
MD(Medicine) MAMS FRCP FACP FICP
FRSSDI FIACM
Professor
Department of Medicine
Sarojini Naidu Medical College
Agra, Uttar Pradesh, India

Pradip Mukhopadhyay MD DM
Professor and Head
Department of Endocrinology and
Metabolism
Institute of Post Graduate Medical
Education and Research
Kolkata, West Bengal, India

Pradnya Gatkal MBBS
2nd Year Resident
Department of Medicine
Vedantaa Institute of Medical
Sciences
Palghar, Maharashtra, India

Preya Parag Rana MBBS
Research Fellow
Department of Sleep Medicine
Cleveland Clinic
Ohio, USA

Ruchi Shah MBBS MD(Dermatology)
MD(Internal Medicine and Rheumatology)
Former Resident Physician
Department of Skin and VD
Baroda Medical College and
SSG Hospital
Vadodara, Gujarat, India

Rutul Gokalani MD
Consultant Diabetologist
Department of Diabetology
Diabetes and Metabolic Physician
AHC Diabetes Clinic
Ahmedabad, Gujarat, India

Sandipta Kumar Panda MBBS
Junior Resident
Department of Medicine,
Sarojini Naidu Medical College
Agra, Uttar Pradesh, India

Santosh B MD(Internal Medicine)
DNB(Endocrinology)
Consultant Endocrinologist
Department of Endocrinology,
Baptist Hospital
Bangalore, Karnataka, India

Sona Mitra DNB(Family Medicine)
Consultant Physician and Clinical Research Associate
Department of General Medicine
Parul Sevashram Hospital
PIMSR, Parul University
Vadodara, Gujarat, India

Sudhir Kumar MD
Consultant Physician
Department of Diabetology
Advanced Medicentre
Bokaro, Jharkhand, India

Suhas Gopal Erande MD(Medicine)
Diabetologist
Department of Medicine
Akshay Hospital
Pune, Maharashtra, India

Sujoy Ghosh MD DM
Professor
Department of Endocrinology and Metabolism
Institute of Post Graduate Medical Education and Research
Kolkata, West Bengal, India

Tithi Shah MBBS MD DVL
Postdoctoral Dermatology Research Fellow
Department of Dermatology
Centre for Blistering Diseases
Boston, MA, USA

Twinkle C Rangnani MBBS MD DVL
Senior Resident
Department of Dermatology
GAIMS Bhuj
Gujarat, India

Viral Thakkar MD
Dermatologist
Department of Dermatology
Dermatology Clinic
Ahmedabad, Gujarat, India

Vishwa Marvania MBBS
3rd Year Resident
Department of Skin and VD
Baroda Medical College
Vadodara, Gujarat, India

Yashika Doshi MD DNB
Assistant Professor
Department of Dermatology
BJ Medical College and Civil Hospital
Ahmedabad, Gujarat, India

Yogesh Marfatia MD(Skin and VD)
Professor (Skin-VD)
Department of Dermatology
SBKS Medical Institute and Research Centre, Vadodara
Gujarat, India

Acknowledgments

The creation of the *RSSDI Atlas of Dermatological Conditions in Diabetes* has been a truly collaborative journey, and we gratefully acknowledge the many individuals and institutions who made this work possible.

We express our deepest appreciation to the Research Society for the Study of Diabetes in India (RSSDI) for its constant encouragement, academic support, and commitment to bridging gaps in diabetes care. This atlas would not have taken shape without the organization's vision to highlight the dermatological dimension of diabetes management.

We place on record our special gratitude to Vijay Vishwanathan, President, RSSDI; Anuj Maheshwari, President Elect, RSSDI; and Sanjay Agrawal, Secretary General, RSSDI, for their unwavering encouragement and guidance at every stage of the atlas development. Their timely inputs and motivation inspired the team to maintain academic rigor and clinical relevance throughout this work.

Our sincere thanks go to the chapter authors and contributors, who combined their clinical wisdom and academic depth to enrich this atlas. We are indebted to the reviewers and peer experts for their critical insights that ensured scientific accuracy and practical utility.

We also acknowledge the invaluable contributions of our dermatology and diabetology colleagues across the country, who, through their clinical observations and case documentation, inspired the content and images that form the foundation of this atlas.

We are especially grateful to M/s Jaypee Brothers Medical Publishers (P) Ltd for taking the onus of publishing this atlas and for their professionalism in bringing this vision to reality with the highest editorial and production standards.

Special gratitude is reserved for the editorial and technical teams, whose tireless efforts in formatting, image processing, and design ensured the highest quality output.

Finally, we remain ever grateful to our patients, who entrusted us with their care. Their experiences, courage, and consent to share clinical images have transformed this atlas into a practical, patient-centered resource for the medical community.

We hope that this atlas will serve as a lasting testament to the power of interdisciplinary collaboration in advancing diabetes care.

NK Singh

Contents

SECTION 1: Introduction and Overview

CHAPTER 1: **Epidemiology of Diabetes and Its Cutaneous Manifestations** — 3
Amit Kumar, Arti Muley

CHAPTER 2: **Normal Skin and Pathogenesis of Skin Changes in Diabetes** — 5
Amit Kumar, Arti Muley

CHAPTER 3: **Common Skin Conditions in Diabetes and their Distribution** — 11
Arti Muley, Akashkumar N Singh

SECTION 2: Dermatologic Conditions Directly Attributed to Diabetes

CHAPTER 4: **Diabetic Dermopathy (Shin Spots) in a Type 2 Diabetic Male** — 19
Suhas Gopal Erande

CHAPTER 5: **Necrobiosis Lipoidica Based on a Skin Biopsy** — 24
Namrata C Manjunath, Chinmayee Anand N, Niraj, Deepak Das

CHAPTER 6: **Bullous Diabeticorum** — 28
Firdous Shaikh, Avina Jain, Abhinav Jain, Armaan Mishra

CHAPTER 7: **Bullous Pemphigoid in a Diabetic Male** — 31
Nipul Vara, Vishwa Marvania, Preya Parag Rana

CHAPTER 8: **Yellow Palms in Diabetes Mellitus: A Case of Carotenoderma** — 34
Arijit Singha, Pradip Mukhopadhyay, Sujoy Ghosh

CHAPTER 9: **Carotenemia in a Patient with Type 2 Diabetes Mellitus** — 36
NK Singh, Akashkumar N Singh, Anuradha Kapoor

CHAPTER 10: **Diabetic Rubeosis Faciei with Palmar Erythema** — 38
Ashma Surani, Bela J Shah

CHAPTER 11: **Finger Pebbles (Huntley's Papules) in a Diabetic Male** — 40
Suhas Gopal Erande

CHAPTER 12: Perforating Dermatosis   42

Nipul Vara, Vishwa Marvania, Preya Parag Rana, Suhas Gopal Erande, Prabhat Kumar Agrawal, Sandipta Kumar Panda, Gaurav Gupta, Anil Patki, Ashma Surani, Firdous Shaikh, Avina Jain

Part A: Perforating Folliculitis in Uncontrolled Diabetes   42

Part B: Acquired Perforating Dermatosis in a Diabetic Female with Chronic Renal Failure   44

Part C: Kyrle's Disease in a Patient of Diabetes Mellitus and Chronic Kidney Disease on Hemodialysis   46

Part D: Acquired Perforating Dermatosis (Reactive Perforating Collagenosis Variant) in Diabetes   48

Part E: Reactive Perforating Collagenosis in a Type 2 Diabetic Female   50

Part F: Pruritic Perforating Dermatosis Associated with Type 2 Diabetes Mellitus   52

SECTION 3: Skin Conditions Associated with or Exacerbated by Diabetes

CHAPTER 13: Psoriasis in a Diabetic Patient   57

Nipul Vara, Vishwa Marvania

CHAPTER 14: Acanthosis Nigricans and Acrochordons (Skin Tags) in Diabetes   59

Suhas Gopal Erande, Anil Patki, Bharat Bhushan Kukreja, Ruchi Shah, Yogesh Marfatia

CHAPTER 15: Lichen Planus in a Diabetic Male with Hypothyroidism   68

Nipul Vara, Vishwa Marvania

CHAPTER 16: Xerosis and Pruritus in Diabetes (Dry Skin and Generalized Itch)   70

J Thadeus

CHAPTER 17: Subacute Eczema with Id Eruption in Metabolic Syndrome and Type 2 Diabetes   73

Rutul Gokalani, Viral Thakkar

SECTION 4: Cutaneous Infections in Diabetes

CHAPTER 18: Fungal Infections   79

Arti Muley, Akashkumar N Singh, Yashika Doshi, Bela J Shah, Ashma Surani, Nipul Vara, Dhaivat Joshi, Armaan Mishra, Firdous Shaikh, Avina Jain

Part A: Dermatophyte Infection in Diabetes (Tinea and Onychomycosis)   79

Part B: Candidiasis and Other Yeast Infections in Diabetes   86

CHAPTER 19: Bacterial Skin Infections in Diabetes   95

Nipul Vara, Vishwa Marvania, Preya Parag Rana, Hiral Shah, J Thadeus, Aarathy Kannan, Akashkumar N Singh, Ankur Kothari, Suhas Gopal Erande, Anil Patki, Ruchi Shah, Yogesh Marfatia

Part A: Acute Paronychia in a Diabetic Male   95

Part B: Erythrasma in a Diabetic Patient   96

Part C: Furunculosis in Diabetic Patients   99

Part D: Fournier's Gangrene in an Undiagnosed Diabetic Male   103

Part E: Carbuncle in a Diabetic Female   105

Part F: Cutaneous Nontuberculous Mycobacterium Infections in Diabetes   106

Part G: Necrotizing Skin and Soft Tissue Infections in Uncontrolled Diabetes   108

CHAPTER 20: Viral Skin Infections in Diabetes: Hemorrhagic Herpes Zoster (Multidermatomal) in an Uncontrolled Diabetic Patient   111

Bela J Shah

SECTION 5: Rare Dermatological Manifestations of Diabetes (Musculoskeletal and Connective Tissue Manifestations in Diabetes)

CHAPTER 21: Diabetic Cheiroarthropathy (Diabetic Hand Syndrome/Stiff Skin Syndrome) in Long-standing Diabetes   115

Suhas Gopal Erande, Anil Patki

CHAPTER 22: Scleredema Diabeticorum (Diabetic Scleroderma)   118

Suhas Gopal Erande

CHAPTER 23: Granuloma Annulare in Diabetes   121

Firdous Shaikh, Avina Jain, Bela J Shah, Akashkumar N Singh, Anuradha Kapoor, Ruchi Shah, Yogesh Marfatia

CHAPTER 24: Eruptive Xanthomas in Uncontrolled Diabetes Mellitus   129

NK Singh, Akashkumar N Singh, Anuradha Kapoor

CHAPTER 25: Abdominal Pseudohernia due to Diabetic Truncal Neuropathy   132

Santosh B

CHAPTER 26: Porphyria Cutanea Tarda in Patients with Type 2 Diabetes Mellitus   134

Suhas Gopal Erande, Anil Patki

SECTION 6: Psychosocial and Cosmetic Skin Conditions in Diabetes

CHAPTER 27: Vitiligo in Diabetes (Autoimmune Pigmentary Changes)   139

Nipul Vara, Vishwa Marvania

CHAPTER 28: Hidradenitis Suppurativa in Diabetes   141

Bharat Bhushan Kukreja

CHAPTER 29: Alopecia in Diabetes Mellitus (Hair Loss Associations)   144

Nipul Vara, Vishwa Marvania

CHAPTER 30: Postinflammatory Hyperpigmentation in Diabetes: Truncal Distribution   147

Suhas Gopal Erande, Anil Patki

SECTION 7: Dermatology of Diabetic Foot

CHAPTER 31: Nonhealing Foot Ulcer in Diabetes Mellitus — 153
Nipul Vara, Vishwa Marvania

CHAPTER 32: Nonhealing Trophic Ulcer in a Diabetic Male — 156
Bela J Shah

CHAPTER 33: Difficult-to-Treat Diabetic Foot Ulcer Complicated by Osteomyelitis — 159
Amalkumar Bhattacharya, Pradnya Gatkal, Dipali Rahirkar, Arjun Khadse, Chaitanya Bhandekar

CHAPTER 34: Maggot Infestation in a Diabetic Foot Ulcer: Clinical Case and Review — 162
Bharat Bhushan Kukreja

CHAPTER 35: Diabetic Toe Gangrene (Dry Gangrene) in Uncontrolled Diabetes — 166
Suhas Gopal Erande, Anil Patki

CHAPTER 36: Diabetic Foot Gangrene with Heel Ulceration and Digital Necrosis — 169
Suhas Gopal Erande, Anil Patki

CHAPTER 37: Extensive Dry Gangrene of the Foot in a Diabetic Smoker — 172
Nipul Vara

SECTION 8: Diagnostic and Special Considerations in Diabetic Dermatology

CHAPTER 38: Insulin Injection Site Reactions — 177
Arti Muley, Akashkumar N Singh, Sona Mitra, Sudhir Kumar, Gururaj B Sattur, Suhas Gopal Erande, Anil Patki, NK Singh, Leena Singh

  Part A: Lipohypertrophy and Lipoatrophy   177

  Part B: Allergic Contact Dermatitis from Insulin Pump Adhesive   182

  Part C: Postinflammatory Hyperpigmentation Following Insulin Injections   184

CHAPTER 39: Cutaneous Adverse Effects of Diabetes Therapies — 187
Yashika Doshi, Bela J Shah, Twinkle C Rangnani, Tithi Shah

  Part A: Gliptin-Induced Bullous Pemphigoid   187

  Part B: Vildagliptin-Induced Bullous Pemphigoid—Blisters Unveiled   189

  Index   193

SECTION 1

Introduction and Overview

▶ Section Outline

Chapter 1: **Epidemiology of Diabetes and Its Cutaneous Manifestations**
Amit Kumar, Arti Muley

Chapter 2: **Normal Skin and Pathogenesis of Skin Changes in Diabetes**
Amit Kumar, Arti Muley

Chapter 3: **Common Skin Conditions in Diabetes and their Distribution**
Arti Muley, Akashkumar N Singh

SECTION 1

Introduction and Overview

- Section Outline

CHAPTER 1

Epidemiology of Diabetes and Its Cutaneous Manifestations

Amit Kumar, Arti Muley

■ INTRODUCTION

Diabetes mellitus (DM), a chronic metabolic disorder characterized by elevated blood glucose levels, is an epidemic of modern times affecting nearly 8.3% of the adult population. It poses a significant global health challenge, with many cases remaining undiagnosed or uncontrolled.[1]

■ GLOBAL PREVALENCE

Globally, the incidence and prevalence of diabetes have been steadily rising over the past few decades, reaching pandemic proportions. The International Diabetes Federation (IDF) estimates that approximately 537 million adults (20–79 years) were living with diabetes in 2021, which is expected to rise to 783 million by 2045.[2] Factors contributing to this increase include aging populations, urbanization, sedentary lifestyles, and unhealthy dietary patterns.[3]

■ PREVALENCE IN INDIA

India stands as a major epicenter of the diabetes epidemic. The prevalence of diabetes in India has shown a significant upward trend in the last few decades. According to the IDF, in 2021, approximately 77 million adults in India were living with diabetes, which is the second-highest globally in terms of the number of people with diabetes.[2] However, more recent studies suggest that the actual prevalence might be even higher. A large national study, the ICMR-INDIAB study, reported a weighted prevalence of diabetes of 11.4% in the adult population across various states of India.[4] This highlights the substantial burden of diabetes on the Indian healthcare system and economy.

The incidence of diabetes, which refers to the number of new cases diagnosed within a specific period, also remains a concern in India. While precise nationwide incidence data is challenging to obtain, regional studies indicate a continuous increase in new cases, particularly in younger age groups.[5] This early onset of diabetes can lead to a higher cumulative risk of developing long-term complications.

■ GLOBAL EPIDEMIOLOGY OF CUTANEOUS INVOLVEMENT IN DIABETES

Diabetes mellitus is known to affect multiple organ systems. While the systemic complications such as cardiovascular disease, neuropathy, and nephropathy are well-documented, the impact of diabetes on the skin is often underestimated despite many reports of dermal conditions associated with either diabetes or the use of antidiabetic drugs. The precise prevalence, however, varies by study and population. Different studies have reported that *30–70% of patients with diabetes develop a skin complication* at some point in their lifetime. A systematic review of multiple studies found that skin manifestations occur in up to 70% of individuals with diabetes.[6] A large literature review noted prevalence ranges from *51.1% up to 97%* in different cohorts of type 1 and type 2 diabetic patients.[7] This wide range may be because of the use of different study methodologies and definitions, as some included only specific dermatoses, while others included a wider range of skin conditions from xerosis (dry skin) to severe infections. Nonetheless, *over half of all diabetes patients experience dermatological signs* of the disease. Both type 1 diabetes mellitus (T1DM) and type 2 diabetes mellitus (T2DM) can have cutaneous complications, but the *burden is greater in T2DM,* given its higher prevalence and the cumulative effects of long-standing hyperglycemia and insulin resistance. Importantly, cutaneous signs can present at any stage—some appear early (even preceding diabetes diagnosis), whereas others correlate with chronic complications.[8]

INDIAN EPIDEMIOLOGY OF CUTANEOUS INVOLVEMENT IN DIABETES

India has one of the largest diabetic populations (>74 million adults in 2021) and a rising prevalence. For example, an observational study in Eastern India (Kolkata) found that *73.9% of diabetic patients had at least one cutaneous lesion.*[9] They also reported more frequent skin manifestations in type 2 diabetics (75.6%) than in type 1 diabetics (41%). Another Indian study from a tertiary center reported skin lesions in ~74% of diabetics, with multiple lesion types in two-thirds of patients.[4] These numbers are higher than the often-cited 30–40% frequency, likely because Indian studies tend to be hospital-based (capturing patients with complications) and because tropical climates expose patients to more infections.

Hospital-based studies on skin involvement in diabetes in India mirror global findings with xerosis, pruritus, fungal and bacterial infections, and diabetic dermopathy being among the most common. Acanthosis nigricans also remains a significant marker for insulin resistance and diabetes across different ethnicities.[10] The prevalence of specific skin conditions might vary slightly across different populations due to genetic, environmental, and lifestyle factors. For example, in a North Indian (Himalayan) study, *xerosis (dry skin) was the most common finding (44%),* attributed to cold, dry weather, whereas in a South Asian tropical setting, *fungal infections and intertrigo are very common.*[4] Despite these variations, the *overall dermatological burden in Indian diabetics is substantial,* negatively impacting quality of life and sometimes indicating coexisting systemic complications. The subsequent chapters provide a comprehensive outlook of cutaneous manifestations of diabetes.

REFERENCES

1. Idf.org [Internet]. (2015). IDF Diabetes Atlas, 6th edition. [online] Available from http://www.idf.org/diabetesatlas/update, 2014 [Last accessed Aug., 2025].
2. International Diabetes Federation. IDF Diabetes Atlas, 10th edition. Brussels, Belgium: International Diabetes Federation; 2021.
3. Roglic G, Davies MJ, Ozougwu C. Global burden of diabetes. Textbook of Diabetes, 5th edition. Chichester, UK: John Wiley & Sons Ltd; 2017. pp. 3-12.
4. Anjana RM, Deepa M, Pradeepa R, Mahanta J, Narain K, Das HK, et al. Prevalence of diabetes and prediabetes in 15 states of India: results from the ICMR-INDIAB population-based cross-sectional study. Lancet Diabetes Endocrinol. 2017;5(8):585-96.
5. https://diabetesjournals.org/care/article/38/8/1441/31181/Incidence-of-Diabetes-and-Prediabetes-and
6. https://www.medigraphic.com/cgi-bin/new/resumenI.cgi?IDARTICULO=117953
7. de Macedo GM, Nunes S, Barreto T. Skin disorders in diabetes mellitus: an epidemiology and physiopathology review. Diabetol Metab Syndr. 2016;8(1):63.
8. Pavlović MD, Milenković T, Dinić M, Misović M, Daković D, Todorović S, et al. The prevalence of cutaneous manifestations in young patients with type 1 diabetes. Diabetes Care. 2007;30(8):1964-7.
9. Chatterjee N, Chattopadhyay C, Sengupta N, Das C, Sarma N, Pal SK. An observational study of cutaneous manifestations in diabetes mellitus in a tertiary care Hospital of Eastern India. Indian J Endocrinol Metab. 2014;18(2):217-20.
10. https://2024.sci-hub.se/6311/c5efe991e0523315a2c1ad76b6b01beb/lima2017.pdf

CHAPTER 2

Normal Skin and Pathogenesis of Skin Changes in Diabetes

Amit Kumar, Arti Muley

INTRODUCTION

Both type 1 diabetes mellitus (T1DM) and type 2 diabetes mellitus (T2DM) have been associated with a plethora of cutaneous manifestations, e.g., cutaneous infection, dry skin, and pruritus, but remain mostly neglected and underdiagnosed. They are highly associated with hyperglycemia and advanced glycation end products (AGEs).[1] Many human and animal studies have reported changes in the biophysical properties of skin in both T1DM and T2DM, but the differences remain poorly defined.[2] These skin changes offer insight into the glycemic status of patients and often represent the first signs of metabolic abnormalities.[3]

STRUCTURE AND FUNCTION OF NORMAL EPIDERMIS

The epidermis is the outermost layer of skin that acts as a physical barrier to the external environment, regulates water loss and also protects from various infections or insults. It is composed of five layers from inside out: (1) The stratum basale: Innermost layer made of cuboidal and columnar cells; (2) The stratum spinosum: Composed of keratinocytes connected by desmosomes which are seen in light microscopy; (3) The stratum granulosum: Keratinocytes with granules; (4) The stratum lucidum: a thin light layer; and (5) The stratum corneum (SC): The outermost skin layer that serves as the major barrier to microbial, chemical, and physical and mechanical insults **(Fig. 1)**.[4-7]

Historically, the stratum corneum has been described to have a "brick and mortar" appearance, with the corneocytes serving as the bricks while the lipids and free fatty acids (FFAs) act as the cementing materials. The corneocytes are made of water and microfibrillar keratin encompassed by a cornified envelope comprising densely crosslinked layers of filaggrin, loricrin, and involucrin. A monolayer of nonpolar lipids is esterified to make the cornified envelope, which shapes the intercellular lipid layers.

Various factors maintain the epidermal barrier, viz., corneocytes, lipids, junction proteins, proteases, and antimicrobial peptides.[9] Keratinocytes, the primary cell type of epidermis, are paramount to maintaining epidermal integrity. They are present in all layers of epidermis, moving through them by means of differentiation and proliferation while being responsible for proper wound repair and immunological response against various pathogens.[10,11]

PATHOGENESIS OF CUTANEOUS CHANGES IN DIABETES

Diabetic dermatoses stem from a *common milieu of metabolic and vascular derangements* caused by

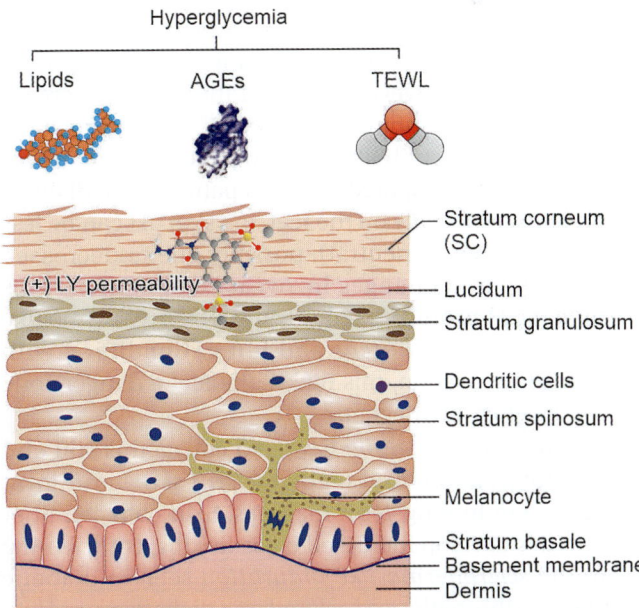

FIG. 1: Structure and regulation of the epidermal barrier.[8]
(AGEs: advanced glycation end-products; TEWL: transepidermal water loss)

chronic hyperglycemia and insulin resistance (IR). It is affected by the same pathological processes that impact other organs in diabetes (e.g., microangiopathy as in retinopathy/nephropathy, and neuropathy). Below, the key pathophysiological mechanisms are discussed individually, though in reality, they *interact and overlap* to produce specific skin conditions.

Hyperglycemia and Advanced Glycation End Products

Chronic hyperglycemia is a fundamental driver of tissue damage in diabetes. Elevated glucose leads to *nonenzymatic glycation* of proteins in the skin and vasculature. Over time, these glycation products cross-link and form irreversible *advanced glycation end products (AGEs)*.[12,13]

Advanced glycation end product compounds such as N-epsilon-carboxy-methyl-lysine (CML), carboxy-ethyl-lysine (CEL), and 5-hydro-5-methylimidazolone (MG-H1) are expressed in tissue and blood plasma.[12] They accumulate in long-lived proteins such as fibrillary collagen, resulting in structural alterations to the skin.[12,13] They also bind to receptor for advanced glycation end-products (RAGE) in diabetes mellitus (DM) patients, resulting in vascular complications.[14] Binding between AGEs and RAGE promotes oxidative stress and inflammatory cascades via the activation of mitogen-activated protein kinases (MAPK), nuclear factor-k-light-chain-enhancer of activated beta cells (NF-β), interleukin 6 (IL-6), and tumor necrosis factor-alpha (TNF-α).[15] These pathological processes have several consequences:

- *Skin pH:* The typical skin pH in healthy subjects is slightly acidic (ranges from 4.1 to 5.8), which inhibits pathogenic bacteria. In T1DM patients, more acidic values have been recorded as compared to the control subjects.[16,17] However, in T2DM models, an increase in skin pH is commonly observed.[18] This explains the increased susceptibility of T2DM patients to cutaneous infections as compared to T1DM patients.[19] In diabetic patients, especially on the feet, the skin pH can be less acidic (closer to neutral), possibly due to decreased sweating and changes in sweat composition. This higher pH promotes colonization by organisms like *Staphylococcus aureus* and fungi. Combined with reduced sensation, this makes the feet a danger zone for the entry of infection.[19]
- *Collagen modification:* Glycated collagen is stiff and less degradable and leads to *"stiff skin"* and joint limitation in long-term diabetes. Skin collagen fiber bundles develop increased cross-linking, contributing to the *scleroderma-like induration* seen in diabetic cheiroarthropathy and scleredema diabeticorum.[13]
- *Stratum corneum barrier:* Although the SC barrier function is poorly defined in diabetic patients, it is known that the correct composition of lipids within the SC is critical for maintaining epidermal homeostasis. Chronic hyperglycemia, oxidative stress, and altered lipid content cause altered hydration status, lipid composition, glycan levels and pH of the barrier, which results in damage to the stratum corneum as observed in animal models in DM studies.[18] Serum lipid abnormalities have been reported in ~75% of DM patients, predisposing them to a variety of lipid-associated complications.[20]
- *Keratinocytes:* Hyperglycemia impairs insulin signaling milieu in both T1DM and T2DM. It is detrimental to the normal proliferation of cells needed for a robust stratum corneum.[21,22] They suppress the proliferation and differentiation of keratinocytes in both human and rodent models, while autonomic neuropathy reduces sweating. Studies have shown *increased transepidermal water loss (TEWL)* in diabetic skin, indicating a compromised barrier that loses moisture more readily. The result is often *xerosis (dry and rough skin)* with increased scaling, possibly explaining the impaired wound healing observed in DM patients.[21,23] Moreover, diabetic stratum corneum may have reduced lipid content and altered fatty acid composition, further impairing barrier function.

Putte et al., in a systematic review, inferred that AGE-accumulation in collagen and elastic fibers in the dermis and vessel walls leads to increased formation of disorganized, shortened and thinned collagen, thereby decreasing the elasticity of the skin and hampering wound healing.[24]

- Disruption and damage to the keratinocytes may also lead to impaired barrier functions of the skin[10,11] in turn leading to increased permeability, increased insult from exogenous substances and higher risk of infections, cascading into many adverse immunological reactions.[25,26]
- Furthermore, *microvascular changes* may reduce the delivery of nutrients (like vitamin A or zinc) to the skin, which are important for keratinocyte health. Some diabetic patients exhibit a *yellowish discoloration* of the skin (thought to be due to glycosylation of proteins or carotene accumulation); while largely benign, it signifies the extent to which metabolic changes can alter skin appearance.

Insulin per se enhances the release of vascular endothelial growth factor (VEGF) from keratinocytes in skin wounds, through *AKT1*-mediated post-transcriptional mechanisms, thereby aiding in wound healing.[27] The decreased wound healing observed in T2DM cases can also be explained by the suppression of *keratinocyte growth factor* (KGF) release seen in T2DM adipose-derived stem cells (ASCs) compared to nondiabetic ASC groups **(Fig. 2)**.[28]

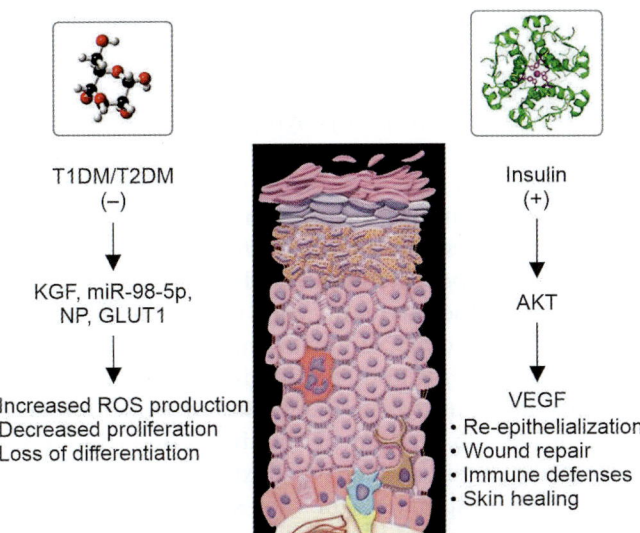

FIG. 2: Altered keratinocyte functions in type 1 diabetes mellitus (T1DM) and type 2 diabetes mellitus (T2DM).[8]
(GLUT1: glucose transporter 1; KGF: keratinocyte growth factor; NP: nonpolar; ROS: reactive oxygen species; VEGF: vascular endothelial growth factor)

- *Impaired repair:* Glycation of epidermal proteins may disturb the normal barrier function. Hyperglycemia directly impairs fibroblast and keratinocyte function. Also, *skin elasticity is reduced* (some diabetic patients appear to have thicker and less pliable skin). These changes contribute to *delayed wound healing and ulcer formation* in the skin.

Insulin Resistance and Hyperinsulinemia

Insulin resistance, characteristic of T2DM, leads to *compensatory hyperinsulinemia* (high circulating insulin levels) as well as elevated levels of insulin-like growth factor (IGF-1).[18] These hormonal changes have direct effects on the skin:
- Excess insulin and IGF-1 bind to growth factor receptors on keratinocytes and dermal fibroblasts, stimulating *hyperplasia of the epidermis and papillomatosis,* manifesting as thick, velvety, hyperpigmented plaques typically on the neck and axillae known as *Acanthosis nigricans (AN),* which is the classic skin finding associated with IR. This is commonly seen in obese type 2 diabetics and even in prediabetes.
- *Acrochordons (skin tags)* are benign fleshy polyps frequently associated with hyperinsulinemia. Insulin and other growth factors may promote their development. These often cluster in the same areas as acanthosis (neck and axilla) and serve as clinical markers of IR.[18]

Insulin resistance is also a component of the metabolic syndrome, which is a proinflammatory state. Resulting chronic inflammation with elevated TNF-α, IL-6, etc., may link IR to certain inflammatory skin conditions. For instance, *psoriasis*—a T-cell mediated inflammatory dermatosis—is strongly associated with metabolic syndrome and diabetes risk. Patients with severe psoriasis have higher odds of developing T2DM, and vice versa, possibly due to shared inflammatory pathways and IR. The presence of AN or multiple skin tags on examination is a red flag for underlying metabolic abnormalities and should prompt evaluation for T2DM or related conditions.[22] Another example is *"hidradenitis suppurativa (HS),"* an inflammatory follicular disease, which is more common in obese, insulin-resistant individuals (some consider it a part of the "metabolic dermatosis" spectrum).

Microangiopathy and Vascular Complications

Advanced glycation end products stimulate inflammation and oxidative stress in vessel walls, damaging the endothelial cells. The oxidative damage, along with other pathways like the polyol pathway and protein kinase C activation, causes *diabetic microangiopathy*—a diffuse dysfunction and loss of capillaries in tissues. In the skin, microangiopathy reduces perfusion and *impairs the skin's ability to respond to injury or metabolic demand,* leading to the following:
- *Reduced skin perfusion:* Even though the skin has a redundant capillary network at rest, diabetic patients lose some of this reserve due to microangiopathy. Hence, under stress (e.g., injury or infection), blood flow may be insufficient to meet the skin's needs. This partly explains why diabetic patients heal poorly and develop ulcers. Areas with end-arterial circulation, like the shin or foot, are especially vulnerable.
- *Diabetic dermopathy:* The *most common microangiopathic skin change* is diabetic dermopathy, presenting as small, round, brown, and atrophic macules usually seen on the anterior shins. These "shin spots" are thought to result from minor trauma in the setting of fragile dermal vasculature. Histologically, there is hemosiderin (iron) deposition and dermal fibrosis, indicating vascular leakage and repair. These lesions are harmless and asymptomatic, but their presence correlates with retinopathy and neuropathy, signaling systemic microvascular disease. Prevalence increases with age and duration of diabetes; roughly 20–50% of long-standing diabetics have dermopathy.[29]
- *Necrobiosis lipoidica (NL):* This is an uncommon but distinctive lesion, often on the shins, where patches of skin become atrophic, yellowish (due to lipid deposition), with an erythematous rim. NL has a

strong female predominance and is more often noted in T1DM. Although rare (only 0.3–1.6% of diabetics develop NL), its *pathogenesis is linked to diabetic microangiopathy*—biopsy shows obliterated vessels and inflammation. Many patients with NL have evidence of other microvascular complications.[30]

- *Bullosis diabeticorum:* Diabetic bullae are spontaneous, noninflammatory blisters on the acral skin (feet and hands) of diabetics. They resemble second-degree burn blisters. The cause is not fully understood; microangiopathy and local ischemia may be the factors responsible for bullae formation in subepidermal planes. They tend to occur in patients with long-standing, uncontrolled diabetes, and neuropathy. While bullae heal spontaneously in a few weeks, they can recur and may become infected secondarily.[30]
- *Macroangiopathy and skin:* Though microangiopathy is the main issue in cutaneous lesions, large-vessel atherosclerosis (which is accelerated in diabetes) also affects the skin's health. Peripheral arterial disease in diabetics leads to *ischemic skin changes* in the legs and feet—e.g., thinning of skin, hair loss on legs, cool extremities, and in severe cases, nonhealing ischemic ulcers or gangrene of toes. Thus, vascular disease at both the micro- and macro-level contributes to diabetic foot complications.[29]

In essence, *diabetes-associated vasculopathy impairs nutrient circulation to the skin,* predisposing to atrophy, ulceration, and poor healing. Recognition of dermatologic signs like dermopathy or necrobiosis should prompt a check for other vascular complications. Good control of blood sugar and blood pressure can slow microangiopathic damage and thus mitigate some of these skin issues.

Neuropathy (Nerve Dysfunction)[31]

Diabetic peripheral neuropathy—affecting sensory, motor, and autonomic nerves—has profound effects on the skin, especially on the feet. *Neuropathy contributes to "diabetic foot"—a confluence of sensory loss, abnormal pressure loading, dry skin, and injury that leads to foot ulcers.* Key aspects of neuropathic pathogenesis include:

- *Sensory neuropathy:* Patients do not feel pain from cuts, blisters, or repetitive pressure. Minor trauma (from ill-fitting footwear, unnoticed foreign objects, etc.) can progress to deep wounds. Pressure points (like the plantar metatarsal heads) develop calluses, which can ulcerate beneath. This is why *neuropathic ulcers* often occur on the soles or edges of the feet. They typically have a painless, punched-out appearance and can go unnoticed until severe.
- *Motor neuropathy:* Damage to motor nerves of the feet leads to small muscle atrophy, claw toe deformities, and altered foot biomechanics. This causes abnormal weight bearing and pressure points on the sole, contributing to the risk of an ulcer. Foot deformities from neuropathy also increase the risk of fissures and corns.
- *Autonomic neuropathy:* Sympathetic nerve damage in the skin results in *anhidrosis (reduced sweating)* in the feet and legs. The loss of sweat, combined with peripheral arterial insufficiency, causes the skin to become *excessively dry and brittle.* Cracks and fissures develop, especially in the heels and toe webs. These fissures are portals for infection (e.g., cellulitis or fungal entry). Autonomic neuropathy may also lead to *increased skin surface pH* and changes in skin flora, fostering infections. Furthermore, autonomic dysfunction causes arterioles in the foot to remain dilated (due to lost vasomotor tone), which paradoxically steals blood away from skin capillaries (the steal syndrome), worsening perfusion in weight-bearing areas.[31]

The culmination of these factors is *diabetic foot ulcer (DFU),* a serious complication. Neuropathy is the primary contributor to the most common type of DFU (the neuropathic ulcer). When neuropathy is combined with microangiopathy and infection, ulcers may progress to deep infections or gangrene. In diabetics, foot ulcers are often polymicrobial infections involving *Candida*, gram-positive cocci, gram-negative rods, etc. If not properly managed, these can lead to osteomyelitis or even necessitate amputation. Thus, *neuropathy's impact on the skin is largely indirect but critical,* setting the stage for painless trauma and poor healing.[32]

Not all neuropathic effects are on the feet—*diabetic truncal neuropathy* can cause localized areas of itching or dysesthesia on the skin (diabetic neuropathic pruritus or cutaneous dysesthesia). And as mentioned, neuropathy contributes to *generalized dry skin,* which can manifest as dullness, flakiness, and itching on the shins and arms of diabetic patients. Managing neuropathy (through glucose control and medications) and *good foot care (moisturizing skin and protective footwear)* are key strategies to prevent these cutaneous sequelae.

Immune Dysregulation and Infections

Diabetes is often considered a state of *immune dysfunction.* Chronic hyperglycemia impairs several aspects of the immune response, which, in turn, makes the skin more susceptible to infections:[32]

- *Neutrophil and phagocyte dysfunction:* Elevated blood glucose impairs neutrophil chemotaxis, adhesion, and phagocytosis. There is also reduced production of cytokines and reactive oxygen species required to kill pathogens. In essence, *white blood cells in diabetics are sluggish and less effective* in containing infections.
- *Circulation impairment:* As noted, microangiopathy and macroangiopathy reduce blood flow. Diminished

circulation means fewer immune cells and nutrients reach the site of injury or infection. It also means decreased oxygen tension, favoring the growth of anaerobic bacteria in wounds.
- *High glucose environment:* Elevated glucose in blood and tissues creates an environment that supports microbial growth. Bacteria can thrive in glucose-rich tissues, and *Candida* yeasts proliferate on skin surfaces where glucose may be elevated (such as sweat or intertriginous areas in hyperglycemic individuals). High glucose can also *glycate immunoglobulins,* potentially reducing their effectiveness.
- *Peripheral neuropathy and barrier:* As discussed, neuropathic dry skin and fissures break the protective barrier, giving microbes easy entry. Additionally, diabetic patients often have colonization with *Staphylococcus* on their skin and nares, predisposing them to staphylococcal infections.

Clinically, this immune dysregulation translates to *frequent and sometimes severe infections* of the skin and soft-tissue in diabetes.[32] Common examples include:
- *Fungal infections: Candida albicans* thrives in high-sugar, moist areas—*candidal intertrigo* in axillae, under breasts, groin folds, and *Candida* paronychia (nailfold infections) are frequent in diabetics. Patients present with erythematous, itchy rashes in folds with satellite pustules typical of candidiasis. *Tinea (dermatophyte) infections* of skin (ringworm) and nails (onychomycosis) are also more persistent in diabetics. *Tinea pedis* (athlete's foot) is especially common and can be a precursor to cellulitis of the skin between toe fissures. Onychomycosis (fungal nails) occurs in up to ~30% of diabetics; if untreated, it can act as a reservoir for repeated foot infection and can increase the risk of ulcers.
- *Bacterial infections:* Diabetics frequently get *staphylococcal infections*—e.g., recurrent boils (furuncles and carbuncles), folliculitis, and impetigo. Cellulitis (a spreading skin infection) often complicate foot ulcers or even minor injuries, and can progress rapidly if not addressed. *Erysipelas* (a form of cellulitis with lymphatic involvement) is also more common. Good glycemic control and skin hygiene help to reduce these risks.
- *Severe and opportunistic infections:* Certain dangerous infections, while rare, are seen almost exclusively in uncontrolled diabetics. One is *Fournier's gangrene,* a necrotizing fasciitis of the perineum often starting from a trivial skin break; diabetes is a major risk factor for this life-threatening infection. Another is *rhinocerebral mucormycosis,* a fulminant fungal infection by *Mucor* species, typically occurring in diabetics with ketoacidosis. Prompt surgical and medical intervention is required in these cases. Diabetic patients are also prone to postsurgical wound infections and have a higher risk of *Mycobacterium* skin infections if they receive injections (e.g., atypical mycobacterial abscess at insulin injection sites, though rare).[32]

CONCLUSION

In conclusion, *diabetes creates an immunocompromised state concerning skin defense. It alters the skin barrier through dryness, changed pH, and slowed epidermal turnover,* making skin more fragile and infection-prone. Regular use of emollients, avoidance of harsh soaps (to maintain skin's acidic mantle), keeping skin clean and moisturized, prompt antiseptic care for cuts, avoiding walking barefoot and prompt treatment of any dermatitis may help in keeping the barrier intact.

REFERENCES

1. Wang YR, Margolis D. The prevalence of diagnosed cutaneous manifestations during ambulatory diabetes visits in the United States. Dermatology. 2006;212:229-34.
2. Kurtalic N, Kurtalic S, Salihbegovic EM. Skin changes in patients with Diabetes Mellitus Type 2 and their impact on quality of life. Mater Sociomed. 2022;32:283-6.
3. Liu J, Wang L, Qian Y, Shen Q, Yang M, Dong Y, et al. Metabolic and genetic markers improve prediction of incident type 2 Diabetes: A nested case-control study in Chinese. J Clin Endocrinol Metab. 2022;107:3120-7.
4. Rotomskis R. Quantum dot migration through natural barriers and distribution in the skin. In: Rotomskis R (Ed). Nanoscience in Dermatology. London: Elsevier; 2016. pp. 307-19.
5. Kadyrov J, Ruiz-Perez L, Benson HAE, Mancera RL. Characterisation of the molecular mechanism of permeation of the prodrug Me-5ALA across the human stratum corneum using molecular dynamics simulations. Int J Mol Sci. 2022;23(24):16001.
6. Sjövall P, Gregoire S, Wargniez W, Skedung L, Luengo GS. 3D molecular imaging of stratum corneum by mass spectrometry suggests distinct distribution of cholesteryl esters compared to other skin lipids. Int J Mol Sci. 2022;23(22):13799.
7. Yoshida M, Numajiri S, Notani N, Sato N, Nomoto K, Arikawa H, et al. Staining of stratum corneum with fluorescent epsilon-poly-L-lysine and its application to evaluation of skin conditions. Skin Res Technol. 2023;29(1):13245.
8. Marks JG, Miller JJ. Lookingbill and Marks' Principles of Dermatology, 5th edition. China: Elsevier Health Sciences; 2013.
9. Natsuga K. Epidermal barriers. Cold Spring. Harb Perspect Med. 2014;4(4):a018218.
10. Bazzoni G, Dejana E. Keratinocyte junctions and the epidermal barrier: how to make a skin-tight dress. J Cell Biol. 2002;156(6):947-9.
11. Feingold KR. Thematic review series: skin lipids. The role of epidermal lipids in cutaneous permeability barrier homeostasis. J Lipid Res. 2007;48(12):2531-46.

12. Singh VP, Bali A, Singh N, Jaggi AS. Advanced glycation end products and diabetic complications. Korean J Physiol Pharmacol. 2014;18(1):1-14.
13. Yokota M, Tokudome Y. The Effect of Glycation on Epidermal Lipid Content, Its Metabolism and Change in Barrier Function. Skin Pharmacol Physiol. 2016;29(5):231-42.
14. Rhee SY, Kim YS. The Role of Advanced Glycation End Products in Diabetic Vascular Complications. Diabetes Metab J. 2018;42(3):188-95.
15. Legiawati L. The Role of Oxidative Stress, Inflammation, and Advanced Glycation End Product in Skin Manifestations of Diabetes Mellitus. Curr Diabetes Rev. 2022;18(3):e200921196637.
16. Báez EA, Shah S, Felipe D, Maynard J, Lefevre S, Chalew SA. Skin advanced glycation end products are elevated at the onset of type 1 diabetes in youth. J Pediatr Endocrinol Metab. 2015;28(1-2):133-7.
17. Mackiewicz-Wysocka M, Araszkiewicz A, Niedzwiedzki P, Schlaffke J, Micek I, Kuczynski S, et al. Skin pH is lower in type 1 diabetes subjects and is related to glycemic control of the disease. Diabetes Technol Ther. 2015;17(1):16-20.
18. Poonja PP, Kiss F. Pathophysiology of the Skin in Type 1 and Type 2 Diabetes and Emerging Therapeutic Opportunities. Int J Diabetes Clin Res. 2024;11:182.
19. Ono S, Imai R, Ida Y, Shibata D, Komiya T, Matsumura H. Increased wound pH as an indicator of local wound infection in second degree burns. Burns. 2015;41(4):820-4.
20. Goguen JM, Leiter LA. Lipids and diabetes mellitus: a review of therapeutic options. Curr Med Res Opin. 2002;18(1):S58-74.
21. Spravchikov N, Sizyakov G, Gartsbein M, Accili D, Tennenbaum T, Wertheimer E. Glucose effects on skin keratinocytes: implications for diabetes skin complications. Diabetes. 2001;50(7):1627-35.
22. Zhang Z, Zi Z, Lee EE, Zhao J, Contreras DC, South AP, et al. Differential glucose requirement in skin homeostasis and injury identifies a therapeutic target for psoriasis. Nat Med. 2018;24(5):617-27.
23. Li M, Zhao Y, Hao H, Dai H, Han Q, Tong C, et al. Mesenchymal stem cell-conditioned medium improves the proliferation and migration of keratinocytes in a diabetes-like microenvironment. Int J Low Extrem Wounds. 2015;14(1):73-86.
24. Van Putte L, De Schrijver S, Moortgat P. The effects of advanced glycation end products (AGEs) on dermal wound healing and scar formation: a systematic review. Scars Burn Heal. 2016;2:2059513116676828.
25. Denda M, Nakatani M. Acceleration of permeability barrier recovery by exposure of skin to 10-30 kHz sound. Br J Dermatol. 2010;162(3):503-7.
26. Yamaguchi K, Mitsui T, Aso Y, Sugibayashi K. Structure-permeability relationship analysis of the permeation barrier properties of the stratum corneum and viable epidermis/dermis of rat skin. J Pharm Sci. 2008;97(10):4391-403.
27. Goren I, Müller E, Schiefelbein D, Gutwein P, Seitz O, Pfeilschifter J, et al. Akt1 controls insulin-driven VEGF biosynthesis from keratinocytes: implications for normal and diabetes-impaired skin repair in mice. J Invest Dermatol. 2009;129(3):752-64.
28. Lafosse A, Dufeys C, Beauloye C, Horman S, Dufrane D. Impact of Hyperglycemia and Low Oxygen Tension on Adipose-Derived Stem Cells Compared with Dermal Fibroblasts and Keratinocytes: Importance for Wound Healing in Type 2 Diabetes. PLoS One. 2016;11(12):e0168058.
29. Ngo BT, Hayes KD, DiMiao DJ, Srinivasan SK, Huerter CJ, Rendell MS. Manifestations of cutaneous diabetic microangiopathy. Am J Clin Dermatol. 2005;6(4):225-37.
30. Edwards E, Yosipovitch G. Skin Manifestations of Diabetes Mellitus. In: Feingold KR, Ahmed SF, Anawalt B (eds). Endotext [Internet]. South Dartmouth (MA): MDText.com, Inc.; 2000.
31. Ghosh K, Das K, Ghosh S, Chakraborty S, Jatua SK, Bhattacharya A, et al. Prevalence of Skin Changes in Diabetes Mellitus and its Correlation with Internal Diseases: A Single Center Observational Study. Indian J Dermatol. 2015;60(5):465-9.
32. Casqueiro J, Casqueiro J, Alves C. Infections in patients with diabetes mellitus: A review of pathogenesis. Indian J Endocrinol Metab. 2012;16(1):S27-36.

CHAPTER 3

Common Skin Conditions in Diabetes and their Distribution

Arti Muley, Akashkumar N Singh

INTRODUCTION

Skin manifestations are among the most frequent but ignored complications in diabetes, affecting a significant proportion of patients. These dermatological signs often reflect the underlying metabolic disturbances and may even precede a diabetes diagnosis.[1] Pathogenetically, diabetic skin disorders can be traced to a core set of interrelated mechanisms: *Chronic hyperglycemia, insulin resistance (IR)*, *microangiopathy, neuropathy, immune dysfunction*, and *skin barrier impairment*. Each of these contributes to a broad spectrum of cutaneous presentations. Following are the most commonly encountered skin conditions in diabetic individuals:

XEROSIS (DRY AND SCALY SKIN)

Xerosis is one of the most common cutaneous manifestations in diabetes, affecting 40–60% of patients in some studies. It typically involves the feet and lower legs and is exacerbated by peripheral neuropathy and dehydration. Generalized pruritus often accompanies the dryness, contributing to discomfort and secondary skin damage.

CUTANEOUS INFECTIONS

Infections represent the *single most frequent* category of skin disorders in diabetic patients, observed in 20–30% of cases.[2] These include:
- *Fungal infections* are especially common due to immune dysfunction and favorable environments, i.e., moist microenvironment in skin folds and feet. These include *Candida intertrigo* **(Figs. 1A and B)**, *dermatophyte (Tinea) infections*, and *onychomycosis*.
- *Bacterial infections* such as *boils (furunculosis), cellulitis*, and *styes* occur recurrently, particularly with poor glycemic control.
- *Viral infections*, notably *herpes zoster*, also have increased prevalence in diabetes.

DIABETIC DERMOPATHY ("SHIN SPOTS")

These small, brown, atrophic macules on the pretibial areas are the *most common diabetes-specific* skin lesion, affecting up to 40% of patients, especially those over 50 years of age. They result from minor trauma in the setting of *diabetic microangiopathy* and often go unnoticed by patients **(Fig. 2)**.

ACANTHOSIS NIGRICANS AND SKIN TAGS

Acanthosis nigricans (AN) presents as velvety, hyperpigmented thickening in intertriginous areas (neck and axillae), and acrochordons (skin tags) often coexist on the neck and axillae **(Figs. 3A and B)**.

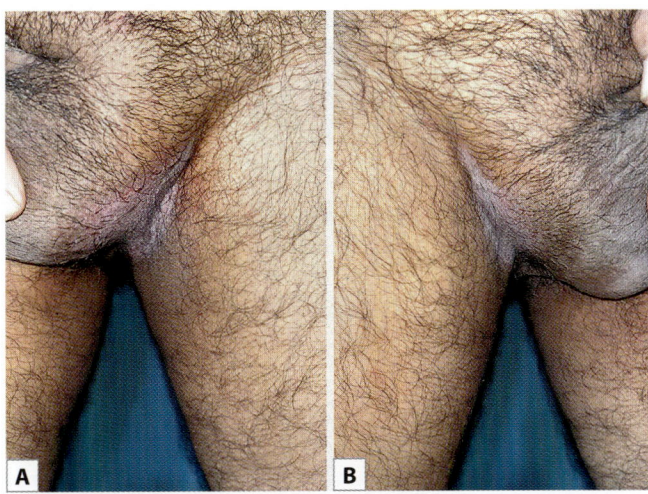

FIGS. 1A AND B: *Candida* intertrigo.

Courtesy: Nipul Vara, Assistant Professor, Department of Skin and VD, Medical College and SSG Hospital, Vadodara.

These are frequently associated with IR and *type 2 diabetes*. Their presence correlates with hyperinsulinemia and obesity (commonly seen in Indian diabetics).[3]

DIABETIC HAND (CHEIROARTHROPATHY)

Seen in up to 30% of long-standing diabetic patients, this condition is characterized by:
- *Waxy skin* on the hands
- *Limited joint mobility*, often demonstrated by a positive "prayer sign"
- It is linked to nonenzymatic glycation of collagen in skin and tendon that can occur in both type 1 and type 2 diabetes, sometimes appearing early in type 1 cases.

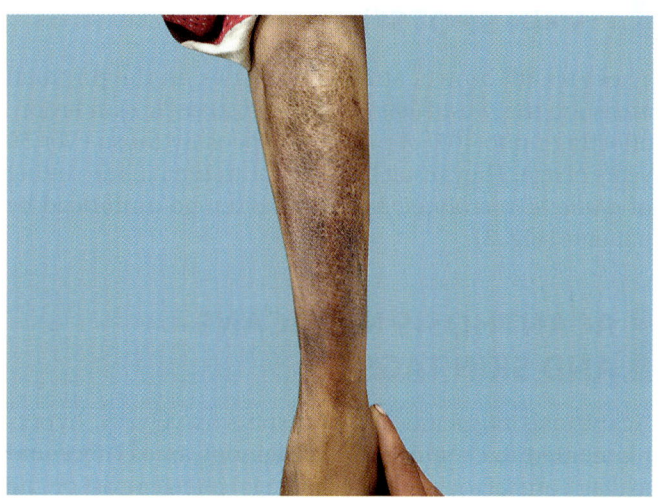

FIG. 2: Diabetic dermopathy.
Courtsey: Nipul Vara, Assistant Professor, Department of Skin and VD, Medical College and SSG Hospital, Vadodara.

OTHER SKIN FINDINGS

Several other cutaneous manifestations may be observed in diabetic individuals:
- Peripheral hair loss (especially on the shins) due to peripheral arterial disease
- Yellowish skin hue or hyperpigmentation
- *Autoimmune skin disorders:* Patients with type 1 diabetes mellitus (DM) (an autoimmune disease) have higher rates of other autoimmune skin disorders such as vitiligo and alopecia areata—these are *associated conditions* rather than caused by hyperglycemia, but their coexistence is epidemiologically notable.
- *Eruptive xanthomas:* Yellow papules resulting from *severe hypertriglyceridemia* in poorly controlled diabetes **(Figs. 4A and B)**

CLINICAL RELEVANCE AND DIAGNOSTIC IMPORTANCE OF CUTANEOUS LESIONS IN DIABETES

The presence of skin lesions often correlates with the *duration and control* of diabetes. Chronic complications such as diabetic dermopathy and foot ulcers become more likely with *longer disease duration*. Poor glycemic control [elevated glycated hemoglobin (HbA1c)] significantly increases the risk of *infections*, as shown in an Eastern India study where infected individuals had markedly higher HbA1c levels.[1]

Importantly, some skin findings—such as *acanthosis nigricans* or *eruptive xanthomas*—may serve as early indicators of *undiagnosed diabetes* or *prediabetes*.[3] Recognizing these dermatological clues is vital for clinicians in early diagnosis and prompting metabolic

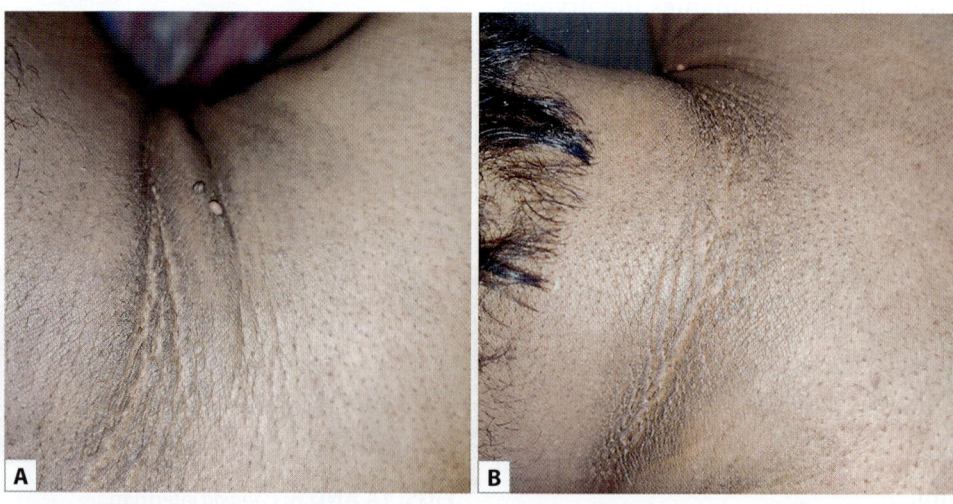

FIGS. 3A AND B: Acanthosis nigricans.
Courtsey: Nipul Vara, Assistant Professor, Department of Skin and VD, Medical College and SSG Hospital, Vadodara.

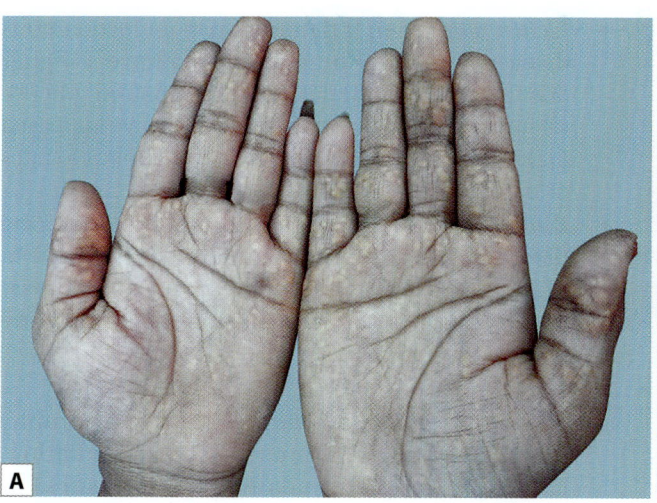 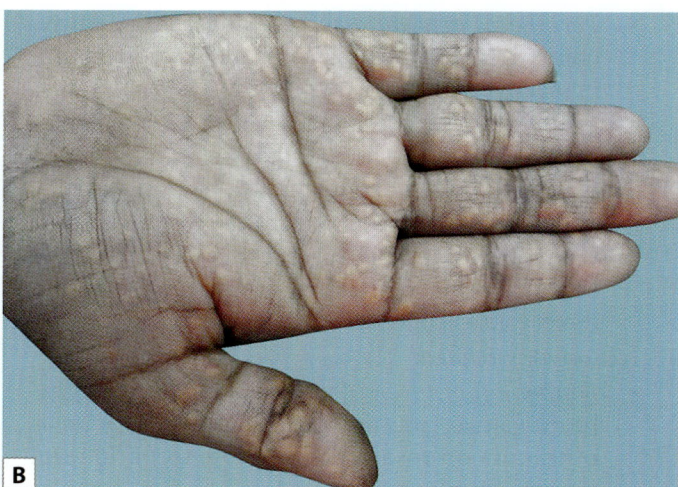

FIGS. 4A AND B: Eruptive xanthomas.
Courtsey: Nipul Vara, Assistant Professor, Department. of Skin and VD, Medical College and SSG Hospital, Vadodara.

control, especially in *India*, where diabetes is frequently underdiagnosed or detected late.[4]

CLASSIFICATION OF DIABETIC CUTANEOUS MANIFESTATIONS

Skin conditions in diabetes can be classified by pathogenesis (underlying cause) or morphology (lesion appearance). A pathogenesis-based approach links skin manifestations to the diabetic environment, helping clinicians understand their mechanisms. Morphological classification, useful for differential diagnosis, complements this by grouping lesions by appearance. Classifying these manifestations based on *underlying pathogenesis* or *morphological appearance* provides a practical framework for clinicians and researchers to better understand and teach the links between diabetes and the skin.

Various authors have proposed alternative classification systems based on clinical observations and research findings, as the spectrum of skin disorders in diabetic patients is broad and continually expanding, with new associations emerging over time. Additionally, the advent of newer antidiabetic therapies has introduced a range of novel cutaneous adverse effects, further complicating dermatologic care in this population. Presented here is a composite classification that synthesizes multiple approaches to offer a comprehensive overview of diabetes-associated skin conditions.

Classification Based on Pathogenesis

- *Hyperglycemia/metabolic-related lesions*:
  - *Diabetic dermopathy*: "Shin spots" due to microvascular changes from chronic hyperglycemia (microangiopathy)
  - *Necrobiosis lipoidica:* Atrophic plaques on shins; linked to microangiopathy and collagen degeneration in uncontrolled diabetes
  - *Diabetic bullae (bullosis diabeticorum):* Spontaneous blisters on acral skin; associated with chronic hyperglycemia and advanced glycation (fragile dermal–epidermal junction).
  - *Eruptive xanthomas:* Crops of yellow papules, usually on extensor surfaces, caused by severe hypertriglyceridemia in poorly controlled diabetes
  - *Diabetic cheiroarthropathy:* Waxy, tight skin on hands, limited joint mobility (prayer sign) due to glycation of collagen [an effect of hyperglycemia/advanced glycation end-products (AGEs)].
  - *Scleredema diabeticorum:* Diffuse induration of upper back/neck skin seen in some type 2 diabetics is thought to relate to glucose-mediated dermal fibrosis.
- IR-related lesions:[3,5]
  - *AN*: Velvety hyperpigmented thickening in neck, axillae; caused by hyperinsulinemia, stimulating epidermal growth.
  - *Acrochordons (skin tags)*: Pedunculated papules in axillae/neck; often coexist with AN as markers of IR.
  - *Hidradenitis suppurativa*: Chronic follicular abscesses in axillae/groin; not caused by diabetes per se, but obesity/IR in type 2 DM predispose to it.
  - *Psoriasis*: An immune-mediated plaque dermatosis; more common in diabetics and obese patients (shared IR and inflammatory pathways)
- *Microangiopathy and ischemia-related*:
  - *Diabetic dermopathy*: (Also listed earlier), the prototype microangiopathic lesion on the shins

- *Peripheral arterial disease lesions:* Thin, shiny, hairless skin on legs; ischemic ulcers or gangrene in severe cases
- *Pressure ulcers:* For example, heel ulcers in diabetics due to both microvascular disease and prolonged pressure (often concomitant with neuropathy)
- *Venous stasis changes:* Diabetes can worsen chronic venous insufficiency changes such as stasis dermatitis and ulcers due to impaired healing. Though not a direct cause, it often coexists in elderly diabetics.
- Neuropathy-related:[6]
  - *Diabetic foot ulcers:* Painless ulcers on weight-bearing areas (sole and metatarsal heads) or areas of trauma on insensate foot; due to peripheral neuropathy plus pressure
  - *Charcot arthropathy:* Joint collapse (often midfoot) due to neuropathy; can lead to rocker-bottom foot and chronic ulceration over bony prominences
  - *Neuropathic edema:* Some diabetics get neuropathy-related swelling of feet, which can further predispose to ulcers.
  - *Anhidrosis and fissures:* Neuropathy-induced dry skin, especially on feet, leading to heel fissures and cracking
- Infection-related lesions:
  - *Candidiasis:* Intertrigo in groins, under breasts; angular cheilitis; vaginal thrush—all more frequent in DM due to fungal overgrowth in high-sugar environment
  - *Dermatophytosis:* Tinea pedis (athlete's foot) and onychomycosis (nail fungus) are particularly common; can be a starting point for bacterial cellulitis.
  - *Bacterial skin infections:* Boils (furuncles), carbuncles, recurrent styes, folliculitis, cellulitis, and erysipelas; they are more frequent and often more severe in diabetics.
  - *Necrotizing fasciitis (e.g., Fournier's gangrene):* Rapidly spreading infection of subcutaneous tissue; diabetes is a major risk factor.
  - *Fungal opportunists:* Mucormycosis (in poorly controlled diabetic ketoacidosis) and *Malassezia* folliculitis, etc., seen in immunosuppressed states such as diabetes
- Autoimmune/associated dermatoses:
  - *Vitiligo:* Depigmented patches on skin caused due to autoimmune destruction of melanocytes. It is seen in type 1 DM as part of autoimmune polyendocrine syndromes.
  - *Alopecia areata:* Autoimmune hair loss in patches; also more common in type 1 DM
  - *Lichen planus:* An inflammatory papulosquamous disease shown in some studies to have a higher occurrence in diabetics or with impaired glucose tolerance. Lichen planus patients also have increased diabetes risk (possibly related to metabolic changes or medications).
  - *Bullous pemphigoid:* An autoimmune blistering disorder that is reported to be more frequent in diabetics (mechanism unclear, possibly cross-reactivity of AGEs with basement membrane proteins).
- *Treatment-related changes:*[7-9]
  - *Insulin injection site changes:* Lipohypertrophy (localized fat and fibrous tissue accumulation, causing a lump at repeated injection sites) or lipoatrophy (depressions due to immune reaction to insulin) can occur. Modern insulin analogs have reduced lipoatrophy incidence, but lipohypertrophy is still common if insulin injection sites are not rotated.
  - *Drug eruptions:* Diabetic patients on multiple medications (e.g., sulfonylureas, metformin, or newer agents) may develop cutaneous drug reactions. For instance, niacin (for dyslipidemia in diabetics) can cause flushing and some sodium–glucose cotransporter-2 (SGLT-2) inhibitors may cause fungal genital infections as a side effect.
  - *Mechanical dermatoses from devices:* Irritant or allergic contact dermatitis from insulin pump adhesives or continuous glucose monitor sensors on the skin

Classification Based on Morphology[1,4]

Classification based on morphology is as follows:
- *Pigmented lesions:* AN and diabetic dermopathy
- *Papulosquamous:* Lichen planus, psoriasis, and granuloma annulare
- *Bullous:* Diabetic bullae and bullous pemphigoid
- *Ulcerative:* Neuropathic ulcers, ischemic ulcers, and pressure ulcers
- *Infective:* Candidiasis, dermatophytosis, and bacterial cellulitis
- *Fibrosing/indurative:* Scleredema and diabetic cheiroarthropathy

Alternative Classification Systems[1-7]

Alternate classification/other classification systems are as follows:
- *Dermatologic lesions associated with but not specific to diabetes (disease markers):* These conditions are more

frequently observed in diabetic patients, but are not exclusive to diabetes:
- Pruritus
- Necrobiosis lipoidica diabeticorum
- Granuloma annulare
- Diabetic dermopathy
- Scleroderma-like syndrome
- Acanthosis nigricans
- Diabetic bullae

- *Skin alterations due to diabetic complications*:
  - Diabetic foot
  - Cutaneous infections are commonly associated with diabetes
    - Furunculosis
    - Carbuncle
    - Pyodermas
    - Candidiasis
    - Dermatophytosis
  - Erythrasma
  - Xanthomatosis
  - Xanthelasma
  - Phycomycosis
  - Malignant otitis externa/media
- *Dermatologic changes associated with neurovascular complications*:[7,10]
  - Macroangiopathy
  - Microangiopathy
  - Diabetic neuropathy
- *Dermatologic complications of diabetes treatment*:[7-9]
  - Reactions related to *oral hypoglycemic agents*
  - Reactions related to *insulin therapy*

- *Endocrine syndromes with skin changes and coexistent diabetes*:[11] Necrolytic migratory erythema (e.g., in glucagonoma)
- *Dermatoses more commonly seen in DM*:[12,13] These are not specific to DM but have an increased prevalence among diabetic patients:
  - Perforating dermatoses
  - Vitiligo
  - Lichen planus
  - Eruptive xanthomas
  - Kaposi's sarcoma
  - Bullous pemphigoid
  - Dermatitis herpetiformis
  - Psoriasis

Cutaneous manifestations are both *common and often inevitable* in the natural course of type 2 DM. These frequently act as a *visible index of the patient's internal metabolic state*, tending to improve with good glycemic control and worsen with poor regulation. From an epidemiological perspective, diabetic dermatoses represent a substantial clinical burden, affecting a significant proportion of patients at some stage of their illness.

In a country like *India*, where diabetes is reaching *epidemic proportions*, early recognition of these skin signs is especially critical. They can serve as *important diagnostic and prognostic clues*, prompting earlier interventions and comprehensive care.

Hence, in managing diabetes, *skin should not be overlooked*—attentive skin examination can yield early clues to systemic disease and prevent minor issues from becoming limb- or life-threatening.

REFERENCES

1. Edwards E, Yosipovitch G. Skin manifestations of diabetes mellitus. In: Feingold KR, Ahmed SF, Anawalt B, Blackman MR, Boyce A, Chrousos G, et al. (Eds). Endotext [Internet]. South Dartmouth (MA): MDText.com, Inc.; 2000.
2. Casqueiro J, Casqueiro J, Alves C. Infections in patients with diabetes mellitus: A review of pathogenesis. Indian J Endocr Metab. 2012;16(11):S27-36.
3. Maaran AT, Prathiba P. Acanthosis nigricans and skin tags as markers of insulin resistance in non-diabetic obese individuals. J Evid Based Med Healthc. 2020;7(6):270-4.
4. Abate MCMO, Aroucha PMT, Nóbrega DVMD, Rocha IPM, Soares SD, Reis AA, et al. Cutaneous manifestations of diabetes mellitus: A narrative review. Einstein (São Paulo). 2025;23:eRW1193.
5. Goyal A, Raina S, Kaushal SS, Mahajan V, Sharma NL. Pattern of cutaneous manifestations in diabetes mellitus. Indian J Dermatol. 2010;55(1):39-41.
6. Dogiparthi SN, Muralidhar K, Seshadri KG, Rangarajan S. Cutaneous manifestations of diabetic peripheral neuropathy. Dermatoendocrinol. 2017;9(1):e1395537.
7. Richardson T, Kerr D. Skin-related complications of insulin therapy: Epidemiology and emerging management strategies. Am J Clin Dermatol. 2003;4(10):661-7.
8. Mederle AL, Dumitrescu P, Borza C, Kundnani NR. Cutaneous Adverse Drug Reactions Associated with SGLT2 Inhibitors. J Clin Med. 2024;14(1):188.
9. Cameli N, Silvestri M, Mariano M, Messina C, Nisticò SP, Cristaudo A. Allergic contact dermatitis, an important skin reaction in diabetes device users: A systematic review. dermatitis. 2022;33(2):110-5.
10. Ngo BT, Hayes KD, DiMiao DJ, Srinivasan SK, Huerter CJ, Rendell MS. Manifestations of cutaneous diabetic microangiopathy. Am J Clin Dermatol. 2005;6(4):225-37.
11. Compton NL, Chien AJ. A rare but revealing sign: necrolytic migratory erythema. Am J Med. 2013;126(5):387-9.
12. Ünlü B, Türsen Ü. Autoimmune skin diseases and the metabolic syndrome. Clin Dermatol. 2018;36(1):67-71.
13. Armstrong AW, Harskamp CT, Armstrong EJ. Psoriasis and the risk of diabetes mellitus: A systematic review and meta-analysis. JAMA Dermatol. 2013;149(1):84-91.

SECTION 2

Dermatologic Conditions Directly Attributed to Diabetes

Section Outline

Chapter 4: Diabetic Dermopathy (Shin Spots) in a Type 2 Diabetic Male
Suhas Gopal Erande

Chapter 5: Necrobiosis Lipoidica Based on a Skin Biopsy
Namrata C Manjunath, Chinmayee Anand N, Niraj, Deepak Das

Chapter 6: Bullous Diabeticorum
Firdous Shaikh, Avina Jain, Abhinav Jain, Armaan Mishra

Chapter 7: Bullous Pemphigoid in a Diabetic Male
Nipul Vara, Vishwa Marvania, Preya Parag Rana

Chapter 8: Yellow Palms in Diabetes Mellitus: A Case of Carotenoderma
Arijit Singha, Pradip Mukhopadhyay, Sujoy Ghosh

Chapter 9: Carotenemia in a Patient with Type 2 Diabetes Mellitus
NK Singh, Akashkumar N Singh, Anuradha Kapoor

Chapter 10: Diabetic Rubeosis Faciei with Palmar Erythema
Ashma Surani, Bela J Shah

Chapter 11: Finger Pebbles (Huntley's Papules) in a Diabetic Male
Suhas Gopal Erande

Chapter 12: Perforating Dermatosis
Nipul Vara, Vishwa Marvania, Preya Parag Rana, Suhas Gopal Erande, Prabhat Kumar Agrawal, Sandipta Kumar Panda, Gaurav Gupta, Anil Patki, Ashma Surani, Firdous Shaikh, Avina Jain

SECTION 2

Dermatologic Conditions and Growth

CHAPTER 4

Diabetic Dermopathy (Shin Spots) in a Type 2 Diabetic Male

Suhas Gopal Erande

Case 1

■ PRESENTATION

A 64-year-old male with a 15-year history of type 2 diabetes mellitus presented with complaints of gradually developing dark patches over the front of both lower legs. The lesions had appeared slowly over the past 6 months. The patient reported no pain, itching, trauma, or history of prior ulceration at the sites.

■ EXAMINATION

On physical examination, multiple well-demarcated, round-to-oval, brownish macules and papules were observed over the anterior aspects of both shins **(Fig. 1)**. The lesions measured between 0.3 and 1.5 cm in diameter and showed central atrophy with peripheral hyperpigmentation. The skin over the lesions appeared thin and mildly scaly. There were no signs of ulceration, active inflammation, or secondary infection.

■ INVESTIGATIONS

- *Neuropathy foot screening:* Revealed altered capillary morphology with mild tortuosity and capillary dropout.
- *Glycemic profile:* Glycated hemoglobin (HbA1c) was found to be 8.1%, indicating poor glycemic control.
- *Ophthalmic evaluation:* Showed early signs of background diabetic retinopathy without macular involvement.
- *Renal parameters:* Urine albumin-to-creatinine ratio (UACR) indicated early microalbuminuria.

Diagnosis

- Diabetic dermopathy (also known as "diabetic shin spots")
- The diagnosis of diabetic dermopathy, also known as "shin spots", was confirmed based on the above clinical findings. It represents a common cutaneous manifestation of long-standing diabetes mellitus and may serve as a cutaneous marker of underlying microvascular complications, analogous to the involvement seen in diabetic retinopathy and nephropathy.[1,2]

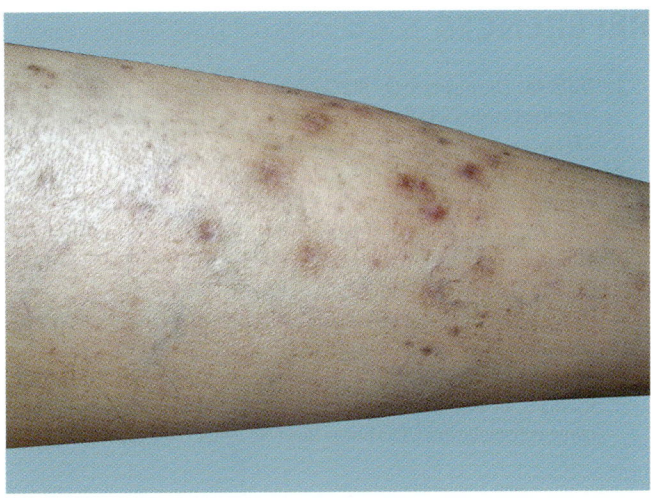

FIG. 1: Dark brown macules and patches over the anterior lower legs in a male patient with type 2 diabetes mellitus.

Differential Diagnoses

- *Stasis dermatitis*: It presents with hyperpigmentation, erythema, and scaling near the ankles, often accompanied by edema.[3]
- *Postinflammatory hyperpigmentation:* It occurs following a history of trauma or preceding inflammation.[3]
- *Lichen planus:* It is characterized by violaceous, flat-topped papules that may be pruritic.[4]
- *Purpura annularis telangiectodes:* It show petechial patches often associated with vasculitis.[5]
- *Necrobiosis lipoidica:* Necrobiosis lipoidica features sharply demarcated plaques with central atrophy and a yellowish hue.[5]

Pathophysiology

- Believed to result from *diabetic microangiopathy*, leading to poor blood flow and subsequent *dermal ischemia*.[2,6]
- Often follows *minor trauma* due to increased skin fragility in diabetes
- Histopathologically, it shows *mild lymphocytic perivascular infiltrate,* hemosiderin deposition, and dermal atrophy.[2]

Management

Dermatology Management

- *No specific treatment* needed in most cases[1,7]
- Application of *emollients* to maintain hydration and barrier function[7]
- Avoidance of trauma to lower legs[2]
- Rarely, cosmetic camouflage for extensive pigmentation[2]

Diabetology/Physician Management

- *Optimize glycemic control* to prevent progression of microvascular complications.[1,8]
- Evaluate for associated *retinopathy, nephropathy, and neuropathy*.[1]
- Educate the patient that lesions are *harmless* and do not require aggressive treatment.[7]
- Encourage foot and leg care to *prevent trauma and secondary infections*.[7]

Prognosis

- Lesions are benign and *do not ulcerate or progress* to malignancy.[2,6]
- Typically *resolve over months to years* but may leave residual pigmentation.[2]
- New lesions may appear even after glycemic control.[8]

> **Clinical Pearls**
> - Seen in *up to 55% of diabetics*, more common in older men.[1,5]
> - Often the *earliest cutaneous* sign of diabetes[1]
> - Should prompt a search for *other microvascular complications* (e.g., fundus examination and urine microalbumin).[1,3]
> - Painless and often symmetrical over bony prominences (tibial region)[2]
> - Also called "*shin spots*" in layman's terminology.[2]

REFERENCES

1. Duff M, Demidova O, Blackburn S, Shubrook J. Cutaneous manifestations of diabetes mellitus. Clin Diabetes. 2008;26(1):27-32.
2. Saxena Pal R, Wal P, Pal Y, Wal A. Recent insights on diabetic dermopathy. Open Dermatol J. 2019;13:8-12.
3. Roslind S, Muhammed K, Kumar KGS. Cutaneous manifestations in patients with type 2 diabetes mellitus and normal controls. J Sci Soc Ther Dermatol. 2020;7(2):95-101.
4. Huntley AC. Cutaneous manifestations of diabetes mellitus. Diabetes Care. 1980;3(1):75-88.
5. Romano G, Moretti G, Di Benedetto A, Giofrè C, Di Cesare E, Russo G, et al. Skin lesions in diabetes mellitus: prevalence and clinical correlations. Diabetes Res Clin Pract. 1998;39(2):101-6.
6. Brzezinski P, Chiriac AE, Pinteala T, Foia L, Chiriac A. Diabetic dermopathy ("shin spots") and diabetic bullae ("bullosis diabeticorum"): two associated cutaneous markers in diabetes mellitus. Clujul Med. 2011;84(1):129-32.
7. Apollo Hospitals. (2025). Diabetic Dermopathy—Causes, Symptoms, Diagnosis, and Treatment. 2025. [online] Available from https://www.apollohospitals.com/diseases-and-conditions/diabetic-dermopathy [Last accessed Aug., 2025].
8. Karra MC, Maheswari PM, Atluri SC, Samanthula H. Dermatological manifestations in diabetes mellitus and its relation with HbA1c levels – An observational study. IP Indian J Clin Exp Dermatol. 2024;10(4):393-7.

Case 2

PRESENTATION

A 48-year-old male presents with a 1-year history of multiple, asymptomatic, and brownish spots on both shins. The lesions have progressively darkened over time and have not been associated with trauma, scratching, or infection. The patient has a long-standing medical background of poorly controlled type 2 diabetes mellitus (12 years, HbA1c 9.6%), hypertension, and dyslipidemia. Compliance with antidiabetic medications (metformin and glimepiride) has been irregular.

EXAMINATION

- On examination, multiple well-demarcated, round-to-oval brown macules and papules with central atrophy and peripheral hyperpigmentation are observed, distributed bilaterally over the anterior tibiae **(Fig. 2)**.
- The lesions are nonscaly, nontender, and not ulcerated, with no surrounding edema or signs of active inflammation.
- Peripheral pulses are intact, and sensory examination is normal.

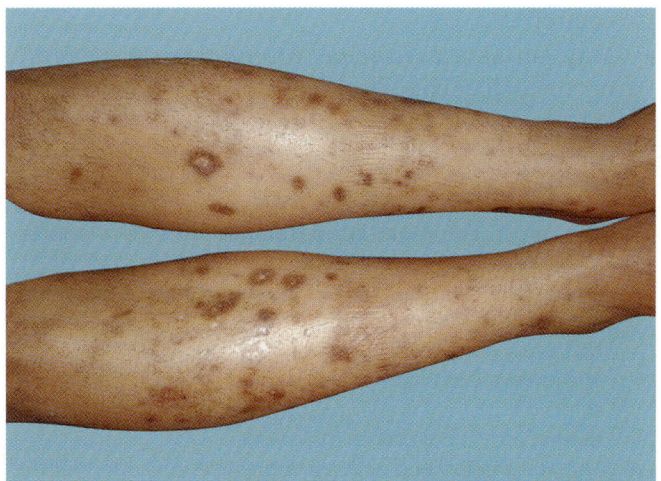

FIG. 2: Multiple well-demarcated, round-to-oval brown macules and papules with central atrophy and peripheral hyperpigmentation distributed bilaterally over the anterior tibiae.

INVESTIGATIONS

To confirm the clinical suspicion and assess the associated systemic status, the following investigations were performed:
- *Glycemic status*:
  - *Glycated hemoglobin (HbA1c):* 9.6% (Reference range: <6.5%)—Suggestive of long-standing and poorly controlled diabetes mellitus
  - *Fasting plasma glucose (FPG):* 165 mg/dL (Reference range: 70–99 mg/dL)—Elevated fasting glucose
  - *Postprandial plasma glucose (PPG):* 250 mg/dL (Reference range: <140 mg/dL)—Elevated postprandial glucose.
- *Lipid profile*:
  - *Low-density lipoprotein (LDL):* 134 mg/dL (Reference range: <100 mg/dL)—Elevated
  - *Triglycerides:* 180 mg/dL (Reference range: <150 mg/dL)—Elevated
- *Urine microalbumin*: 46 mg/g (Reference range: <30 mg/g)—Suggestive of early nephropathy
- *Monofilament test*: Normal—No clinical evidence of neuropathy.
- *Additional dermatological assessment*:
  - *Dermoscopy:* Shows central atrophy with a pigment network, perilesional hyperpigmentation, and sparse perifollicular pigmentation.
  - *Histopathology (if performed):* Epidermal atrophy, increased dermal collagenization, mild perivascular lymphocytic infiltrate, and dermal hemosiderin deposition (no evidence of vasculitis).

PATHOPHYSIOLOGY

In diabetic dermopathy, chronic hyperglycemia leads to microangiopathy and subsequent changes within the skin:
- Capillary basement membrane thickening and endothelial dysfunction
- Reduced perfusion and tissue hypoxia in the lower extremities
- Extravasation of red blood cells with deposition of hemosiderin within the dermis
- Impaired wound healing and vulnerability to minor, unnoticed trauma in the shin area, promoting persistence and recurrence of lesions[1,2]

DIAGNOSIS

Diabetic Dermopathy (Shin Spots)

A clinical diagnosis based on the characteristic morphology and distribution of the lesions over the shins in a patient with long-standing and poorly controlled diabetes mellitus.[3,4]

Systemic Correlation

- Diabetic dermopathy is seen in approximately 30–60% of patients with longstanding type 2 diabetes mellitus.[10,11]
- It is strongly associated with other microvascular complications of diabetes, including:
  - Retinopathy
  - Nephropathy
  - *Peripheral neuropathy* (often present subclinically despite absence of overt clinical signs)
- The presence of these lesions is closely linked to the duration and severity of hyperglycemia.[1,4]

DIFFERENTIAL DIAGNOSIS

- *Necrobiosis lipoidica:* Yellow, waxy plaques with telangiectasia and central atrophy, typically located on the shins and associated with long-standing diabetes.
- *Pigmented purpuric dermatoses:* Characterized by petechiae and "cayenne-pepper" spots, often pruritic and presenting on the lower legs.
- *Stasis dermatitis:* Usually unilateral with associated edema, lipodermatosclerosis, and hyperpigmentation due to chronic venous insufficiency.
- *Lichen planus:* Presents as pruritic, violaceous, polygonal lesions with a characteristic flat-topped surface and Wickham striae.
- *Postinflammatory hyperpigmentation:* Develops following eczema, trauma, or other inflammatory skin conditions, presenting as dark patches in the affected area.

MANAGEMENT

Dermatologist Management

- No specific therapy required for most cases.
- Reassure patient about the benign and selflimiting nature of the condition.
- *Supportive skin care*:
  - Use moisturizers or emollients to reduce dryness.
  - Apply broadspectrum sunscreen to prevent pigment intensification.
- *Cosmetic options (if desired)*:
  - Topical retinoids (e.g., tretinoin 0.025%)
  - Azelaic acid (15–20%) or Kojic acid for lightening hyperpigmentation[5,6]

Diabetologist/Physician Management

- Optimize glycemic control with intensification of therapy (oral agents or insulin as required).
- *Address associated comorbidities*: Hypertension and dyslipidemia.
- *Screen for microvascular complications*:
  - Fundoscopy for diabetic retinopathy
  - Urine albumin assessment for nephropathy
  - Foot examination for early neuropathy
- *Provide patient education on foot care*:
  - Gentle cleaning and inspection of skin
  - Avoid trauma or friction in affected areas

PROGNOSIS

- Benign and nonprogressive
- Individual lesions may *persist for years* or gradually fade.
- New lesions can develop with ongoing poor glycemic control.
- May act as a *cutaneous biomarker* for systemic microvascular complications.[1,3]

> **Clinical Pearls**
> - The most common dermatologic sign of diabetes mellitus.[1]
> - Frequently overlooked but may correlate with silent retinopathy or nephropathy.[3]
> - No biopsy required in classical presentations.[1,3]
> - The presence of bilateral, atrophic brown macules over the shins in a diabetic patient should be considered "diabetic dermopathy" until proven otherwise.[1,3]
> - The progression and activity of these lesions often mirror the patient's glycemic control.[1]

REFERENCES

1. Nigam PK, Saxena AK. Diabetic dermopathy: A cutaneous marker of microangiopathy in diabetes mellitus. Indian J Dermatol. 2019;64(5):379-84.
2. Sanad EM, ElFangary MM, Sorour NE, ElNemisy NM. Skin manifestations in Egyptian diabetic patients: a case-series study. Egypt J Dermatol Venerol. 2013;33(2):56-62.
3. Dinneen SF, Bruckner A, Kirby B, Rogers S, McCulloch DK. Diabetic dermopathy: A marker for microangiopathy. Clin Endocrinol. 1995;43(5):593-8.
4. Singh R, Akhtar N, Chauhan A, Singh A. Histopathological and clinical correlation of diabetic dermopathy. J Clin Diagn Res. 2015;9(6):WC01-WC03.
5. Kumar S, Dogra D, Gupta S. Dermoscopic features of diabetic dermopathy. Clin Dermatol Rev. 2021;5(1):21-4.
6. DiNardo JC. Skin manifestations of diabetes. Clin Dermatol. 2023;41(2):212-9.

CHAPTER 5

Necrobiosis Lipoidica Based on a Skin Biopsy

Namrata C Manjunath, Chinmayee Anand N, Niraj, Deepak Das

Case 1

■ PRESENTATION

A 62-year-old retired female teacher presented with multiple red, raised, and dark lesions, some of which had ulcerated, over both lower legs and thigh. The lesions had gradually evolved over 2 years.

■ CLINICAL HISTORY

The patient first noticed red papules on her lower limbs and left thigh, which overtime ulcerated and developed a shiny, atrophic surface. She reported intermittent mild-to-moderate itching and burning pain localized to the lesions but denied any systemic symptoms. Her occupational history included many years of prolonged standing. She had a 2-year history of type 2 diabetes mellitus managed with oral hypoglycemic agents.

■ EXAMINATION

Multiple well-defined erythematous brown plaques and ulcers with shiny surfaces were present on both the lower leg **(Fig. 1)** and the left thigh **(Fig. 2)**. There were no signs of systemic infection or other dermatoses.

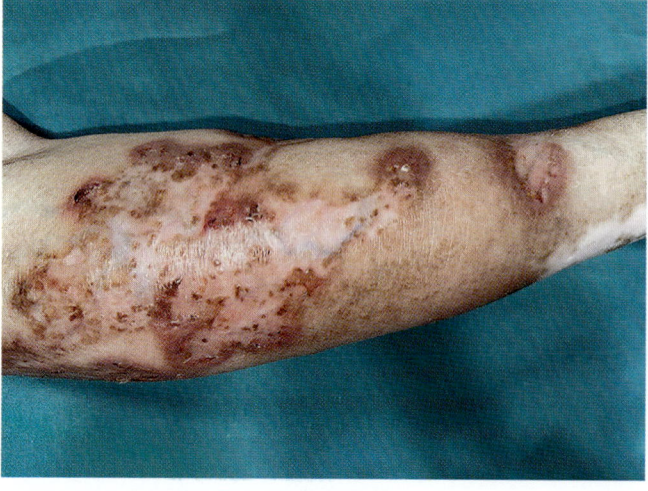

FIG. 1: Multiple red, raised, and dark lesions with areas of ulceration over the lower leg in a female patient.

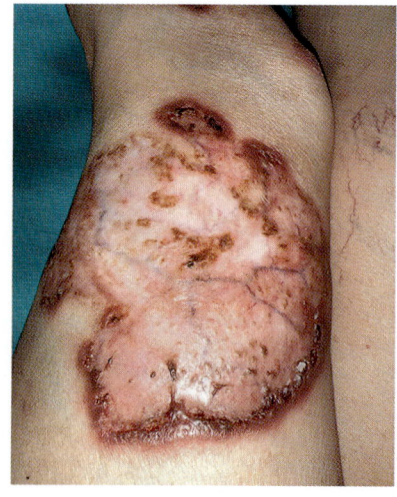

FIG. 2: Multiple red, raised, and dark lesions with areas of ulceration over the left thigh in a female patient.

LABORATORY FINDINGS

- *Fasting blood sugar (FBS)*: 112 mg/dL
- *Postprandial blood sugar (PPBS)*: 145 mg/dL
- *Glycated hemoglobin (HbA1c)*: 6.7%
- *Urine routine*: Within normal limits
- *Erythrocyte sedimentation rate (ESR)*: 40 mm/h (elevated)

HISTOPATHOLOGY

Microscopic examination of the skin biopsy revealed:
- Irregular acanthosis and mild spongiosis of the epidermis
- Increased dermal fibrosis and areas of necrobiosis (collagen degeneration)
- Dense lymphohistiocytic infiltrate with multinucleated giant cells forming granuloma-like structures
- Inflammation extending into the subcutaneous tissue
- No caseous necrosis; Ziehl–Neelsen stain was negative for acid–fast bacilli

These findings are consistent with necrobiosis lipoidica (NLD), particularly the presence of necrobiotic collagen, granulomatous inflammation, and fibrosis, with the absence of infectious organisms.

DIAGNOSIS

Necrobiosis lipoidica was confirmed by clinical features and skin biopsy.[1,2]

DIFFERENTIAL DIAGNOSES

- *Pyoderma gangrenosum*: Rapidly progressive, painful ulcerative lesions, and usually with a violaceous border
- *Lupus vulgaris*: Chronic cutaneous tuberculosis; ruled out by negative Ziehl–Neelsen stain
- *Epidermolysis bullosa acquisita*: Chronic bullous dermatosis; direct immunofluorescence is necessary for diagnosis.
- *Bullous pemphigoid*: It is characterized by tense bullae but lacks necrobiotic histology
- *Squamous cell carcinoma*: It is characterized by chronic ulcerated nodules with cytological atypia, not seen in this case[3]

MANAGEMENT

Dermatologic Treatment

- Topical halobetasol propionate 0.05% combined with fusidic acid 2% cream applied nightly for 2 months
- Oral doxycycline 100 mg/day for anti-inflammatory and immunomodulatory effects
- Low-dose aspirin 75 mg/day to improve microcirculatory perfusion[4,5]

Monitoring

- Regular follow-up to assess wound healing and glycemic control
- Ongoing wound care advice

Response

After 2 months of therapy, the patient showed a reduction in ulcer size and erythema, indicating good clinical improvement.[2]

Prognosis

Necrobiosis lipoidica is a chronic dermatologic complication of diabetes that can be difficult to manage once established. Although not life-threatening, it can significantly affect quality of life due to ulceration, pigmentation, and cosmetic disfigurement. Long-term outcomes depend on early recognition, effective glycemic control, and timely dermatologic intervention.[1,2,5]

> **Clinical Pearls**
>
> ▶ Necrobiosis lipoidica often begins as erythematous papules that progress to atrophic, shiny plaques.[1]
> ▶ There is a strong association with diabetes mellitus; cutaneous lesions may precede the diagnosis of diabetes in some patients.[4]
> ▶ Histopathology is the gold standard for diagnosis, demonstrating necrobiosis, granulomatous inflammation, and fibrosis.[1,2]
> ▶ Early dermatological evaluation and strict glycemic control are essential to prevent progression and ulceration.[6,7]
> ▶ Skin findings such as NLD may serve as external markers of underlying systemic metabolic dysfunction.[4,7]

Case 2

PRESENTATION

A 38-year-old male with a 10-year history of well-controlled type 2 diabetes mellitus presented with a solitary lesion on the posterior aspect of his right lower leg. The lesion began as a small reddish patch several months ago and gradually enlarged, developing central atrophy and a shiny surface. The patient reported occasional mild itching and tenderness but denied significant pain. There was no history of trauma, immunosuppressant, or anticoagulant use. He worked in an office setting with minimal physical strain.

EXAMINATION

- A single, well-demarcated, reddish-brown to yellow plaque was noted on the posterior right lower leg (**Fig. 3**).
- The lesion had a shiny, atrophied central area.
- No ulceration or signs of secondary infection were observed.
- Peripheral sensation was intact, and there were no clinical signs of venous insufficiency.
- No similar lesions were present elsewhere

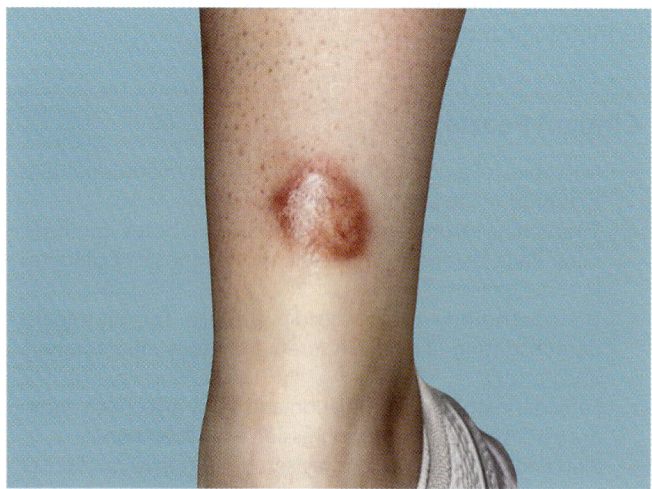

FIG. 3: A single, well-demarcated, and reddish-brown to yellow plaque on the posterior aspect of the right lower leg.

INVESTIGATION

- Laboratory studies, including fasting and postprandial blood glucose, were performed to assess glycemic status.
- No evidence of systemic immunosuppression or coagulation abnormality was identified.

DIAGNOSIS

The clinical features—sharply demarcated, atrophic, and shiny plaque on the lower leg in a patient with long-standing diabetes—were diagnostic of necrobiosis lipoidica.[8,9]

DIFFERENTIAL DIAGNOSIS

- *Granuloma annulare*: It presents as annular lesions, often without central atrophy.[8]
- *Cutaneous sarcoidosis*: It can resemble NLD but lacks the typical shiny, atrophic center.[8]
- *Stasis dermatitis*: It is associated with venous insufficiency and lacks the distinct atrophic features of NLD.
- *Tinea corporis*: It is a fungal infection that usually has raised border and scales.[8]

MANAGEMENT

Topical Therapy

- Potent corticosteroids (e.g., clobetasol propionate) to reduce inflammation[8]
- Topical calcineurin inhibitors (e.g., tacrolimus 0.1% ointment) as steroid-sparing agents for long-term use[8,10]

Systemic Therapy

- Pentoxifylline and aspirin may improve microcirculation in select cases.[8]
- Methotrexate or other immunosuppressants for refractory, progressive, or ulcerative lesions.[8,10,11]

Metabolic and Supportive Care

- Optimize glycemic control to prevent progression[12]
- Employ wound care protocols for ulcerated lesions (appropriate dressings, hygiene)[13]
- Advise smoking cessation to enhance vascular health[8]

Prognosis

Necrobiosis lipoidica is chronic and unpredictable. Lesions may remain stable, enlarge, or ulcerate over time. Spontaneous resolution is rare. Early intervention and optimal diabetes control can limit disease progression.

Secondary infections and ulcerations are potential complications, especially in advanced or neglected cases.[1,12-14]

Clinical Pearls

- Sharply demarcated, reddish-brown to yellow plaques with shiny, atrophic centres[8]
- Predominantly affects shins and lower legs[8,9]
- Strong association with long-standing diabetes mellitus[8,12]
- Central atrophy, telangiectasia, and occasional ulceration are the hallmark features[8]
- Poor glycemic control and smoking may accelerate progression[12]

REFERENCES

1. Thomas M, Khopkar US. A clinicopathological study of necrobiosis lipoidica in the Indian scenario. Indian Dermatol Online J. 2013;4(4):288-91.
2. Naumowicz M, Modzelewski S, Macko A, Łuniewski B, Baran A, Flisiak I. A breakthrough in the treatment of necrobiosis lipoidica? Update on treatment, etiopathogenesis, diagnosis, and clinical presentation. Int J Mol Sci. 2024;25(6):3482.
3. Johnson E, Patel MH, Brumfiel CM, Severson KJ, Bhullar P, Boudreaux B, et al. Histopathologic features of necrobiosis lipoidica. J Cutan Pathol. 2022;49(8):692-700.
4. Romano G, Moretti G, Di Benedetto A, Giofrè C, Di Cesare E, Russo G. Skin lesions in diabetes mellitus: prevalence and clinical correlations. Diabetes Res Clin Pract. 1998;39(2):101-6.
5. Erfurt-Berge C, Seitz AT, Rehse C, Wollina U, Schwede K, Renner R. Update on clinical and laboratory features in necrobiosis lipoidica: a retrospective multicentre study of 52 patients. Eur J Dermatol. 2012;22(6):770-5.
6. Boulton AJ, Meneses P, Ennis WJ. Diabetic foot ulcers: a framework for prevention and care. Wound Repair Regen. 1999;7(1):7-16.
7. Edwards E, Yosipovitch G. Skin manifestations of diabetes mellitus. In: Feingold KR, Anawalt B, Boyce A, et al., editors. Endotext [Internet]. South Dartmouth (MA): MDText.com, Inc.; updated 2025 Mar 21. Available from: https://www.ncbi.nlm.nih.gov/books/NBK481900/
8. Reid SD, Ladizinski B, Lee K, Baibergenova A, Alavi A. Update on necrobiosis lipoidica: a review of etiology, diagnosis, and treatment options. J Am Acad Dermatol. 2013;69(5):783-91.
9. Dissemond J. Necrobiosis lipoidica diabeticorum. N Engl J Med. 2012;366(26):2502.
10. Nihal A, Caplan AS, Rosenbach M, Damsky W, Mangold AR, Shields BE. Treatment options for necrobiosis lipoidica: a systematic review. Int J Dermatol. 2023;62(12):1529-37.
11. Basoulis D, Fragiadiki K, Tentolouris N, Sfikakis PP, Kokkinos A. Anti-TNF-α treatment for recalcitrant ulcerative necrobiosis lipoidica diabeticorum: a case report and literature review. Metabolism. 2016;65(4):569-73.
12. Mistry BD, Alavi A, Ali S, Mistry N. A systematic review of the Relationship between glycemic control and necrobiosis lipoidica diabeticorum. Int J Dermatol. 2017;56(12):1319-27.
13. Young T. Understanding necrobiosis lipoidica diabeticorum. Wounds UK. 2019;15(1):49-54.
14. Ionescu C, Petca A, Dumitrașcu MC, Petca RC, Ionescu Miron AI, Șandru F. The intersection of dermatological dilemmas and endocrinological complexities: understanding necrobiosis lipoidica – a comprehensive review. Biomedicines. 2024;12(2):337.

CHAPTER 6

Bullous Diabeticorum

Firdous Shaikh, Avina Jain, Abhinav Jain, Armaan Mishra

Case 1

■ PRESENTATION

A 60-year-old male factory worker presented with a sudden onset of fluid-filled blisters over the lower legs and dorsal aspects of both feet. The blisters had appeared spontaneously 2 weeks prior to consultation, with no history of preceding trauma, burns, or chemical exposure. Initial treatment with oral antihistamines for a presumed allergic reaction was ineffective. The blisters gradually increased in size and number, and some ruptured, leaving behind shallow erosions. There was no associated pain, itching, fever, or other systemic symptoms. The patient reported standing for long periods due to occupational demands.

■ EXAMINATION

- Multiple tense and flaccid bullae were observed on the lower legs and dorsum of both feet **(Figs. 1A and B)**. Some of the blisters were intact, while others had ruptured, resulting in superficial erosions and serous crusting.
- The lesions were nontender with no signs of erythema, warmth, or purulent discharge.
- The surrounding skin appeared healthy.
- The peripheral pulses were intact and symmetrical.
- There was no peripheral neuropathy or signs of vascular compromise.

■ INVESTIGATIONS

- *Glycated hemoglobin (HbA1c)*: 9.8%—indicating newly diagnosed and poorly controlled type 2 diabetes mellitus
- *Serum creatinine*: 1.0 mg/dL—within normal limits
- *Complete blood count*: Within normal range

■ DIAGNOSIS

Bullous diabeticorum is associated with newly detected type 2 diabetes mellitus.[1,2]

■ DIFFERENTIAL DIAGNOSES

- *Bullous pemphigoid*: It is excluded due to the absence of widespread involvement, pruritus, erythema, and a negative Nikolsky's sign.[2]

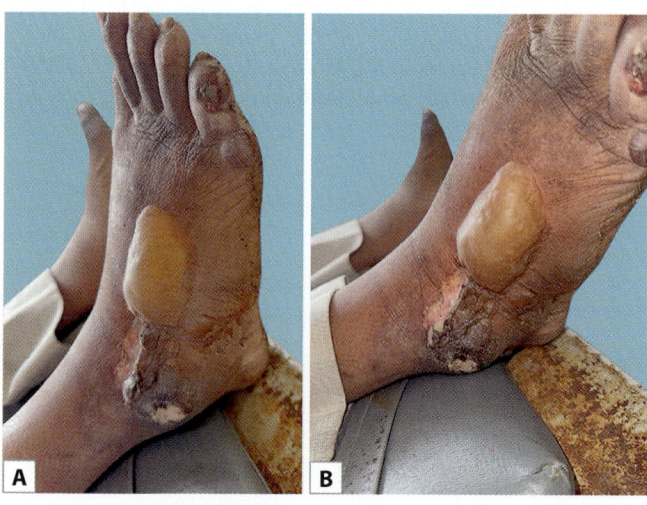

FIGS. 1A AND B: Multiple tense and flaccid bullae on the lower legs and dorsum of both feet.

- *Diabetic foot ulcers*: They are ruled out as the lesions were primarily bullous rather than ulcerative at onset.[3]
- *Infectious bullae*: They are considered but deemed unlikely in the absence of purulence, cellulitis, or systemic signs of infection.[4]

■ MANAGEMENT

Dermatologist

- Recognized the characteristic appearance of the bullae and suspected underlying diabetes.[5]
- Recommended urgent blood glucose testing and specialist referral.
- *Advised basic wound care*:
  - Sterile dressing for both intact and ruptured bullae
  - Topical mupirocin for erosions to prevent secondary infection[2]

Diabetologist

- *Initiated glucose-lowering therapy*:
  - Metformin + gliclazide extended release (30/500 mg) twice daily
  - Insulin glargine 12 units at bedtime
- Prescribed multivitamins with zinc to support skin healing.

- Educated the patient on foot care, wound care, and signs of infection.
- Emphasized the importance of strict glycemic control to prevent recurrence.[4]

Prognosis

Bullous diabeticorum typically resolves spontaneously within 2–4 weeks if secondary infection is avoided.[1,6] Poor glycemic control, however, increases the risk of recurrence, infection, or delayed healing.[2] Long-term management centers on maintaining optimal blood sugar levels and preventive foot care.[7]

> **Clinical Pearls**
>
> ▶ Rapid onset of large, painless bullae, primarily on the feet and lower legs.[3]
> ▶ Most commonly seen in individuals with long-standing or poorly controlled diabetes but may also occur at initial diagnosis.[6]
> ▶ Lesions often heal spontaneously but may rupture and become infected if not properly managed.[5]
> ▶ Important to distinguish from autoimmune and infectious bullous diseases.[2]
> ▶ Peripheral neuropathy and microangiopathy are frequently associated.[4]

Case 2

■ PRESENTATION

A man in his 40s presented with a sudden-onset, painless blister over the dorsum of his left foot, which had persisted for approximately 2 weeks. He denied any history of trauma, burns, or insect bites. The blister was tense, fluid-filled, and nonprogressive, with no associated pruritus, pain, or warmth. The patient was a known case of type 2 diabetes mellitus and was admitted due to the frequent noncompliance with his prescribed medications.

■ EXAMINATION

- Single, tense, and clear bulla over the dorsum of the left foot **(Fig. 2)**
- Surrounding skin appeared normal and without erythema, tenderness, or signs of infection.
- Peripheral pulses were palpable and symmetric.
- No edema or evidence of vascular insufficiency

■ DIAGNOSIS

- Bullosis diabeticorum (diabetic bulla)
- A spontaneous, noninflammatory blistering disorder is seen in patients with poorly controlled diabetes mellitus.[1,3,4,6]

■ DIFFERENTIAL DIAGNOSES

The main differentials to consider include:
- *Bullous pemphigoid*: It typically presents as tense, pruritic bullae often in a generalized distribution and is confirmed by biopsy and direct immunofluorescence.[5-7]
- *Frictional blisters*: These are usually found at sites of repeated mechanical trauma, such as from ill-fitting footwear.[2]
- *Edema or stasis bullae*: These are associated with fluid overload or chronic venous insufficiency.[6]

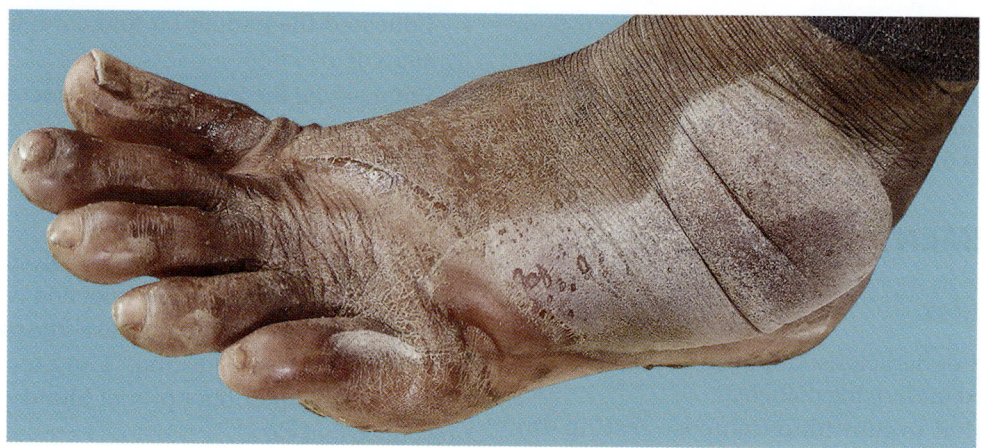

FIG. 2: A sudden-onset, painless blister over the dorsum of the left foot in a middle-aged man.

- *Bullous drug eruptions*: These eruptions may occur following recent changes in medication and can present with systemic symptoms.[6]

MANAGEMENT

- Supportive care is the cornerstone, as the condition is typically self-limiting.[1,3,6]
- For large bullae, aseptic aspiration of fluid may be performed to reduce the risk of accidental rupture and secondary infection.[2,6]
- Apply sterile dressings to protect intact or drained bullae.[1,6]
- Use topical or systemic antibiotics only if there are signs of secondary infection.[1,6]
- Optimize blood glucose levels to promote healing and minimize recurrence.[1,3,6]

PROGNOSIS

Bullosis diabeticorum usually heals spontaneously within 2–6 weeks, often without residual scarring. The main complication is secondary bacterial infection if the blister is not properly protected. Recurrence is possible, especially in patients with poor glycemic control.[1,3,6]

Clinical Pearls

- Sudden appearance of painless, tense bullae on acral sites (feet and hands) in individuals with diabetes.[1,3,6]
- Typically occurs in patients with long-standing or poorly controlled diabetes.[1,3,6]
- Absence of trauma, infection, or systemic symptoms.[1,3,6]
- Although benign and self-limiting, it may indicate underlying microvascular complications such as neuropathy or nephropathy.[1,3,6]

REFERENCES

1. Gupta V, Gulati N, Bahl J, Bajwa J, Dhawan N. Bullosis Diabeticorum: Rare Presentation in a Common Disease. Case Rep Endocrinol. 2014;2014:862912.
2. Onalaja-Underwood AA, Hurley MY, Sokumbi O. Diagnosis and Management of Bullous Disease. Clin Geriatr Med. 2024;40(1):37-74.
3. Chouk C, Litaiem N. Bullosis Diabeticorum. [Updated 2024 Jan 10]. In: StatPearls [Internet]. Treasure Island (FL): StatPearls Publishing; 2025 Jan. Available from: https://www.ncbi.nlm.nih.gov/books/NBK539872/
4. Senneville É, Albalawi Z, van Asten SA, Abbas ZG, Allison G, Aragón-Sánchez J et al. IWGDF/IDSA guidelines on the diagnosis and treatment of diabetes-related foot infections (IWGDF/IDSA 2023). Diabetes Metab Res Rev. 2024;40(3):e3687.
5. Lipsky BA, Baker PD, Ahroni JH. Diabetic bullae: 12 cases of a purportedly rare cutaneous disorder. Int J Dermatol. 2000;39(3):196-200.
6. Basarab T, Munn SE, McGrath J, Russell Jones R. Bullosis diabeticorum. A case report and literature review. Clin Exp Dermatol. 1995;20(3):218-20.
7. Allen GE, Hadden DR. Bullous lesions of the skin in diabetes (bullosis diabeticorum). Br J Dermatol. 1970;82(3):216-20.

CHAPTER 7

Bullous Pemphigoid in a Diabetic Male

Nipul Vara, Vishwa Marvania, Preya Parag Rana

■ PRESENTATION

A 68-year-old male with a 17-year history of type 2 diabetes mellitus and a 5-year history of hypertension presented with the chief complaints of gradually progressive itchy red lesions that developed into tense bullae over the past 3 weeks. The lesions involved the abdomen, groin, thighs, and arms, with no mucosal or ocular involvement.

His diabetes management had been irregular, with inconsistent use of metformin and glimepiride, and he had never been on insulin. His hypertension was managed with amlodipine 5 mg once daily. He led a sedentary lifestyle.

■ EXAMINATION

The following points were noted on examination:
- The patient was overweight [body mass index (BMI = 29 kg/m^2)].
- Blood pressure was 138/84 mm Hg and heart rate was 78 beats/minute.
- Pedal edema was present without lymphadenopathy.
- Neurologically, he had decreased vibration sense in both feet.
- Cutaneous examination revealed multiple tense bullae on both erythematous and normal skin, with several ruptured blisters and erosions **(Fig. 1)**.
- Nikolsky's sign was negative.
- There was no mucosal or ocular involvement.

■ INVESTIGATIONS

The following investigations were advised, and the results were as follows:
- *Glycemic profile*:
  - *Glycated hemoglobin (HbA1c):* 9.4%
  - *Fasting blood glucose:* 176 mg/dL
  - *Postprandial blood glucose:* 260 mg/dL
- *Complete blood count (CBC):* Mild leukocytosis with total white blood cell (WBC) count of 12,000/mm^3
- *Liver function test (LFT) and renal function tests (RFT):* Within normal limits
- *Urine analysis and diabetic foot screening:* Advised
- *Skin biopsy:* Skin biopsy and direct immunofluorescence (DIF) were performed to confirm the suspected diagnosis of bullous pemphigoid (BP):
  - Histopathology showed a subepidermal blister with an eosinophilic infiltrate.

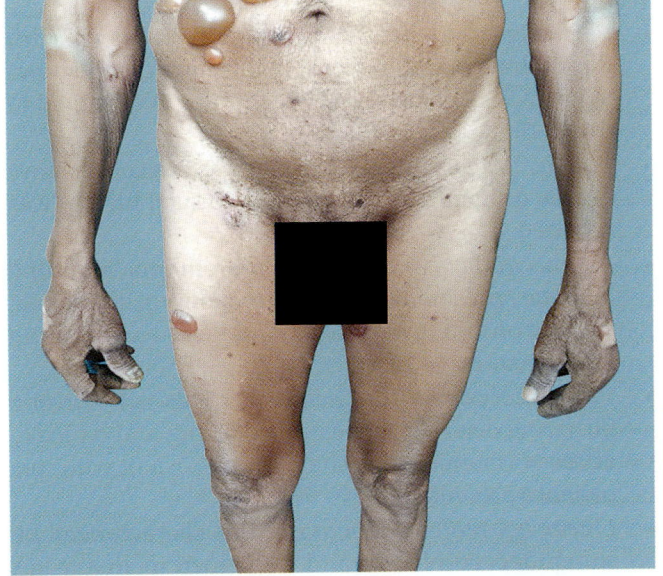

FIG. 1: Multiple tense bullae over normal and erythematous skin on the abdomen, thighs, and upper limbs in a male patient with uncontrolled diabetes.

- Direct immunofluorescence revealed linear immunoglobulin G (IgG) and complement (C3) deposits along the basement membrane zone, which is confirmatory for BP.[4]

PATHOPHYSIOLOGY

Bullous pemphigoid is a chronic autoimmune subepidermal blistering disorder. It is characterized by autoantibodies directed against BP180 (type XVII collagen) and BP230, proteins anchoring the epidermis to the dermis.[1]
- The formation of IgG autoantibodies activates C3 and neutrophils/eosinophils, leading to subepidermal blister formation.[2]
- Bullous pemphigoid is more common in the elderly and is associated with:
    - Neurological disorders (e.g., Parkinson's and stroke)
    - Hypertension and chronic kidney disease
    - Diabetes mellitus, possibly due to glycation-induced antigenic modifications[3]

DIAGNOSIS

Bullous pemphigoid in a patient with uncontrolled type 2 diabetes mellitus.

DIFFERENTIAL DIAGNOSES

- *Pemphigus vulgaris:* This typically presents with flaccid bullae and mucosal involvement, and shows a positive Nikolsky's sign, which was not observed in this patient.
- *Bullous drug eruption:* This requires a recent history of new drug intake; in this case, no such history was reported.
- *Bullous diabeticorum:* This is seen in long-standing diabetes; presents with painless, nonpruritic bullae, usually on the lower limbs, and lacks surrounding inflammation.
- *Epidermolysis bullosa acquisita:* This is a chronic blistering disorder that causes scarring and typically arises at trauma-prone sites; not consistent with this patient's presentation.
- *Linear IgA bullous dermatosis:* It is characterized by subepidermal blisters and confirmed by linear IgA deposition on direct immunofluorescence.

MANAGEMENT

Dermatological Management

Dermatological management includes:
- *Systemic corticosteroids*: Prednisolone 40 mg/day, tapering based on response
- Topical potent steroids for localized lesions
- Tetracycline + nicotinamide or doxycycline as steroid-sparing options[5]
- Monitoring for secondary infection and skincare measures
- *In recalcitrant or severe cases:* Methotrexate, azathioprine, or rituximab

Diabetology/Physician Management

Diabetology/physician management is as follows:
- *Initiated on basal-bolus insulin regimen due to*:
    - Uncontrolled glucose
    - Anticipated steroid-induced hyperglycemia
- Advised frequent self-monitoring of blood glucose (SMBG)
- *Referral to:*
    - Diabetes educator for insulin technique
    - Dietitian for glycemic optimization
- Screening for microvascular complications

PROGNOSIS

Prognosis is as follows:
- Bullous pemphigoid generally has a good prognosis with appropriate treatment.
- However, in diabetic patients, delayed healing, superadded infections, and hyperglycemia from steroids complicate outcomes.
- Insulin therapy often becomes mandatory to control glucose during systemic steroid use.

Clinical Pearls

▶ Bullous pemphigoid in diabetics may present atypically and may be confused with bullous diabeticorum.
▶ Direct immunofluorescence is mandatory for confirmation.
▶ Steroids worsen glycemic control—always anticipate insulin initiation.
▶ Optimal interdisciplinary care between dermatologists and diabetologists improves outcomes.

REFERENCES

1. Schmidt E, Zillikens D. Modern diagnosis of autoimmune blistering skin diseases. Autoimmun Rev. 2010;10(2):84-9.
2. Di Zenzo G, Della Torre R, Zambruno G, Borradori L. Bullous pemphigoid: From the clinic to the bench. Clin Dermatol. 2012;30(1):3-16.
3. Kalinska-Bienias A, Kowalewski C, Jagielski P, Kowalczyk E, Woźniak K, Łupińska A, et al. Bullous pemphigoid and diabetes mellitus: A systematic review and meta-analysis. Clin Dermatol. 2021;39(5):812-20.
4. Pohla-Gubo G, Hintner H. Direct and indirect immunofluorescence for the diagnosis of bullous autoimmune diseases. Dermatol Clin. 2011;29(3):365-72.
5. Wojnarowska F, Kirtschig G, Highet AS, Venning VA, Khumalo NP; British Association of Dermatologists. Guidelines for the management of bullous pemphigoid. Br J Dermatol. 2002;147(2):214-21.

CHAPTER 8

Yellow Palms in Diabetes Mellitus: A Case of Carotenoderma

Arijit Singha, Pradip Mukhopadhyay, Sujoy Ghosh

■ PRESENTATION

A 52-year-old man with a 5-year history of type 2 diabetes mellitus presented for assessment of persistently elevated blood glucose levels. He had recently observed a gradual yellowish discoloration of both palms over the preceding 3 months. The discoloration was asymptomatic—there was no itching, scaling, rash, or thickening. He explicitly denied consuming foods rich in carotene, such as carrots, pumpkin, sweet potatoes, spinach, or egg yolk. There was no evidence of jaundice, hypothyroidism, or use of dietary supplements.

■ EXAMINATION

Examination findings are as follows:
- Bilateral yellow-orange pigmentation of the palms **(Fig. 1)**
- Soles, sclera, and oral mucosa were unaffected.
- No clinical signs of systemic illness or dermatological disorders.

■ LABORATORY FINDINGS

Laboratory findings are as follows:
- *Fasting plasma glucose:* 146 mg/dL
- *Postprandial plasma glucose:* 332 mg/dL
- *Glycated hemoglobin (HbA1c):* 8.8%
- *Total bilirubin:* 0.73 mg/dL (Direct: 0.25 mg/dL)
- *Aspartate transaminase (AST):* 25.6 U/L and *alanine transaminase (ALT):* 38.4 U/L
- *Thyroid profile:* Within normal limits
- *Lipid profile:* Total cholesterol 258 mg/dL and triglycerides 180 mg/dL
- No microvascular complications were identified upon screening

■ DIAGNOSIS

Carotenoderma (also known as xanthoderma) secondary to poorly controlled type 2 diabetes mellitus.[1]

■ DIFFERENTIAL DIAGNOSES

Differential diagnoses are:
- Excessive intake of carotenoid-rich foods or supplements
- Hypothyroidism
- Nephrotic syndrome
- Chronic liver disease
- Anorexia nervosa
- Rare metabolic disorders (e.g., β-carotene mono-oxygenase deficiency)
- Diabetes mellitus, due to altered carotenoid metabolism[1,2]

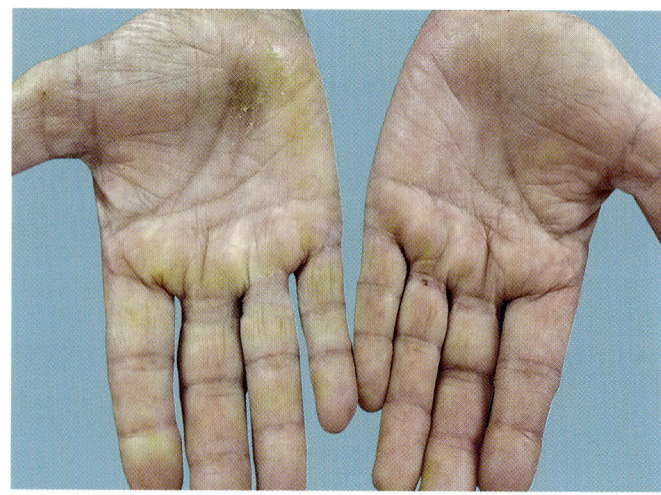

FIG. 1: Bilateral yellow-orange pigmentation of the palms in both hands.

PATHOPHYSIOLOGY

Carotenoderma is defined by a yellow-orange hue of the skin, most apparent on the palms, soles, and nasolabial folds, resulting from the accumulation of carotenoids within the stratum corneum.[1,3] Unlike jaundice, this pigmentation characteristically spares the sclera and mucous membranes, and is often more prominent under artificial lighting.[1,2] In diabetes, impaired hepatic and duodenal conversion of β-carotene to vitamin A is proposed as a key mechanism. Additionally, advanced glycation end-products may interfere with normal carotenoid metabolism, promoting cutaneous deposition.[4] Carotenoderma is classified as:

- *Primary:* Due to excessive dietary or supplemental carotenoid intake
- *Secondary:* Associated with metabolic conditions such as diabetes, hypothyroidism, or chronic kidney disease[1,4] Notably, up to 10% of individuals with diabetes may develop this condition, underscoring the importance of recognizing cutaneous markers of metabolic dysregulation.[4]

MANAGEMENT

Management includes the following:

Dermatology/Nutritional Management

- No specific dermatological intervention is necessary.
- Dietary assessment is important to exclude inadvertent carotenoid overconsumption.
- Patients should be reassured about the benign and reversible course of the condition.
- Cosmetic concerns may be addressed, but aggressive interventions are unwarranted.

Diabetology/Physician Management

- Focus on optimizing glycemic control, including review and adjustment of oral hypoglycemic agents or consideration of insulin therapy.

- After 3 months, the patient's HbA1c improved to 6.8%, with marked reduction in palmar discoloration.[5]
- Lipid-lowering therapy, such as statins, may be indicated for dyslipidemia.
- Continued surveillance for diabetes complications (foot, eye, and renal screening) is advised.
- Improvement in both pigmentation and glycemic indices further supports the benign and self-limiting nature of carotenoderma in diabetes.[5,6]

PROGNOSIS

Carotenoderma is a harmless and reversible condition, with significant improvement following better glycemic and lipid control. Its presence may serve as an early dermatological clue to underlying metabolic imbalance, and its resolution can be a useful indicator of therapeutic success.[5,6]

> **Clinical Pearls**
>
> ▶ Carotenoderma is a benign, self-limiting, and uncommon cutaneous manifestation associated with underlying diabetes mellitus. It typically improves with good glycemic control.
> ▶ Presents as yellow discoloration localized to the palms and soles, with sparing of the sclera and mucous membranes.
> ▶ The discoloration is often more noticeable under artificial light.
> ▶ Differentiation from jaundice is essential, as jaundice involves scleral icterus and is usually accompanied by systemic symptoms.
> ▶ Carotenoderma is frequently underrecognized in diabetes clinics.
> ▶ Identifying and resolving this sign can serve as a useful clinical indicator of the importance of achieving metabolic control.

REFERENCES

1. Haught JM, Patel S, English JC 3rd. Xanthoderma: A clinical review. J Am Acad Dermatol. 2007;57(6):1051-8.
2. Soundararajan V, Charny JW, Bain MA, Tsoukas MM. Orange diseases of the skin. Clin Dermatol. 2019;37(5):520-7.
3. Hess AF, Myers VC. Carotinemia: A new clinical picture. JAMA. 1919;73(23):1743-5.
4. Priyadarshani AMB. Insights of hypercarotenaemia: A brief review. Clin Nutr ESPEN. 2018;23:19-24.
5. Lin JN. Yellow palms and soles in diabetes mellitus. N Engl J Med. 2006;355(14):1486.
6. Chhabra P, Bhasin DK. Yellow palms and soles: Think beyond hyperbilirubinemia. Perm J. 2017;21:17-34.

CHAPTER 9

Carotenemia in a Patient with Type 2 Diabetes Mellitus

NK Singh, Akashkumar N Singh, Anuradha Kapoor

■ PRESENTATION

A 40-year-old male laborer presented with a gradually increasing yellow–orange discoloration of the palms, soles, and nails over the past month. He denied any associated itching, jaundice, weight loss, or other systemic symptoms. There was no history of consuming carotene-rich foods, nor any use of topical agents or medications that could cause pigmentation. He had a known diagnosis of type 2 diabetes mellitus but reported poor adherence to both medication and dietary advice.

■ EXAMINATION

- On physical examination, a distinct yellow–orange discoloration was observed over palms, soles, and fingernails **(Fig. 1)**. The skin was otherwise normal in texture, with no thickening, desquamation, or inflammation.

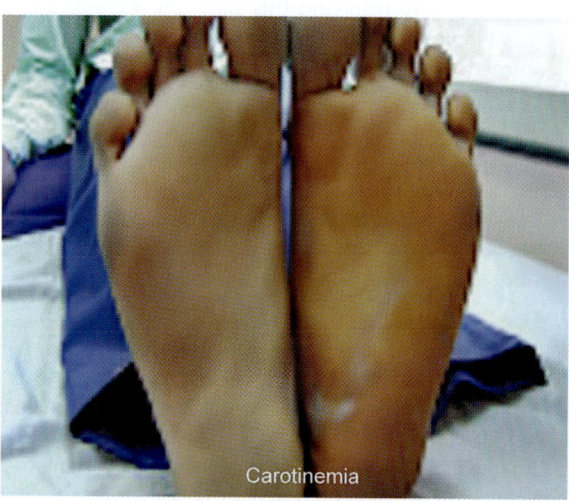

FIG. 1: A distinct yellow–orange discoloration observed over the palms, soles, and fingernails in patient with type 2 diabetes mellitus (T2DM).

- The sclerae were clear, with no evidence of jaundice.
- There were no mucosal pigmentary changes or signs suggestive of systemic disease.

■ INVESTIGATIONS

- Investigations revealed significantly elevated fasting and postprandial blood glucose levels. His glycated hemoglobin (HbA1c) was 10.6%, indicating chronic poor glycemic control.
- Thyroid function tests and liver function tests were within normal limits.
- The absence of scleral icterus and normal liver parameters helped exclude jaundice.

■ DIAGNOSIS

Diagnosis was carotenemia associated with poorly controlled type 2 diabetes mellitus. Although serum carotene levels were not measured, the diagnosis was supported clinically by the exclusion of other common causes of skin pigmentation.

■ DIFFERENTIAL DIAGNOSIS

- *Jaundice:* It is characterized by involvement of the sclerae (icterus), abnormal liver function tests, and systemic symptoms. In this case, sparing of the sclerae and normal liver function ruled out jaundice.[1]
- *Lycopenemia:* It presents with a reddish-orange skin hue due to excessive intake of tomatoes or red fruits.
- *Type III hyperlipoproteinemia:* It leads to palmar xanthomas, particularly in diabetic patients with dyslipidemia.
- *Hypothyroidism:* Impaired conversion of carotene to vitamin A can result in carotenemia, often coexisting with diabetes.

- *Drug-induced pigmentation:* Medications such as quinacrine, sorafenib, and certain topical agents may cause similar discoloration.
- *Exogenous pigment exposure:* Contact with turmeric or industrial dyes can also produce yellowish skin changes.[2]

PATHOPHYSIOLOGY

Carotenemia arises due to the deposition of beta-carotene within the stratum corneum, most notably in areas with thicker skin or higher sebum production, such as the palms, soles, and nasolabial folds. In diabetic individuals, several mechanisms contribute to the following:

- Impaired conversion of carotene to retinol, often related to insulin resistance and hepatic dysfunction
- Hyperlipidemia, frequently seen in diabetes, facilitates increased transport and deposition of carotenoids in the skin.[3]
- Advanced glycation end-products (AGEs) from chronic hyperglycemia may further impart a yellow-brown skin tone.[4]
- Diabetic patients may consume more carotene-rich foods as part of dietary modifications or due to dietary monotony.[5]

MANAGEMENT

Dermatological Approach

- No specific topical therapies are needed.
- Clinical photographs should be taken for documentation and follow-up.
- Careful examination and history are essential to exclude other causes of pigmentation.
- Patients should be reassured regarding the benign nature of carotenemia.[4]

Diabetological/Physician Approach

- Achieving optimal glycemic control is paramount. The patient was initiated on:
  - Metformin 1,000 mg/day
  - Glimepiride 2 mg/day
  - Dapagliflozin 10 mg/day
- Lipid profile assessment revealed mild dyslipidemia, prompting the addition of rosuvastatin 10 mg/day.
- Dietary evaluation confirmed no excessive carotenoid intake, but a balanced diabetic diet was reinforced.
- On follow-up at 6 weeks, the pigmentation had begun to diminish, and by 3 months, it had resolved completely, with HbA1c improving to 7.2%.[6,7]

PROGNOSIS

The outlook is excellent once glycemic and lipid parameters are controlled. Skin pigmentation typically resolves within 4–12 weeks following correction of metabolic abnormalities. There is no risk of vitamin A toxicity, as the conversion of beta-carotene to vitamin A is self-regulated. Recurrence is possible if glycemic or dietary control lapses.[3,7]

Clinical Pearls

- ▶ Carotenemia in diabetic patients is harmless but may serve as a visible indicator of suboptimal metabolic control.[8]
- ▶ Always examine the sclerae to differentiate carotenemia from jaundice.[1]
- ▶ The condition may be underrecognized in individuals with darker skin tones.[5]
- ▶ Carotenemia can be a useful tool to motivate patients toward better dietary and glycemic management.
- ▶ Photographic documentation aids in monitoring progress during follow-up.[2]

REFERENCES

1. Lin JN. Images in clinical medicine: Yellow palms and soles in diabetes mellitus. N Engl J Med. 2006;355(14):1486.
2. Chhabra P, Bhasin DK. Yellow Palms and Soles: Look beyond the eyes. Perm J. 2017;21:17-034.
3. Hoerer E, Dreyfuss F, Herzberg M. Carotenemia, skin color and diabetes mellitus. Acta Diabetol Lat. 1975;12(3-4):202-7.
4. Edigin E, Asemota IR, Olisa E, Nwaichi C. Carotenemia: A case report. Cureus. 2019;11(7):e5218.
5. Ul Bari A. Carotenemia in an African lady. Indian J Dermatol. 2009;54(S1):71-3.
6. Julka S, Jamdagni N, Verma S, Goyal R. Yellow palms and soles: A rare skin manifestation in diabetes mellitus. Indian J Endocrinol Metab. 2013;17(Suppl1):S299-300.
7. Kapsetaki ME. Diet-induced carotenodermia: a literature review. Int J Dermatol. 2024;63(2):161-8.
8. Rabinowitch IM. Carotinaemia and diabetes. Can Med Assoc J. 1928;18(5):527-30.

CHAPTER 10

Diabetic Rubeosis Faciei with Palmar Erythema

Ashma Surani, Bela J Shah

PRESENTATION

A 49-year-old male employed as a construction worker arrived at the dermatology outpatient department, reporting persistent generalized itching for several months. He had a known history of type 2 diabetes mellitus for 15 years, managed with both insulin and oral hypoglycemic agents. There was no record of alcohol consumption or other systemic complaints.

EXAMINATION

- On clinical examination, the patient displayed marked facial redness, especially over the cheeks and nasal bridge, consistent with rubeosis faciei **(Fig. 1)**.
- Both palms demonstrated erythema, most noticeably over the hypothenar areas **(Fig. 2)**.
- Extensive dryness of the skin (xerosis) and scratch marks (excoriations) were observed on the back. No additional notable skin lesions were detected.

INVESTIGATIONS

Laboratory investigations revealed:
- *Random blood glucose:* 360 mg/dL
- *Glycated hemoglobin (HbA1c):* 12.3%, reflecting inadequate glycemic control
- *Urinalysis:* Presence of glucose and absence of ketones
- *Complete blood count, liver and renal function tests, and thyroid profile:* All within normal parameters

DIAGNOSIS

Diabetic rubeosis faciei with palmar erythema.

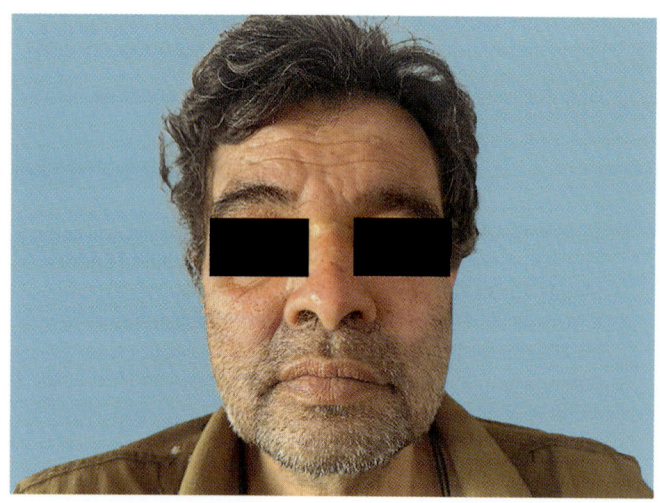

FIG. 1: Marked facial redness over the cheeks and nasal bridge, consistent with rubeosis faciei.

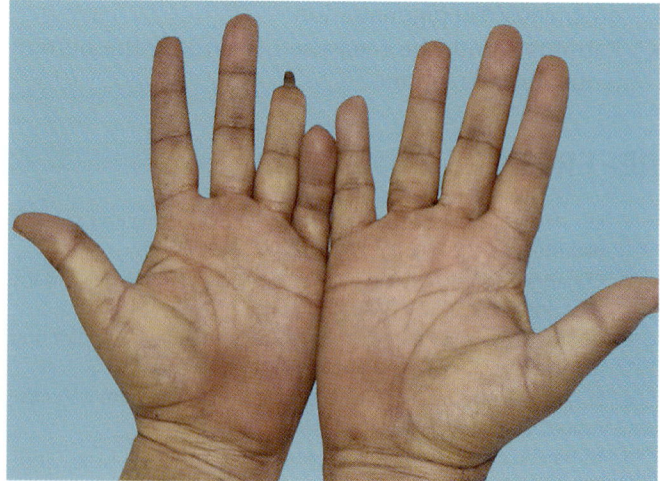

FIG. 2: Erythema of both palms, most prominent over the hypothenar areas.

DIFFERENTIAL DIAGNOSIS

For Facial Erythema

- *Rosacea:* Typically presents with papules and pustules, which were not observed in this patient.[1]
- *Photo-induced facial changes:* Usually associated with actinic damage on sun-exposed skin.[2]
- *Topical steroid-induced facial damage (TSDF):* Characterized by skin thinning and telangiectasia, generally seen in patients with a history of topical steroid application, which was not reported here.[2]

For Palmar Erythema

- *Hepatic disease:* Ruled out based on normal liver function tests[3]
- *Polycythemia vera and thyrotoxicosis:* No clinical or laboratory evidence to support these diagnoses.[3]

MANAGEMENT

Dermatological Approach

- Application of topical emollients to manage xerosis and minimize further scratching[2]
- Use of second-generation antihistamines for symptomatic relief from pruritus[2]

Management by Diabetologist or Physician

- Reinforcement of strict blood glucose control and reassessment of the antidiabetic regimen[2]
- Lifestyle counseling, emphasizing dietary modifications, weight reduction, and moderation of alcohol and caffeine intake[2]

FURTHER EVALUATION

- Screening for microalbuminuria to detect early diabetic nephropathy[4]
- Fundoscopic examination to exclude diabetic retinopathy[4]

PROGNOSIS

Facial and palmar erythema are likely to improve with optimized glycemic control and lifestyle adjustments, such as reducing alcohol and caffeine intake. However, some microvascular alterations may persist if they have been present for a prolonged period.[1,3]

> ### Clinical Pearls
>
> ▸ Rubeosis faciei is characterized by persistent facial redness, often resulting from diabetic microangiopathy and chronic dilation of small blood vessels.[1]
> ▸ This dermatological sign is commonly linked to advanced microvascular complications of diabetes, including retinopathy, nephropathy, and neuropathy.[4,5]
> ▸ In diabetic patients, palmar erythema is generally attributed to microvascular changes rather than liver dysfunction.[3]
> ▸ These lesions are usually asymptomatic, underscoring the need for clinical awareness to facilitate early identification and intervention for underlying diabetic complications.[6,7]

REFERENCES

1. Ngan V, Freeman S. Rubeosis faciei diabeticorum: A cutaneous manifestation of diabetes mellitus. Australas J Dermatol. 1993;34(2):63-6.
2. Hu S, Lan CCE, Yu HS. Skin manifestations of diabetes mellitus. Kaohsiung J Med Sci. 2020;36(1):11-7.
3. Pavlovic MD, Kacar SD, Djurovic M, Duric M. Palmar erythema in diabetes mellitus: A microvascular complication? Diabetes Res Clin Pract. 2001;52(2):137-9.
4. Yosipovitch G, Hodak E, Vardi P, Shraga I, Karp M, Sprecher E, et al. The prevalence of cutaneous manifestations in IDDM patients and their association with diabetes risk factors and microvascular complications. Diabetes Care. 1998; 21(4):506-9.
5. Romano G, Morello C, Di Benedetto A, Romeo G, Di Cesare E, Spinella R, et al. Skin lesions in diabetes mellitus: prevalence and clinical correlations. Diabetes Res Clin Pract. 1998;39(2):101-6.
6. Demirseren DD, Emre S, Akoglu G, Arpacı D, Arman A, Metin A, et al. Relationship between skin diseases and extracutaneous complications of diabetes mellitus: clinical analysis of 750 patients. Am J Clin Dermatol. 2014;15(1):65-70.
7. Bhat YJ, Gupta V, Kudyar RP. Cutaneous manifestations of diabetes mellitus. Int J Diabetes Dev Ctries. 2006;26(4):152-5.

CHAPTER 11

Finger Pebbles (Huntley's Papules) in a Diabetic Male

Suhas Gopal Erande

■ PRESENTATION

A 36-year-old obese male, known case of type 2 diabetes mellitus, presented with asymptomatic, raised, skin-colored papules on the dorsal aspect of his fingers. The onset appeared gradual, though the exact duration was not specified. The patient denied any joint stiffness, itching, or systemic symptoms. There was no history of inflammatory or infectious skin disease.

■ EXAMINATION

On examination, multiple firm and skin-colored papules were observed over the dorsal surfaces of the fingers **(Fig. 1)**. These lesions were:
- Discrete and firm in consistency
- Located predominantly near the interphalangeal joints
- Symmetrically distributed on both hands
- Nontender and nonpruritic
- Not associated with scaling, redness, or signs of inflammation

The overall appearance was consistent with *Huntley's papules* (also known as *finger pebbles*), a benign cutaneous finding linked to diabetic thick skin.

■ INVESTIGATION

While this condition is primarily diagnosed clinically, the following routine investigations are recommended to assess metabolic status and rule out complications:
- *Glycated hemoglobin (HbA1c):* To evaluate the degree of glycemic control.
- *Body mass index (BMI) and waist circumference:* To assess obesity status.
- *Metabolic profile:* Including fasting lipids, liver function, renal function, and screening for other diabetes-related complications.

There is no need for a skin biopsy unless the diagnosis is unclear. Management focuses on optimal diabetes control and weight reduction through dietary changes, physical activity, and lifestyle modification.

■ DIAGNOSIS

Huntley's Papules (Diabetic Finger Pebbles)

- A cutaneous marker of *diabetic thick skin syndrome* (also called diabetic cheiroarthropathy)
- Considered a *benign and early skin sign* of long-standing or poorly controlled diabetes.[1-3]

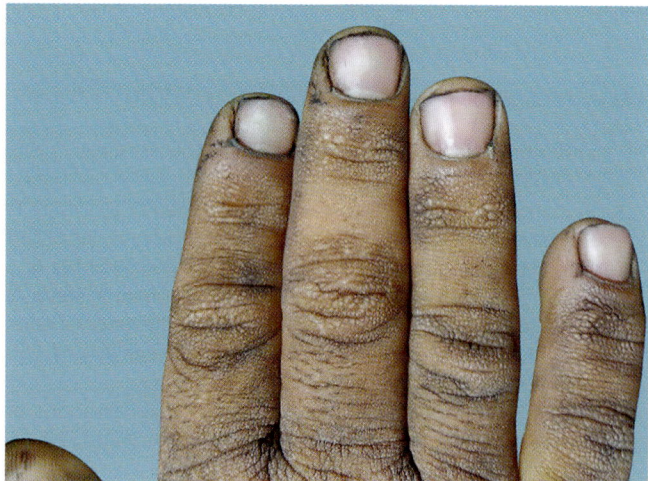

FIG. 1: Multiple firm and skin-colored papules over the dorsal surfaces of the fingers.

DIFFERENTIAL DIAGNOSES

- *Lichen nitidus*: Small and shiny papules in clusters, usually on genitalia, trunk, and limbs.[4,5]
- *Keratosis pilaris*: Follicular papules, mostly on arms and thighs.[4,5]
- *Papular mucinosis:* Waxy papules, usually more diffuse, with systemic associations.[4,6]
- *Flat warts:* Slightly elevated and skin-colored lesions often caused by HPV.[4,5]
- *Early knuckle pads:* Firm plaques over joints, usually familial or trauma-related.[4,5]

PATHOPHYSIOLOGY

- Huntley's papules are attributed to *glycosylation of collagen and other dermal proteins* in long-standing diabetes.
- This leads to *dermal fibrosis,* skin thickening, and the development of papules.
- Often associated with *limited joint mobility* and *diabetic cheiroarthropathy*, which may restrict finger extension.
- Their presence may precede or coexist with other thick skin syndromes in diabetes.[1-3,6]

MANAGEMENT

Dermatologic Management

- No specific treatment is required for the papules themselves.
- Educate the patient about the *cosmetic benignity* of lesions.
- Encourage use of *emollients or keratolytics* (urea or salicylic acid creams) for associated dryness or thickening.[1,2,6]

Physician/Diabetologist Management

- *Optimize glycemic control:* Essential to prevent progression of connective tissue complications.
- Encourage *weight loss* through dietary changes and physical activity.
- *Screen for diabetic cheiroarthropathy*: Look for limited joint mobility, prayer sign, and skin thickening.
- Consider referral to physiotherapy if *range of motion is affected.*[1,2,4-8]

PROGNOSIS

- Papules themselves are benign and asymptomatic.
- Often indicate a *systemic collagen glycosylation process,* which may lead to more significant mobility impairment over time.
- Improvement seen with *strict glycemic control and weight reduction.*[1-3,6]

Clinical Pearls

▶ Huntley's papules are an *early cutaneous marker* of collagen glycation in diabetes.[1,2]
▶ Always assess for *diabetic cheiroarthropathy* in patients with finger papules.[1-3]
▶ Consider *these papules as a warning sign* for more extensive connective tissue involvement.[1,6]
▶ Educate the patient about the *noninfectious and nonscarring nature* of the condition.[1,2]

REFERENCES

1. Huntley AC. The cutaneous manifestations of diabetes mellitus. J Am Acad Dermatol. 1982;7(4):427-55.
2. Duff M, Demidova O, Blackburn S, Shubrook J. Cutaneous manifestations of diabetes mellitus. Clin Diabetes. 2015;33(1):40-8.
3. Guarneri C, Guarneri F, Borgia F, Vaccaro M. Finger pebbles in a diabetic patient: Huntley's papules. Int J Dermatol. 2005;44(9):755-6.
4. Bhat YJ, Ragunatha S, Inamadar AC. Cutaneous disorders in 500 diabetic patients attending a diabetic clinic. Indian J Dermatol. 2011;56(2):160-4.
5. Nigam PK, Pande S. Pattern of dermatoses in diabetics. Indian J Dermatol Venereol Leprol. 2003;69(2):83-5.
6. Sibbald RG, Schachter RK. The skin and diabetes mellitus. Int J Dermatol. 1984;23(9):567-84.
7. Bhargava P, Mathur SK. Insulin resistance and skin tags. Dermatology. 1997;195(2):184.
8. Kahana M, Grossman E, Feinstein A. Skin tags: A cutaneous marker for diabetes mellitus. Acta Derm Venereol. 1987;67:175-7.

CHAPTER 12

Perforating Dermatosis

*Nipul Vara, Vishwa Marvania, Preya Parag Rana, Suhas Gopal Erande,
Prabhat Kumar Agrawal, Sandipta Kumar Panda, Gaurav Gupta,
Anil Patki, Ashma Surani, Firdous Shaikh, Avina Jain*

Part A: Perforating Folliculitis in Uncontrolled Diabetes

PRESENTATION

A 61-year-old male with a 15-year history of type 2 diabetes mellitus presented with pruritic and painful raised lesions over his upper back and shoulders **(Fig. 1)**, persisting for 1 month. His diabetes control was suboptimal, with a recent glycated hemoglobin (HbA1c) of 9.6%. The skin changes began as small papules, which gradually evolved into crateriform plugs. There was no preceding trauma, no new medications, and no evidence of systemic illness. The patient also had established diabetic peripheral neuropathy.

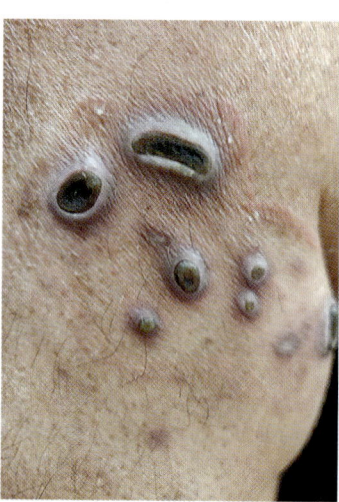

FIG. 1: Multiple umbilicated papules and nodules with central keratotic plugs distributed over the shoulder and upper back. Lesions are crateriform, with dark central cores suggestive of perforating folliculitis.

EXAMINATION

- Cutaneous evaluation revealed numerous erythematous to skin-colored papules and nodules, each centered around a follicle with a prominent central keratin plug **(Fig. 1)**.
- The lesions were symmetrically distributed across the upper back and shoulders. There was no clinical evidence of secondary infection, such as purulent discharge, crusting, or surrounding cellulitis.

DIAGNOSIS

Perforating folliculitis associated with poorly controlled type 2 diabetes mellitus.[1,2]

DIFFERENTIAL DIAGNOSES

- *Kyrle's disease:* Features larger, deeply crateriform lesions, frequently associated with underlying renal pathology.[1,3]
- *Reactive perforating collagenosis:* Typically follows minor trauma and is more prevalent among younger individuals.[3]
- *Elastosis perforans serpiginosa:* Characterized by annular or arcuate lesions, most often on the neck and arms.[1]
- *Acquired perforating dermatosis (APD):* An umbrella term encompassing all perforating dermatoses in adults with diabetes and/or renal dysfunction.[4,5]

- *Folliculitis decalvans:* Predominantly affects the scalp, leading to scarring alopecia.[1]
- *Secondary bacterial folliculitis:* Lacks the hallmark central plugs and perforation on histopathology.[1]

PATHOPHYSIOLOGY AND DIABETES LINK

Perforating dermatoses are defined by the transepidermal elimination (TEE) of dermal substances such as collagen or elastin through the epidermis.[1]

In perforating folliculitis, necrotic follicular debris is expelled via the follicular epithelium as a result of inflammation and aberrant repair mechanisms.[1,5]

Diabetes mellitus contributes to this process through several mechanisms:
- Microvascular disease and compromised blood supply
- Impaired wound healing
- Enhanced oxidative stress and accumulation of advanced glycation end products (AGEs), which modify collagen and extracellular matrix proteins.[2,5]
- Acquired perforating dermatoses, including perforating folliculitis, are observed in up to 11% of patients with diabetes and chronic kidney disease.[5,6]

MANAGEMENT

Dermatological Approaches

- *Topical keratolytics:* Salicylic acid (3–6%) and urea creams (10–20%) to promote desquamation.[1,4]
- *Topical corticosteroids:* To control inflammation and alleviate pruritus.[1]
- *Topical retinoids:* Tretinoin to normalize follicular keratinization.[1]
- *Antiseptic washes:* For the prevention of secondary infection.[1]
- *Phototherapy:* Narrowband ultraviolet A (UVB) or psoralen plus ultraviolet A (PUVA) for resistant or widespread cases.[4]
- *Antibiotics:* Reserved for cases with secondary infection.[1]

Physician/Diabetology Approaches

- *Glycemic optimization*:
  - Patient's education regarding self-monitoring of blood glucose
  - Adjustment of antidiabetic therapy, including insulin titration or addition of glucagon-like peptide-1 (GLP-1) receptor agonists.[2]
- *Screening for complications*: Renal function assessment and fundus examination[2]
- *Foot and skin care*: Advise avoidance of trauma, regular use of emollients, and maintenance of skin hygiene.[2]

PROGNOSIS

- The disease often follows a chronic, relapsing course, particularly if glycemic control and renal function are not optimized.[5]
- Lesions may heal with scarring or postinflammatory hyperpigmentation.
- Achieving better glycemic control has been shown to decrease the development of new lesions.[2,5]

> **Clinical Pearls**
> - Perforating folliculitis should be suspected in diabetic patients presenting with folliculocentric, umbilicated lesions, especially on the trunk and extensor surfaces.[2]
> - Always assess for renal involvement, as many patients may have underlying chronic kidney disease.[5]
> - Transepidermal elimination is a diagnostic hallmark and may necessitate skin biopsy for confirmation[1]
> - Long-term management of glycemic status and renal function is crucial for preventing recurrence.[2,5]

REFERENCES

1. Lynde CB, Pratt MD. Acquired perforating dermatosis: association with diabetes and renal failure. CMAJ. 2009;181(8):479-81.
2. Mima Y, Ohtsuka T, Ebato I, Nishie R, Uesugi S. A Case of Acquired Reactive Perforating Dermatosis with Complete Resolution of Eruptions on Upper and Lower Limbs During the Treatment of Diabetes Mellitus and Peripheral Artery Disease. Case Rep Dermatol. 2023;15(1):1-6.
3. Khalidi M, Frikh R, Hjira N, Boui M. Acquired perforating dermatosis in renal dialysis and diabetic patient: A case report. Our Dermatol Online. 2021;12(1):39-41.
4. Rapini RP. Acquired perforating dermatosis. In: Bologna JL, Schaffer JV, Cerroni L (Eds). Dermatology, 4th edition. Amsterdam, Netherlands: Elsevier Saunders; 2017. pp. 1428-30.
5. Rapini RP. Perforating Diseases. In: Dermatology, Vol. 1 and 2, fifth edition. Amsterdam, Netherlands: Elsevier; 2024. pp. 1707-13.
6. Faver IR, Daoud MS, Su WP, Gibson LE. Acquired perforating dermatosis: a clinicopathologic study of forty-one cases associated with diabetes mellitus and chronic renal failure. J Am Acad Dermatol. 1994;30(4):575-80.

Part B: Acquired Perforating Dermatosis in a Diabetic Female with Chronic Renal Failure

■ PRESENTATION

A 56-year-old female with a known history of type 2 diabetes mellitus and chronic renal failure, likely on hemodialysis, presents with multiple pruritic, hyperkeratotic papules that have central adherent crusts. The lesions are predominantly located on the extensor surfaces of the limbs and trunk. She experiences moderate to severe pruritus. Associated comorbidities include diabetic nephropathy and probable uremia. The duration of symptoms is not specified but is presumed chronic. Lesions are often surrounded by erythema or pigmentation and may show signs of excoriation or secondary infection due to scratching.

■ EXAMINATION

On inspection, the skin reveals hyperkeratotic, umbilicated papules with central crusts. These lesions are commonly distributed over the extensor limbs **(Fig. 1)**, trunk, and occasionally the scalp. Some lesions may be surrounded by erythema or postinflammatory pigmentation. Evidence of excoriation and secondary infection from scratching is often present.

The morphology and distribution are typical for acquired perforating dermatosis in patients with diabetes and chronic kidney disease.

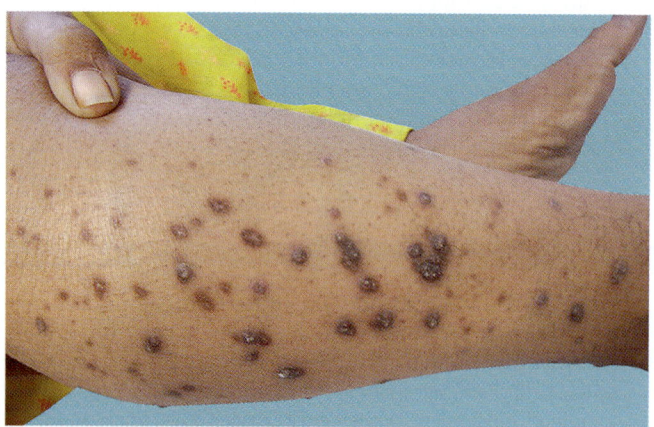

FIG. 1: Hyperkeratotic, umbilicated papules with central crusts, over extensor limbs.

■ INVESTIGATIONS

Laboratory investigations should include:
- *Renal function tests* such as urea, creatinine, and electrolytes to assess the degree of renal impairment.
- *Glycemic status* should be evaluated with glycated hemoglobin (HbA1c) and fasting or postprandial glucose levels.
- *A complete blood count* is necessary to rule out secondary infection.
- *Serum calcium, phosphate, and parathyroid hormone levels* should be checked to assess for chronic kidney disease—mineral bone disorder.
- *Nutritional assessment,* including zinc and vitamin levels, is recommended.
- *Histopathological examination* of skin lesions typically shows a central crater filled with keratotic debris and transepidermal extrusion of basophilic collagen bundles or elastic fibers, with surrounding dermal inflammatory infiltrate and fibrosis.

■ DIAGNOSIS

Acquired perforating dermatosis (APD): The clinical and histopathological findings are consistent with the APD, a group of perforating disorders most commonly seen in adults with long-standing diabetes mellitus and renal failure.[1-3]

■ DIFFERENTIAL DIAGNOSIS

- *Prurigo nodularis:* Discrete hyperkeratotic nodules due to chronic scratching, no central keratin plug.
- *Lichen planus hypertrophicus:* Pruritic, violaceous plaques with Wickham striae.
- *Folliculitis:* Inflammatory papules/pustules centered on follicles
- *Scabies:* Burrows, nocturnal pruritus, and family history
- *Kyrle's disease:* Often grouped with APD; perforating collagenosis variant.[4,5]

PATHOPHYSIOLOGY

Acquired perforating dermatosis is characterized by the transepidermal elimination of altered dermal substances, such as collagen or elastin. Chronic scratching and the presence of uremic toxins contribute to dermal matrix degeneration. Diabetes-associated microangiopathy impairs tissue repair and facilitates lesion formation. The condition is prevalent in patients on hemodialysis or with end-stage renal disease.[1,2,4,6]

MANAGEMENT

Dermatological Management

- *Topical corticosteroids* (such as clobetasol propionate 0.05%) to reduce inflammation and pruritus
- *Oral antihistamines* (like levocetirizine or hydroxyzine) for symptomatic relief, and
- *Keratolytics* (such as salicylic acid or urea) to soften the papules
- *Phototherapy,* including narrow-band ultraviolet B (NB-UAB) or psoralen and ultraviolet A (PUVA), may be beneficial in refractory cases.
- Topical retinoids and allopurinol are rarely used but may help in resistant cases.[2,5,7]

Diabetology/Physician Management

- Systemic management involves tight glycemic control with insulin or optimized oral hypoglycemics.
- Monitoring and correction of uremia or dialysis adequacy, and
- Addressing parathyroid hormone, calcium, and phosphate balance
- Screening for secondary bacterial infection and providing appropriate antibiotics, as well as
- Nutritional supplementation to address deficiencies (zinc and vitamins A/D/E) is also important.[2,4,7]

PROGNOSIS

Acquired perforating dermatosis is a chronic and relapsing condition. Lesions often recur despite treatment, and the primary goals are symptom control (especially pruritus) and prevention of secondary infection. Partial improvement can be achieved with better glycemic and renal management.[2,5]

> **Clinical Pearls**
>
> ▶ There is a strong association between acquired perforating dermatosis and long-standing diabetes with chronic kidney disease.
> ▶ Lesions often develop after persistent scratching or trauma, a phenomenon known as the "Koebner effect".
> ▶ Transepidermal elimination is the hallmark of histopathological feature.
> ▶ The disorder is more common in dialysis patients with inadequate control of metabolic waste and is frequently under-recognized or misdiagnosed as prurigo or folliculitis.[1,2,4,7]

REFERENCES

1. Rapini RP, Hebert AA, Drucker CR. Acquired perforating dermatosis: Evidence for combined transepidermal elimination of both collagen and elastin. Arch Dermatol. 1989;125(8):1074-8.
2. Saray Y, Seçkin D, Bilezikçi B. Acquired perforating dermatosis: Clinicopathological features in twenty-two cases. J Eur Acad Dermatol Venereol. 2006;20(6):679-88.
3. Faver IR, Daoud MS, Su WP. Acquired reactive perforating collagenosis: Report of six cases and review of the literature. J Am Acad Dermatol. 1994;30(4):575-80.
4. Lipsker D. Acquired perforating dermatosis. In: Griffiths CEM, Barker J, Bleiker T, Chalmers R, Creamer D (Eds). Rook's Textbook of Dermatology, 9th edition. United States: WileyBlackwell; 2016.
5. Mills KM, Jones S. Acquired perforating dermatosis: An updated review. Clin Dermatol. 2021;39(2):295-303.
6. Kanitakis J. Perforating dermatoses: Classification, histopathology and clinical associations. Am J Dermatopathol. 2006;28(6):517-26.
7. Sánchez NP. Transepidermal elimination: A review of its mechanisms and role in skin disorders. Dermatol Clin. 2010;28(1):55-9.

Part C: Kyrle's Disease in a Patient of Diabetes Mellitus and Chronic Kidney Disease on Hemodialysis

■ PRESENTATION

A 52-year-old male, employed as a primary school teacher, presented with a 3-month history of papulonodular, reddish-brown lesions on both lower limbs. He reported severe pruritus, scaling, and the appearance of new lesions at sites of minor trauma, consistent with the Koebner phenomenon. There was no history of pain, fever, abdominal symptoms, pedal edema, or dyspnea.

Medical History

- His medical background included type 2 diabetes mellitus for 15 years, hypertension for 5 years, and chronic kidney disease on maintenance hemodialysis for the past 3 years.
- His medications included subcutaneous insulin and amlodipine 10 mg daily, with no additional drugs.

■ EXAMINATION

On examination, multiple papules and nodules (0.2–1 cm in diameter), reddish-brown with silvery scales and central depressions, were observed on both flexor and extensor surfaces of the lower limbs **(Figs. 1 and 2)**. Systemic examination was unremarkable.

■ LABORATORY INVESTIGATIONS

- Laboratory investigations revealed a glycated hemoglobin (HbA1c) of 9.2%, serum urea of 128 mg/dL, and creatinine of 5.2 mg/dL. Other routine tests, including complete blood count, liver function tests, ECG, and two-dimensional (2D) echocardiography, were within normal limits.
- Ultrasonography of the abdomen showed bilaterally small kidneys with loss of corticomedullary differentiation, while other organs appeared normal.

■ DIAGNOSIS

- The clinical and investigative findings were suggestive of Kyrle's disease.[1-3]
- A diagnosis of Kyrle's disease was confirmed by histopathology, which demonstrated epidermal hyperplasia with downward invagination into the dermis, marked hyperkeratosis, a prominent keratotic plug, and absence of collagen fibers in the epidermis.[1-3]

■ DIFFERENTIAL DIAGNOSES

Kyrle's disease is a primary perforating dermatosis, most commonly seen in association with chronic systemic

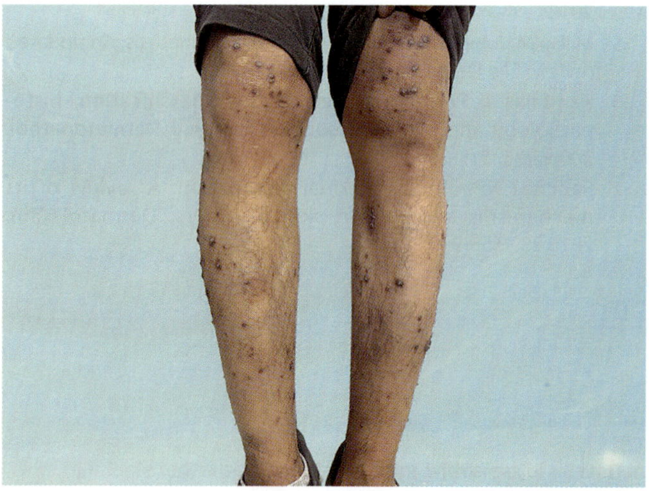

FIG. 1: Showing papulonodular reddish-brown lesions on bilateral lower limbs (anterior aspect).

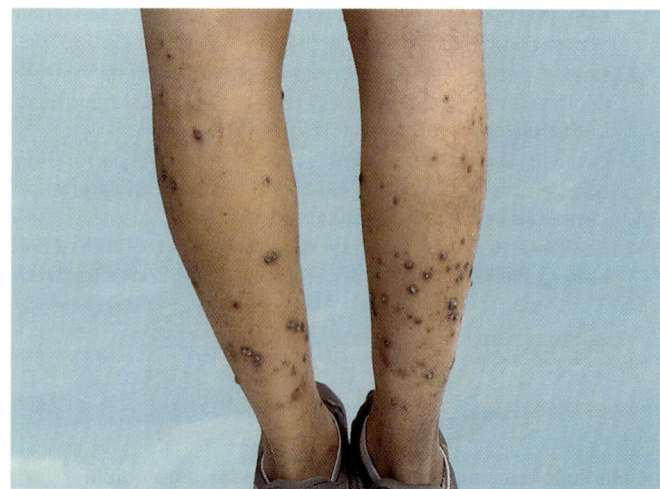

FIG. 2: Showing papulonodular reddish-brown lesions on bilateral lower limbs (posterior aspect).

diseases such as diabetes mellitus and chronic renal failure.[1] The main differential diagnoses include:
- *Acquired perforating collagenosis (APC):* Characterized by transepidermal elimination of collagen fibers.[2,3]
- *Perforating folliculitis (PF):* Involves follicular plugging and elimination of degenerated material.[2,3]
- *Elastosis perforans serpiginosa (EPS):* Defined by elimination of abnormal elastic fibers.[2,3]
- *Secondary perforating dermatoses:* Such as granuloma annulare and psoriasis.[2,3]

Histopathological differentiation is crucial; Kyrle's disease is identified by keratinous debris, whereas, APC is defined by elimination of collagen.[4,5]

MANAGEMENT

Dermatological Management

- *Topical therapy*:
  - Topical retinoids (e.g., tretinoin 0.05%)
  - Keratolytic agents like salicylic acid
  - Topical corticosteroids to reduce inflammation
  - Emollients to manage xerosis.[5]
- *Systemic therapy*:
  - Oral antihistamines (e.g., levocetirizine) for pruritus
  - Systemic retinoids (e.g., isotretinoin) in resistant cases
  - Antibiotics such as doxycycline or clindamycin for secondary infection
  - Immunomodulators (e.g., allopurinol and tacrolimus) in chronic or refractory cases.[5]
- *Other modalities*:
  - Phototherapy with narrow-band ultraviolet B (NB-UVB)
  - *Surgical options:* CO_2 laser, cryotherapy, or electrocautery for recalcitrant lesions.[5]

PHYSICIAN/DIABETOLOGY MANAGEMENT

- *Glycemic optimization*:
  - Intensification of insulin therapy to achieve target HbA1c (<7%)
  - Regular monitoring and adjustment of the antidiabetic regimen.[1]
- *Renal optimization*:
  - Strict adherence to the hemodialysis schedule
  - Correction of the uremic milieu [blood urea nitrogen (BUN): 128 mg/dL, creatinine: 5.2 mg/dL][1]
- *Lifestyle and supportive care*:
  - Avoidance of trauma and scratching
  - Comprehensive skin care, foot care, and regular follow-up[1]

PROGNOSIS

Kyrle's disease is chronic and relapsing, with a high rate of recurrence, particularly in patients with long-standing diabetes and end-stage renal disease. Lesions may increase in size and frequency with age progression. Although Kyrle's disease itself is not life-threatening, the prognosis and overall life expectancy are determined by the underlying systemic disorder.[1] The disease can have significant cosmetic and psychological effects.[1]

> **Clinical Pearls**
> - There is strong association with diabetes mellitus and chronic renal failure, especially in patients on hemodialysis.[1]
> - Presents as intensely pruritic, hyperkeratotic, umbilicated papules and nodules, predominantly on extensor surfaces.[1]
> - Koebner phenomenon is frequently observed.[1]
> - Histopathological examination is essential for distinguishing Kyrle's disease from other perforating dermatoses.[4,5]
> - Management is often challenging and requires a multidisciplinary approach with strict metabolic control.[5]

REFERENCES

1. Ngan V, Tai A, MacCallum P, Smithson S. Kyrle Disease. DermNet NZ. 2022.
2. Macca L, Vaccaro F, Li Pomi F, Borgia F, Irrera N, Vaccaro M. Kyrle disease: a case report and literature review. Eur Rev Med Pharmacol Sci. 2023;27:10705-15.
3. Schreml S, Hafner C, Eder F, Landthaler M, Burgdorf W, Babilas P. Kyrle disease and acquired perforating collagenosis secondary to chronic renal failure and diabetes mellitus. Case Rep Dermatol. 2011;3(3):209-11.
4. Rice AS, Zedek D. Kyrle Disease. StatPearls [Internet]. Treasure Island (FL): StatPearls Publishing; 2023.
5. Forouzandeh M, Stratman S, Yosipovitch G. The treatment of Kyrle's disease: a systematic review. J Eur Acad Dermatol Venereol. 2020;34(7):1457-63.

Part D: Acquired Perforating Dermatosis (Reactive Perforating Collagenosis Variant) in Diabetes

■ PRESENTATION

A 51-year-old man with a 15-year history of type 2 diabetes mellitus presents with multiple umbilicated, hyperkeratotic papules and nodules on the lower limbs, and dorsum of the foot. The lesions have central keratotic plugs and are associated with postinflammatory hyperpigmentation and atrophic scarring. The patient reports intense pruritus and occasional pain, with new lesions appearing at scratch-prone sites, suggesting Koebnerization and a chronic relapsing clinical course.

■ EXAMINATION

- On examination, the patient has multiple hyperkeratotic, umbilicated papules and nodules, ranging from 2 to 8 mm, with central crusting. The lesions are located mainly on the extensor surfaces of the legs **(Fig. 1)** and thigh **(Fig. 2)**.
- Features such as Koebnerization, postinflammatory hyperpigmentation, and depressed scars are noted.

■ INVESTIGATIONS

To confirm the clinical suspicion and assess systemic involvement, the following investigations were performed:

Laboratory Tests

- *Glycated hemoglobin (HbA1c):* 9.2% (indicating poorly controlled diabetes).
- *Serum creatinine/estimated glomerular filtration rate (eGFR):* Mildly reduced, suggesting early nephropathy.
- *Urine microalbumin:* Present (indicative of microalbuminuria)
- *Additional screening:* Evaluated for chronic kidney disease, hypothyroidism, and hypertension

Histopathology (Punch Biopsy)

- Cup-shaped epidermal invagination filled with necrotic debris
- Transepidermal elimination of dermal collagen and occasional elastic fibers
- Perivascular lymphohistiocytic infiltrate
- Confirms reactive perforating collagenosis, a subtype of acquired perforating dermatosis

Imaging

Doppler ultrasound: Normal vascular status, excluding macrovascular etiology.

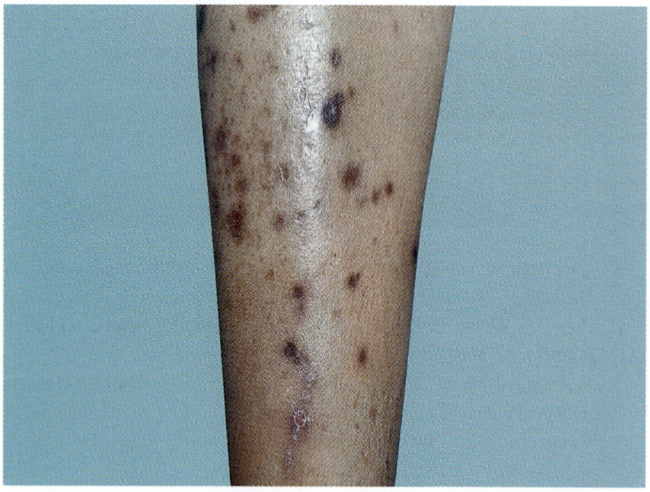

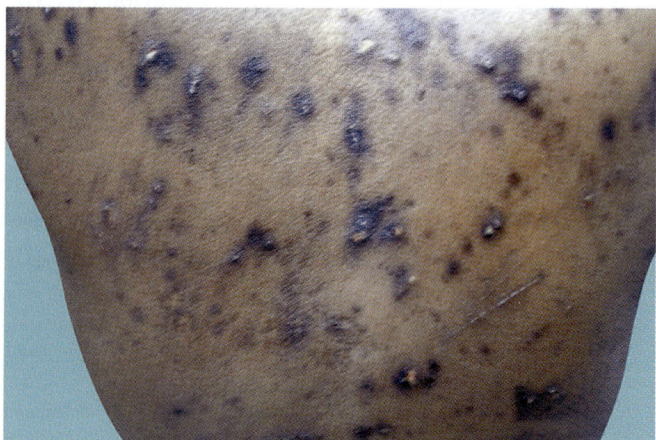

FIG. 2: Multiple hyperkeratotic, umbilicated papules and nodules with central crusting on the thigh.

FIG. 1: Multiple hyperkeratotic, umbilicated papules and nodules with central crusting on the extensor surface of lower limbs.

■ PATHOPHYSIOLOGY

The pathogenesis of reactive perforating collagenosis is multifactorial, involving structural changes in the dermis and external triggering factors:

- Transepidermal elimination of altered dermal connective tissue, including collagen and elastin, occurs through epidermal channels.[1,2]
- Chronic microangiopathy in diabetes leads to dermal hypoxia and subsequent collagen degeneration.[1,3]
- Pruritus and repeated trauma (Koebner phenomenon) further aggravate lesion formation.[1,4] Advanced glycation end-product (AGE) deposition and oxidative damage disrupt the dermal structure, promoting elimination.[1-3]
- Chronic kidney disease and other metabolic derangements may exacerbate these changes through the accumulation of toxins.[1,5]

■ DIAGNOSIS

Reactive Perforating Collagenosis (Acquired Perforating Dermatosis)

The diagnosis is primarily clinical, supported by the characteristic morphology and distribution of lesions.[1-3] It is confirmed by histopathology, which shows transepidermal elimination of collagen and elastin.[1,2,4] The clinical context of long-standing, poorly controlled diabetes, and chronic kidney disease further supports the diagnosis.[1,3,5]

Diabetes Correlation

Acquired perforating dermatoses (APDs) are frequently observed in patients with both type 1 and type 2 diabetes mellitus, especially in middle-aged adults with long-standing disease and poorly controlled blood glucose levels.[1-3] These lesions are closely associated with microvascular complications such as retinopathy, nephropathy, and neuropathy.[1,4] The prevalence of perforating dermatoses is estimated to be as high as 65% among diabetic patients presenting with such skin changes.[1,2,5] Chronic kidney disease (present in approximately 30–60% of these patients) often coexists, exacerbating the skin manifestations due to the accumulation of uremic toxins.[1,2,5]

■ DIFFERENTIAL DIAGNOSIS

- *Kyrle disease:* Similar hyperkeratotic papules, but usually larger and more generalized, with distinct histopathology.[1,4]
- *Perforating folliculitis:* Lesions centered around hair follicles, with transepidermal elimination confined to follicular openings.[1,2]
- *Prurigo nodularis and lichen planus:* Pruritic, hyperkeratotic papules that may require biopsy to rule out the presence of a central keratotic plug and transepidermal elimination.[1-3]
- *Diabetic dermopathy:* Flat, atrophic brown macules without keratotic plugs, making it a distinct clinical entity.[1,5]

■ MANAGEMENT

Dermatologist Management

Topical therapy: High-potency corticosteroids for reducing local inflammation; emollients and keratolytics (e.g., salicylic-urea preparations) to soften hyperkeratotic lesions.[1-3]

- *Antipruritics:* Nonsedating antihistamines (e.g., loratadine) to break the itch-scratch cycle.[1,4]
- *Second-line treatments:*
  - Intralesional corticosteroids, topical retinoids (tazarotene), and imiquimod[1,2,4]
  - Phototherapy [narrow-band ultraviolet B (NB-UVB) or psoralen and ultraviolet A (PUVA)] for extensive or refractory lesions[1,2,5]
  - Systemic therapy, such as allopurinol, doxycycline, and oral retinoids; biologics (e.g., dupilumab and nemolizumab) for refractory cases[1,2,5]

Diabetologist/Physician Management

- *Glycemic control:* Aim for the HbA1c < 7% to minimize microvascular complications.[1,3,4]
- *Systemic optimization:* Monitor and manage associated conditions such as chronic kidney disease and hypertension.[1,2,5]
- *Preventive measures:* Minimize trauma and scratching through behavioral counseling, regular moisturization, and patient's education.[1,2,3]

■ PROGNOSIS

Chronic relapsing course; lesions may heal with hyperpigmented or atrophic scars.[1,2,4] Early intervention reduces lesion burden; untreated cases remain symptomatic.[1,3,5] No malignant transformation reported.[1,2]

Clinical Pearls

▶ In diabetic patients with pruritic, umbilicated papules, especially on extensor legs, consider APD.[1-3]
▶ Biopsy is essential to confirm transepidermal elimination.[1,2,4]
▶ Control pruritus aggressively to prevent new lesions via Koebnerization.[1,4]
▶ Address underlying diabetes and chronic kidney disease to improve skin outcomes.[1,2,5]

REFERENCES

1. García-Malinis AJ, Sánchez-Valle E, Sánchez-Salas MP, Del Prado E, Coscojuela C, Gilaberte Y. Acquired perforating dermatosis: clinicopathological study of 31 cases. J Eur Acad Dermatol Venereol. 2017;31(10):1757-63.
2. Wang MF, Mei XL, Wang L, Lin-Feng L. Clinical characteristics and prognosis of acquired perforating dermatosis: a case report. Exp Ther Med. 2020;19(6):3634-40.
3. Zhang LW, Wu J, Xu RH, Chen T. Acquired reactive perforating collagenosis in a patient with diabetes. Cleveland Clinic J Med. 2024;91(4):213-4.
4. Saray Y, Seçkin D, Bilezikçi B. Clinicopathological features in 22 cases. J Eur Acad Dermatol Venereol. 2006;20(6):679-88.
5. González-Lara L, Gómez-Bernal S, Vázquez-López F, Vivanco-Allende B. Acquired perforating dermatosis: report of 8 cases. Actas Dermosifiliogr. 2014;105(4):372-9.

Part E: Reactive Perforating Collagenosis in a Type 2 Diabetic Female

PRESENTATION

A 55-year-old obese female [body mass index (BMI): 32 kg/m²], homemaker, presented with severe pruritic eruptions involving both lower limbs, buttocks, and the right forearm for the past 8 months. There was no personal or family history of similar dermatologic issues. She had a 7-year history of type 2 diabetes mellitus, managed with metformin and voglibose.

EXAMINATION

On examination, multiple discrete umbilicated papules with central adherent keratotic plugs were observed, predominantly over the shins and buttocks **(Fig. 1)**, with a few on the right forearm. There were no signs of secondary infection, ulceration, or lichenification.

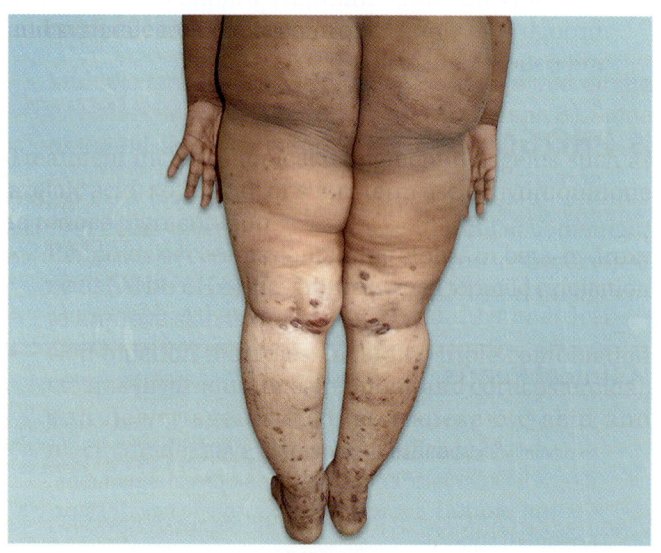

FIG. 1: Multiple discrete umbilicated papules with central adherent keratotic plugs are observed over the shins and buttocks.

INVESTIGATIONS

Laboratory Findings

Laboratory investigations revealed:
- Fasting blood glucose of 188 mg/dL and glycated hemoglobin (HbA1c) of 8.8%.
- Other blood parameters, including CBC, liver, renal, and thyroid function tests, were within normal limits.
- Viral markers (HBV, HCV, and HIV) were negative.

Skin Biopsy

Skin biopsy demonstrated epidermal hyperplasia with a cup-shaped central depression containing keratin and cellular debris, along with transepidermal elimination of collagen fibers, confirming reactive perforating collagenosis (RPC).

DIAGNOSIS

Reactive perforating collagenosis—an acquired perforating dermatosis frequently associated with poorly controlled diabetes mellitus.[1,2]

DIFFERENTIAL DIAGNOSIS

- *Folliculitis:* Typically presents with follicle-centered pustules and lacks the central keratotic plug.[3]
- *Prurigo nodularis:* Characterized by hyperkeratotic nodules, often due to chronic scratching.[3]
- *Kyrle's disease:* Features larger papules with keratin plugs and more extensive transepidermal elimination on histopathology.[3]
- *Perforating granuloma annulare:* Usually annular with granulomatous inflammation and elastin extrusion in the dermis.[3]

PATHOPHYSIOLOGY

Reactive perforating collagenosis belongs to the group of acquired perforating dermatoses (APD), most commonly seen in patients with diabetes mellitus and/or chronic kidney disease (CKD).[1,4] The hallmark is transepidermal elimination of altered collagen fibers through the epidermis.[2] Proposed mechanisms include microangiopathy and accumulation of advanced glycation end-products (AGEs) causing dermal injury, pruritus-induced trauma (Koebner phenomenon), delayed wound healing resulting in abnormal collagen repair and extrusion, and the involvement of inflammatory mediators such as interleukin 1 (IL-1), tumor necrosis factor alpha (TNF-α), and matrix metalloproteinases (MMPs).[1,5-7]

MANAGEMENT

Dermatological Management

- Oral doxycycline (100 mg daily) for anti-inflammatory and antimicrobial effects[7]
- Topical retinoids (e.g., tretinoin 0.025%) to promote epidermal turnover[7]
- Second-generation antihistamines (e.g., levocetirizine) to control pruritus[7]
- Emollients and urea-based creams to maintain the skin barrier[7]
- Patient's education to minimize scratching and trauma[7]
- In recalcitrant cases, phototherapy [narrow-band ultraviolet B (NB-UVB) or psoralen and ultraviolet A (PUVA)], allopurinol, or oral retinoids may be considered.[6,7]

Diabetology/Physician Management

- Intensification of antidiabetic therapy for optimal glycemic control[5,7]
- Nutrition counseling for weight management and awareness of the glycemic index[5]
- Regular screening for microvascular complications (retinopathy, nephropathy, and neuropathy)[5]
- Periodic follow-up every 3 months for HbA1c and metabolic panel monitoring[5]

PROGNOSIS

With improved glycemic control and appropriate dermatologic therapy, lesions generally resolve within 3–6 months, though residual postinflammatory hyperpigmentation is common.[5,7] Recurrences may occur with poor glycemic control or repeated trauma from scratching. Importantly, these lesions are benign and do not progress to systemic disease.[5]

> **Clinical Pearls**
>
> ▶ Lesions typically affect extensor surfaces, presenting as keratotic papules with central umbilication.[1,2]
> ▶ Most commonly involve the lower limbs, gluteal region, and forearms.[1,2]
> ▶ More prevalent in overweight or poorly controlled type 2 diabetic patients[5]
> ▶ *Histological hallmark*: Cup-shaped epidermal invagination with transepidermal elimination of collagen.[2,3]
> ▶ Reactive perforating collagenosis is part of the spectrum of perforating dermatoses, including Kyrle disease, acquired perforating collagenosis, elastosis perforans serpiginosa, and perforating folliculitis.[3,4]

REFERENCES

1. Saray Y, Seçkin D, Bilezikçi B. Acquired perforating dermatosis: clinicopathological features in twenty-two cases. J Eur Acad Dermatol Venereol. 2006;20(6):679-88.
2. Faver IR, Daoud MS, Su WP. Acquired perforating dermatosis: a clinicopathologic study of forty-one cases. J Am Acad Dermatol. 1994;30(4):575-80.
3. Rapini RP, Herbert AA, Drucker CR. Acquired perforating dermatosis: evidence for combined transepidermal elimination of both collagen and elastic fibers. Arch Dermatol. 1989;125(8):1074-8.
4. Satti MB, Al-Amoudi NS. Perforating dermatoses: a clinicopathologic study. Int J Dermatol. 2007;46(4):380-4.
5. Wollina U, Hansel G, Köstler E. Acquired reactive perforating dermatosis in diabetes mellitus. J Eur Acad Dermatol Venereol. 2001;15(6):522-4.
6. Dominguez-Cherit J, Vega-Memije ME, Hojyo-Tomoka MT. Acquired perforating dermatosis: response to allopurinol. J Am Acad Dermatol. 1992;27(2 Pt 2):354-5.
7. Faver IR, Daoud MS, Su WP. Acquired reactive perforating collagenosis. J Am Acad Dermatol. 1994;30(4):575-80.

Part F: Pruritic Perforating Dermatosis Associated with Type 2 Diabetes Mellitus

■ PRESENTATION

A 35-year-old male working in a corporate setting presented with severe itching and lesions distributed across his face **(Fig. 1)**, upper torso **(Fig. 2)**, and both lower limbs.[1-3] Over the last 8 months, these lesions had progressively increased in number. The patient noted that the lesions would eventually perforate and heal, leaving behind areas of hyperpigmentation. He denied experiencing any systemic symptoms such as fever or joint discomfort.

Medical History

- Type 2 diabetes mellitus (duration: 5 years)
- Hypertension (duration: 5 years)
- Dyslipidemia (duration: 5 years)

Medications

- Gliclazide + Metformin 80/500 mg twice daily
- Metoprolol 25 mg once daily
- Empagliflozin 10 mg once daily
- Rosuvastatin 40 mg once daily
- Insulin glargine 12 units at bedtime

■ EXAMINATION

Physical examination revealed numerous umbilicated papules and nodules, each with a central crust or perforation and surrounding hyperpigmentation. The lesions were predominantly found on the face **(Fig. 1)**, upper trunk, and lower legs **(Figs. 2 and 3)**. There was no evidence of secondary infection.

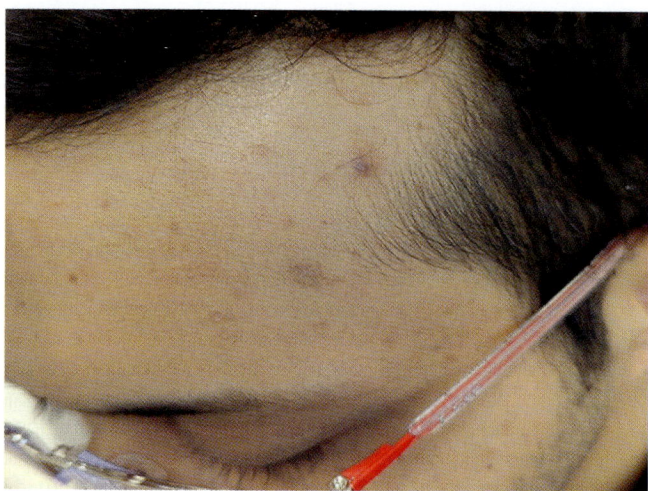

FIG. 1: Numerous umbilicated papules and nodules with central crusting and perifocal hyperpigmentation are seen over the face.

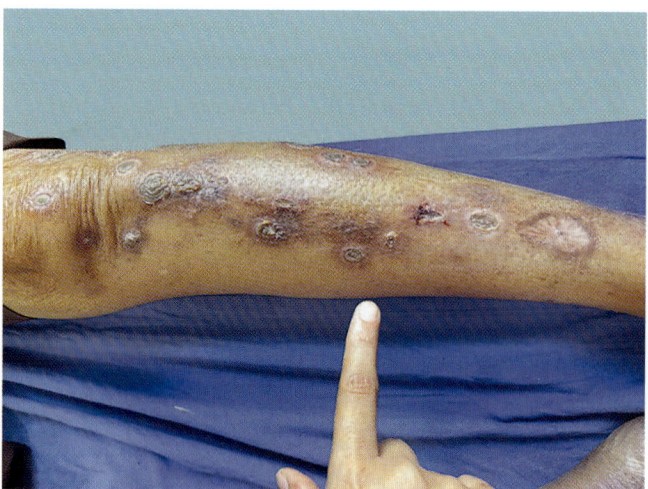

FIG. 2: Multiple crusted, umbilicated papules, and nodules with surrounding hyperpigmentation noted over the anterior aspect of the lower limbs.

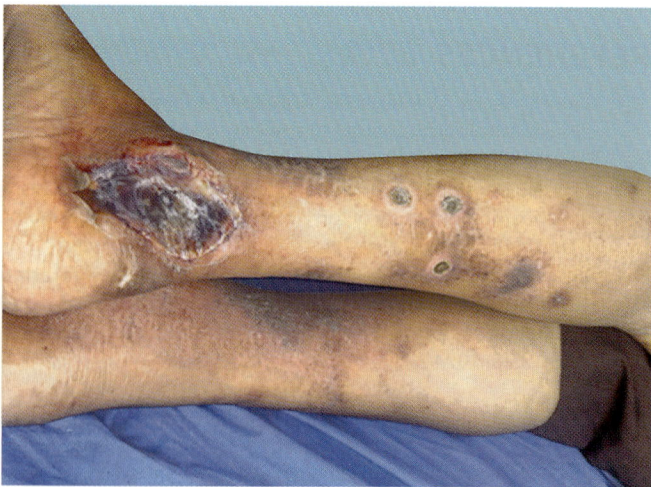

FIG. 3: Scattered umbilicated lesions with central perforation and prominent hyperpigmentation present over the posterior aspect of the lower limbs.

DIAGNOSIS

The clinical picture was consistent with pruritic perforating dermatosis (Kyrle's disease) in the context of type 2 diabetes mellitus, hypertension, and dyslipidemia.

DIFFERENTIAL DIAGNOSIS

- *Kyrle's disease (pruritic perforating dermatosis):* Most probable, given the distinctive perforating skin lesions and the patient's diabetic background.[3]
- *Secondary bacterial infection:* Considered unlikely due to the absence of pus or systemic symptoms.[1]
- *Lichen planus:* Ruled out, as the lesions were not flat-topped or violaceous.[1]
- *Folliculitis:* Typically presents with pustules, not perforating papules.[1]

MANAGEMENT

Dermatological Management

- The diagnosis was confirmed clinically.
- Topical corticosteroids were prescribed to alleviate inflammation and pruritus.
- Oral antihistamines were started for symptomatic relief from itching.
- Keratolytic agents, such as salicylic acid creams, were recommended to facilitate resolution of lesions.
- The importance of optimal glycemic control was emphasized to reduce the risk of recurrence.[4]

Physician/Diabetologist Management

- *Initial laboratory results:* Glycated hemoglobin (HbA1c) 11.5%, fasting glucose 280 mg/dL, postprandial glucose 310 mg/dL, and serum creatinine 0.8 mg/dL.
- *Diabetes therapy was intensified:* Insulin glargine was increased to 16 units at night.
- Dapagliflozin 10 mg + Sitagliptin 100 mg + Metformin 500 mg once daily was added.
- Glimepiride + Metformin 2/500 mg three times daily was started.
- Metoprolol and rosuvastatin were continued.
- The patient was hesitant to initiate bolus insulin.
- Counseling was provided regarding hypoglycemia prevention and management.
- Follow-up was advised in 2 weeks with fasting and postprandial glucose, urine routine, and microscopy.[1]

At follow-up, fasting glucose was 146 mg/dL, postprandial was 184 mg/dL, and urine analysis was unremarkable. Lifestyle changes, including a low-glycemic index diet and regular exercise, were reinforced. Further investigations were planned after 3 months: HbA1c, lipid profile, renal and liver function tests, microalbuminuria, and retinal screening for diabetic retinopathy.[1]

PROGNOSIS

With improved glycemic control and targeted dermatological therapy, the frequency and severity of skin lesions generally decrease. Nevertheless, postinflammatory hyperpigmentation may remain. The long-term outlook depends on consistent diabetes management and prevention of recurrences.[5]

> **Clinical Pearls**
>
> ▶ The presence of pruritic, perforating lesions (umbilicated papules with central keratotic plugs) is characteristic of Kyrle's disease, especially in individuals with diabetes or chronic kidney disease.[6]
> ▶ Multiple comorbidities, such as diabetes, hypertension, and dyslipidemia, contribute to increased skin fragility and delayed wound healing.[1]
> ▶ Prompt dermatological intervention and strict metabolic control are essential for minimizing recurrences and enhancing quality of life.[7]

REFERENCES

1. Saray Y, Seçkin D, Bilezikçi B. Acquired perforating dermatosis: clinicopathological features and possible pathogenetic mechanisms. Int J Dermatol. 2006;45(6):693-9.
2. Rapini RP, Herbert AA, Drucker CR. Acquired perforating dermatosis: evidence for combined transepidermal elimination of both collagen and elastic fibres. ArchDermatol. 1989;125(8):1074-8.
3. Angelopoulos TJ, Kubilus J. Kyrle's disease and perforating dermatoses. Dermatol Clin. 2010;28(3):475-81.
4. Faver IR. Acquired perforating dermatosis: report of six cases and a review of the literature. J Am Acad Dermatol. 1988;19(5 Pt 1):808-14.
5. Patterson JW. The perforating disorders. In: Patterson JW (Ed). University of Virginia. Weedon's Skin Pathology, 5th edition. Netherland: Elsevier; 2020. pp. 432-6.
6. Chen MT, Cohen PR. Pruritic papules with central keratotic cores in a diabetic patient: Kyrle disease. Cutis. 2012;89(5):223-6.
7. Morgan MB, Stevens GL, Somach S, Tannenbaum M. Acquired perforating dermatosis: a clinicopathologic study emphasizing the spectrum of histologic findings. Am J Dermatopathol. 2001;23(6):446-9.

SECTION 3

Skin Conditions Associated with or Exacerbated by Diabetes

▶ Section Outline

Chapter 13: Psoriasis in a Diabetic Patient
Nipul Vara, Vishwa Marvania

Chapter 14: Acanthosis Nigricans and Acrochordons (Skin Tags) in Diabetes
Suhas Gopal Erande, Anil Patki, Bharat Bhushan Kukreja, Ruchi Shah, Yogesh Marfatia

Chapter 15: Lichen Planus in a Diabetic Male with Hypothyroidism
Nipul Vara, Vishwa Marvania

Chapter 16: Xerosis and Pruritus in Diabetes (Dry Skin and Generalized Itch)
J Thadeus

Chapter 17: Subacute Eczema with Id Eruption in Metabolic Syndrome and Type 2 Diabetes
Rutul Gokalani, Viral Thakkar

CHAPTER 13

Psoriasis in a Diabetic Patient

Nipul Vara, Vishwa Marvania

■ PRESENTATION

A 62-year-old male with a 15-year history of type 2 diabetes mellitus presented with suboptimal glycemic control (HbA1c—9.2%). He is a retired office clerk and is currently on metformin 500 mg three times daily and glimepiride 2 mg once daily. There is no known family history of psoriasis. He complained of pruritic, scaly, erythematous plaques on the trunk, limbs, and scalp, with a chronic course and intermittent exacerbations and remissions.

■ EXAMINATION

- Multiple well-demarcated, scaly, erythematous plaques were observed on the trunk **(Fig. 1)**, limbs **(Fig. 2)**, and scalp.
- The lesions demonstrated pinpoint bleeding upon scratching (Auspitz sign positive).
- No evidence of psoriatic arthritis or other systemic involvement was noted.

■ INVESTIGATIONS

The clinical presentation was highly suggestive of psoriasis.

A skin biopsy may be performed for histopathological confirmation in atypical cases, but was not deemed necessary here due to the classic clinical findings.

■ DIAGNOSIS

In a patient with pre-existing type 2 diabetes mellitus, the diagnosis of chronic plaque psoriasis was made.

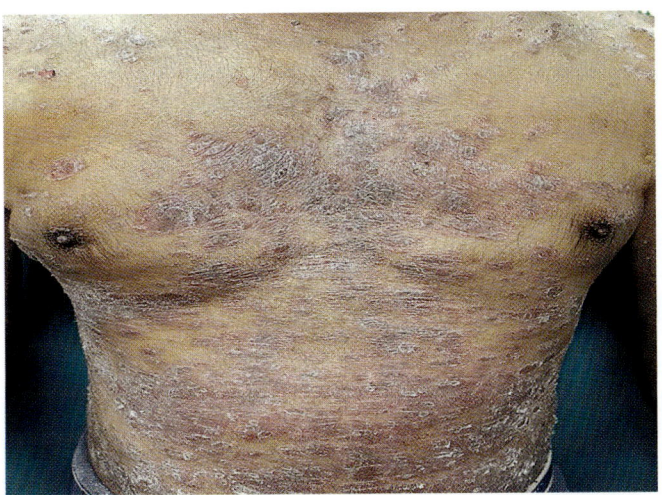

FIG. 1: Numerous erythematous plaques with prominent silvery-white scaling distributed across the chest and abdomen.

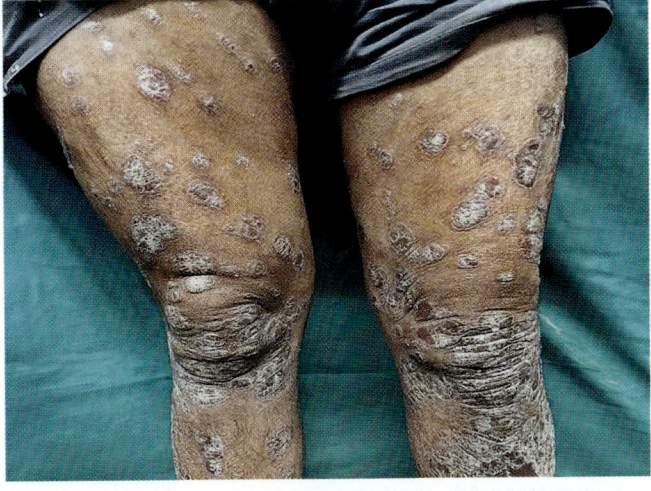

FIG. 2: Hyperkeratotic, sharply demarcated plaques affecting both knees and lower legs, showing marked scaling and lichenification.

DIFFERENTIAL DIAGNOSIS

- *Tinea corporis:* Characterized by central clearing and an active, advancing border; potassium hydroxide (KOH) examination positive
- *Seborrheic dermatitis:* Presents with greasy, yellowish scales localized to seborrheic regions
- *Lichen simplex chronicus*: Exhibits localized skin thickening due to persistent scratching
- *Early cutaneous T-cell lymphoma*: Patch-stage lesions may resemble psoriasis.
- *Pityriasis rubra pilaris*: Features include areas of sparing and follicular papules.

PATHOPHYSIOLOGY

Psoriasis is a persistent inflammatory dermatosis marked by excessive keratinocyte proliferation and immune dysregulation, particularly involving Th1 and Th17 lymphocyte pathways.[1] Type 2 diabetes mellitus is similarly associated with chronic inflammation, heightened oxidative stress, and insulin resistance—mechanisms also implicated in psoriasis.[2] Both conditions share risk factors such as obesity, metabolic syndrome, and genetic susceptibility, notably HLA-Cw6.[3] Inflammatory mediators in psoriasis can further impair insulin sensitivity, potentially worsening hyperglycemia in diabetic individuals.[4] Biomarkers including tumor necrosis factor-alpha (TNF-α), interleukin-6 (IL-6), and adiponectin are elevated in both disorders.[5] Additionally, both diseases confer an increased risk of cardiovascular morbidity.[4]

MANAGEMENT

Dermatological Approach

- *Topical therapies:*
    - Potent corticosteroids (e.g., clobetasol propionate)
    - Combination of calcipotriol and betamethasone
    - Salicylic acid 6% for scalp involvement and thick plaques
- *Systemic agents (use with caution in diabetes):*
    - *Methotrexate*: Requires close monitoring of hepatic and renal function, particularly in diabetics
    - *Apremilast*: Generally considered safe in patients with diabetes
    - *Biologic agents*: Anti-TNF (etanercept), IL-17 inhibitors (secukinumab); metabolic safety assessment advised[6]
- *Phototherapy:* Narrowband ultraviolet B (UVB) or psoralen plus ultraviolet A therapy (PUVA) therapy for stable, widespread psoriasis

Diabetology/Physician Approach

- *Optimize glycemic management*: Intensify antidiabetic therapy; consider adding a dipeptidyl peptidase-4 (DPP-4) inhibitor, which is safe in psoriasis
- *Evaluate comorbidities:* Screen lipid profile, blood pressure, and cardiovascular risk
- *Lifestyle modification:* Recommend weight reduction through diet and physical activity, benefiting both conditions[7]
- *Avoid medications that can aggravate psoriasis:* Beta-blockers, lithium, and antimalarial drugs

PROGNOSIS

Psoriasis is a chronic, relapsing disorder. Improved glycemic control is associated with milder psoriasis severity.[3] Poorly managed cases of both diseases increase the risk of cardiovascular complications and psychological comorbidities such as depression.[4]

> ### Clinical Pearls
> - *Auspitz* sign: Pinpoint bleeding upon removal of scales
> - *Koebner phenomenon:* New lesions developing at sites of trauma
> - Thick, silvery scales predominantly on extensor surfaces
> - Psoriasis is a multisystem disease; patients should be screened for diabetes, dyslipidemia, and metabolic syndrome.[2]

REFERENCES

1. Rendon A, Schäkel K. Psoriasis pathogenesis and treatment. Int J Mol Sci. 2019;20(6):1475.
2. Takeshita J, Grewal S, Langan SM, Mehta NN, Ogdie A, Van Voorhees AS, et al. Psoriasis and comorbid diseases. J Am Acad Dermatol. 2017;76(3):377-90.
3. Armstrong AW, Harskamp CT, Armstrong EJ. Psoriasis and metabolic syndrome: a systematic review and meta-analysis of observational studies. J Am Acad Dermatol. 2013;68(4):654-62.
4. Boehncke WH, Boehncke S, Tobin AM, Kirby B. The 'psoriatic march': a concept of how severe psoriasis may drive cardiovascular comorbidity. Exp Dermatol. 2011;20(4):303-7.
5. Coimbra S, Oliveira H, Reis F, Belo L, Rocha S, Quintanilha A, et al. Interleukin (IL)-22, IL-17, and IL-23 levels in patients with psoriasis before and after systemic treatment. Br J Dermatol. 2010;163(6):1282-90.
6. Boehncke WH. Systemic inflammation and cardiovascular comorbidity in psoriasis patients: causes and consequences. Front Immunol. 2018;9:579.
7. Love TJ, Qureshi AA, Karlson EW, Gelfand JM, Choi HK. Prevalence of the metabolic syndrome in psoriasis: results from the National Health and Nutrition Examination Survey, 2003–2006. Arch Dermatol. 2011;147(4):419-24.

CHAPTER 14

Acanthosis Nigricans and Acrochordons (Skin Tags) in Diabetes

Suhas Gopal Erande, Anil Patki, Bharat Bhushan Kukreja, Ruchi Shah, Yogesh Marfatia

Case 1: Facila Acanthosis Nigricans

■ PRESENTATION

A 38-year-old overweight South Asian male presented with gradual darkening and thickening of the skin over the forehead and periocular region for the past 1.5 years. The lesions developed insidiously without associated itching, pain, or scaling. He has a history of prediabetes [fasting plasma glucose (FPG) = 112 mg/dL, glycated hemoglobin (HbA1c) = 6.1%], hypertension, and dyslipidemia. There is a family history of diabetes in first-degree relatives. His body mass index (BMI) is 28.5 kg/m². On questioning, he reported similar changes over the posterior neck and axillae.

■ EXAMINATION

- On inspection, there were hyperpigmented, velvety plaques on the central forehead extending toward the glabella and periorbital areas **(Fig. 1)**.
- The lesions were bilateral, symmetrical, and without erythema, fissuring, scaling, or mucosal involvement.
- Classical acanthosis nigricans (AN) patches were also present over the axillae and posterior neck folds. There were no signs of hirsutism or other endocrine stigmata.

■ INVESTIGATION

- Laboratory investigations revealed *FPG* of 112 mg/dL and *HbA1c* of 6.1%, confirming prediabetes.
- *Fasting insulin* was elevated at 23 µIU/mL, *with a homeostatic model assessment for insulin resistance (HOMA-IR)* of 6.3, indicating significant IR.
- *The lipid profile* showed triglycerides of 198 mg/dL and high-density lipoprotein (HDL) of 36 mg/dL, consistent with atherogenic dyslipidemia.
- *Thyroid function tests and liver function tests* were within normal limits, helping to rule out endocrine or hepatic causes.
- *On dermoscopy,* net-like pigment reticulation with a sulcus-crista pattern and hyperpigmented ridges was noted.
- *Histology,* if performed, would reveal hyperkeratosis, papillomatosis, and basal layer hyperpigmentation without significant dermal inflammation.

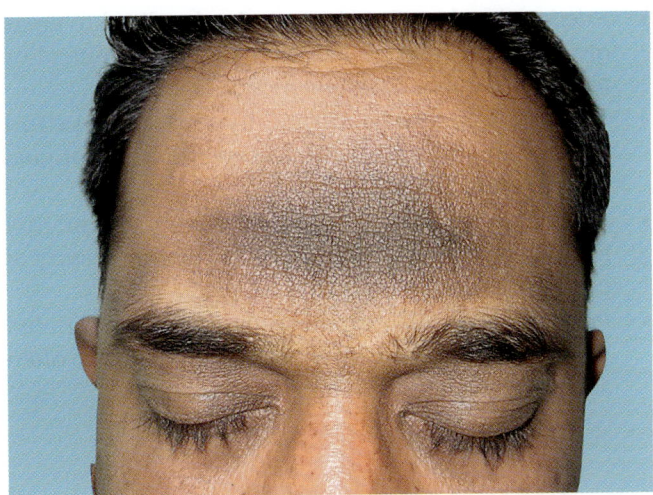

FIG. 1: Hyperpigmented, velvety plaques observed on the central forehead, extending toward the glabella and periorbital regions.

PATHOPHYSIOLOGY

Facial acanthosis nigricans (FAN) develops as a cutaneous marker of underlying metabolic dysfunction, particularly IR. The key driver is hyperinsulinemia, which stimulates the proliferation of epidermal keratinocytes and dermal fibroblasts by binding to insulin-like growth factor-1 (IGF-1) receptors. This leads to epidermal thickening, papillomatosis, and basal layer hyperpigmentation.[1,2] South Asian populations may exhibit facial AN at lower BMI thresholds compared to other groups, reflecting a heightened susceptibility to IR and metabolic syndrome at relatively modest levels of adiposity.[3]

DIAGNOSIS

Facial acanthosis nigricans—a cutaneous marker of IR and metabolic syndrome—is increasingly reported in South Asian populations. Its presence should prompt evaluation for prediabetes and associated metabolic derangements.[1-3]

DIFFERENTIAL DIAGNOSIS

Several conditions can mimic the clinical appearance of FAN. A careful history and examination help in distinguishing these:
- *Melasma*—presents as smooth, macular hyperpigmentation often induced by sun exposure; typically affects the cheeks, forehead, and upper lip.
- *Lichen planus pigmentosus*—features grayish-brown patches with a predilection for sun-exposed areas; associated with histological interface dermatitis.
- *Frictional melanosis*—pigmentation localized to areas of repeated rubbing, such as the lateral forehead or temples; history of habitual friction is key.
- *Addison's disease*—diffuse hyperpigmentation accompanied by systemic features such as fatigue, hypotension, and weight loss.
- *Postinflammatory hyperpigmentation*—pigmentation following prior dermatitis, acne, or trauma; history of preceding skin inflammation is typical.
- *Paraneoplastic AN*—rapidly progressive, widespread hyperpigmentation with mucosal involvement, often associated with internal malignancies.

CLINICAL CORRELATION WITH METABOLIC SYNDROME

Facial acanthosis nigricans may precede the onset of type 2 diabetes mellitus by several years and serves as an early clinical marker of IR. It is closely linked with key components of the metabolic syndrome, highlighting the need for timely intervention:
- Obesity and central adiposity
- Fatty liver disease [nonalcoholic fatty liver disease, (NAFLD)]
- Polycystic ovary syndrome (in women)
- Early cardiometabolic risk in males[1,3-6]

MANAGEMENT

The management of FAN requires a dual approach—addressing both the cutaneous changes and the underlying metabolic derangements.

Dermatologic Treatment

- *Topical retinoids:* Tretinoin 0.05% cream applied at night may help to reduce epidermal thickening.[6]
- *Keratolytics:* Agents such as ammonium lactate 12% or salicylic acid can soften hyperkeratotic plaques.
- *Depigmenting agents:* Azelaic acid or kojic acid may aid in reducing hyperpigmentation.
- *Procedures:* Chemical peels (glycolic acid or trichloroacetic acid) and microdermabrasion may be considered for resistant cases.

Diabetologist/Physician Management

- *Metformin:* 500–1,000 mg/day can improve insulin sensitivity and may contribute to the gradual resolution of skin changes.[1,6]
- *Lifestyle modification:* A structured program including caloric restriction, aerobic exercise, and resistance training is essential to improve IR.
- *Dietary counseling:* Adoption of a low-carbohydrate or Mediterranean-style diet supports weight reduction and metabolic control.
- *Risk factor control:* Concurrent management of hypertension and dyslipidemia is important to reduce overall cardiometabolic risk.

PROGNOSIS

- Gradual improvement with weight loss and insulin sensitization
- Early recognition of FAN can *prevent progression to overt diabetes*
- Cosmetic regression encourages patient compliance.

> **Clinical Pearls**
> ▶ Facial acanthosis nigricans is a visible, noninvasive clue to IR in metabolic syndrome.
> ▶ Always examine the neck and axillae when facial hyperpigmentation is observed.
> ▶ Facial acanthosis nigricans in South Asians is disproportionately high—even at nonobese BMI levels.
> ▶ Do not overlook rapid or mucosal involvement—screen for malignancy if suspected.
> ▶ Early metformin and lifestyle changes may prevent type 2 diabetes mellitus and reduce cutaneous changes.

Case 2 | Acanthosis Nigricans on Other Parts of Body

PRESENTATION

Acanthosis nigricans typically presents as symmetrical, dark brown to black, velvety plaques, most often located on the posterior neck, axillae, groin, knuckles, and elbows. While usually asymptomatic, some patients may experience associated skin tags or an unpleasant odor. The condition tends to develop slowly and chronically. Its onset often reflects the underlying systemic issue. Early recognition provides an opportunity for lifestyle modifications and metabolic intervention.[7-9] Patient history may reveal:
- Weight gain or central obesity
- Features of IR or metabolic syndrome
- Strong family history of diabetes
- Onset before or around puberty in children (suggesting a metabolic cause)
- In adults, sudden and extensive AN may point to an underlying malignancy (e.g., gastric adenocarcinoma).[9,10]

Location: Posterior neck (nape)

Appearance: Faint brownish discoloration is visible only on close inspection. Skin remains smooth with minimal thickening. No raised plaques or pronounced velvety texture. Involvement is limited to the nape, with no extension to lateral or anterior neck surfaces.

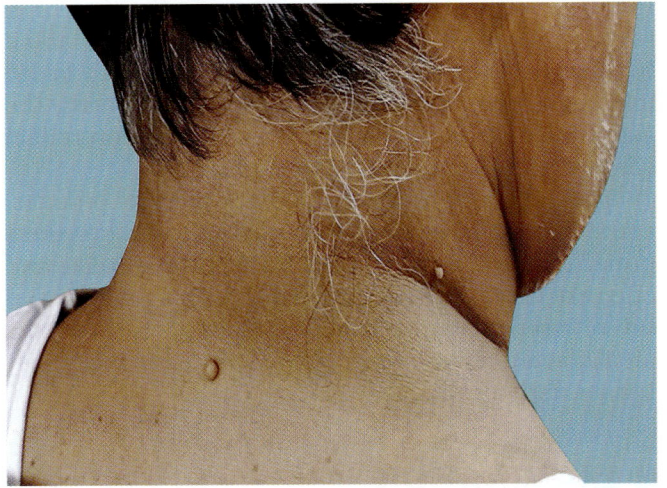

FIG. 2: Grade 1 acanthosis nigricans.

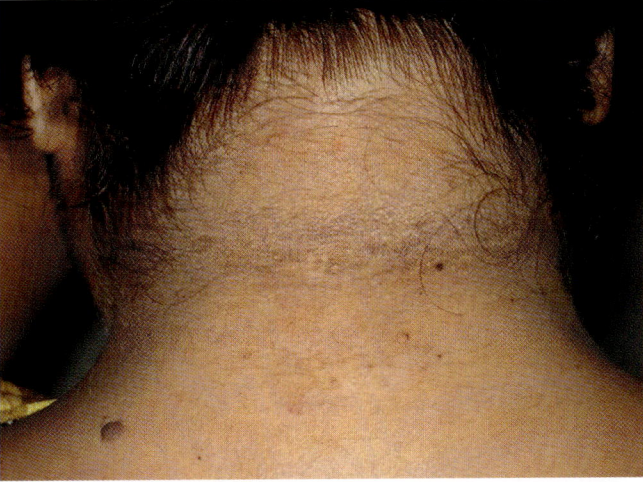

FIG. 3: Grade 2 acanthosis nigricans.

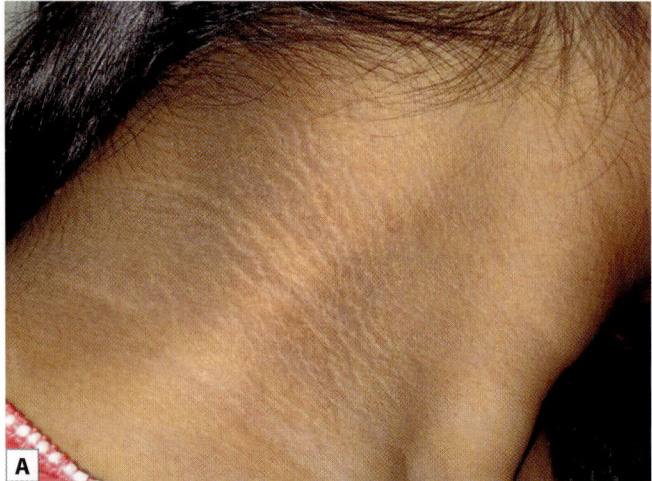
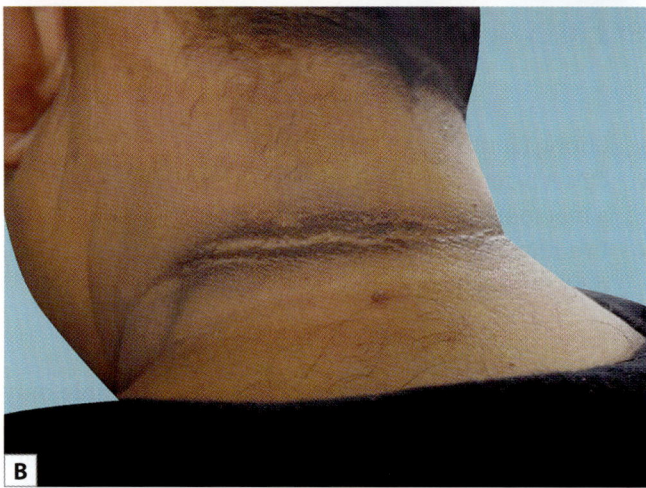
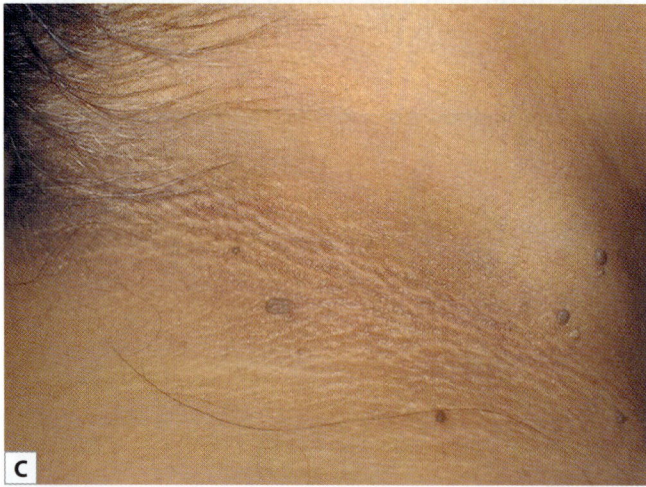

FIG. 4A TO C: Grade 3 acanthosis nigricans.

The lesion is confined to the posterior neck at the base of the skull, showing mild-to-moderate uniform brownish discoloration. The skin appears velvety with slight thickening, but there is no extension to the lateral or anterior surfaces of the neck. The pigmentation is easily visible on casual inspection, distinguishing it from Grade 1. However, the extent of involvement is not sufficient to qualify as Grade 3. Overall, the changes are evident but remain localized to the midline and posterior aspect of the neck.

The pigmentation is prominently visible and extends laterally across the sides of the neck, beyond the midline. The skin shows dark hyperpigmentation with noticeable thickening, giving it a coarse and velvety appearance. This grade is characterized by involvement that is no longer limited to the nape or base of the skull but reaches the lateral margins of the neck. The lesion is visible even from a distance and does not require close inspection. However, there is no extension to the anterior neck, which differentiates it from Grade 4.

Thick and dark pigmentation is visible across the posterior neck, with lateral spread that does not reach the anterior surface. The lesion appears as a sharply demarcated, horizontal band with a velvety and corrugated texture. The severity and distribution suggest chronicity and underlying metabolic significance.

The lesion shows thick and dark pigmentation that is easily visible without close inspection. It extends across the nape with lateral spread but does not involve the anterior neck. Located over the mid-to-lower posterior cervical area, the pigmentation is dark brown to black, sharply defined, and forms a horizontal band. The skin is markedly thickened with a velvety, corrugated texture, indicating chronicity and possible underlying metabolic dysfunction.

Pigmentation and thickening extend laterally and are visible from the anterior aspect **(Fig. 5C)**, confirming circumferential neck involvement. The skin is coarsely textured with pronounced ridges, indicating high severity. All three views **(Figs. 5A to C)** show marked hyperpigmentation, thickened velvety skin, and raised folds across the posterior, lateral, and anterior neck. The extensive distribution and deep pigmentation reflect chronicity and significant metabolic burden.

Thickened, dark brown to black, velvety plaques, and linear folds with rough texture and papillomatous projections are seen, typically involving the axillae and often extending to the antecubital and popliteal fossae. In severe cases, hyperpigmented lesions may also affect the areolar and umbilical regions, and in rare instances, may involve the entire body.

■ EXAMINATION

A detailed skin examination is essential, especially in obese individuals or those with features of metabolic syndrome.

Chapter 14: Acanthosis Nigricans and Acrochordons (Skin Tags) in Diabetes

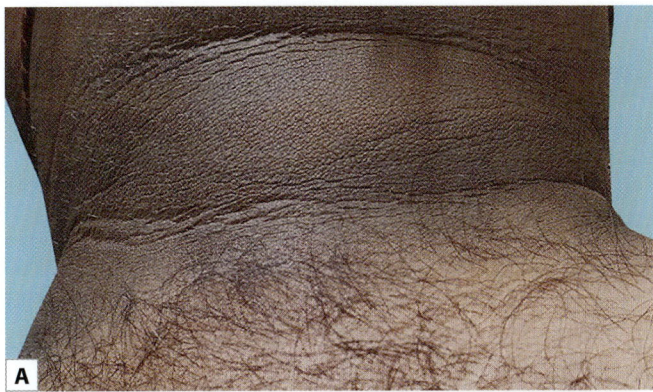
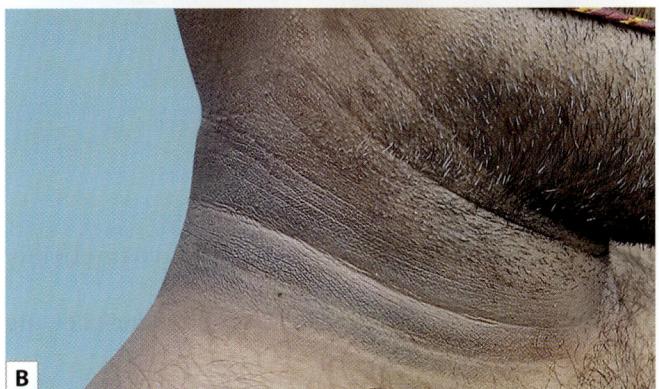
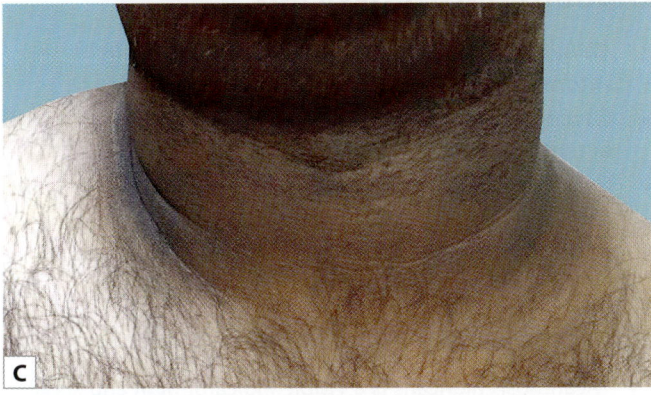

FIGS. 5A TO C: Grade 4 acanthosis nigricans. (A) Acanthosis nigricans (nape of neck); (B) Acanthosis nigricans (lateral view); (C) Acanthosis nigricans (front view)

Grading AN is useful for documenting severity and tracking progression over time (1), see **Table 1**. **Figures 6A and B** show acanthosis nigricans in other areas.

Other Findings

- Skin tags (acrochordons) are frequently associated.
- Velvety texture and papillomatosis
- Broad involvement of axillae, groin, and popliteal/antecubital fossae

TABLE 1: Grading (Burke Scale).		
Grade	Description	
0	No visible lesion	
1	Subtle pigmentation, visible only upon close inspection	Figure 2
2	Involvement of posterior neck only, ≤3 inches wide	Figures 3A to C
3	Extension to lateral margins of the neck, 3–6 inches	Figures 4A to C
4	Anterior extension >6 inches, visible from the front	Figures 5A to C

■ INVESTIGATIONS

The following investigations should be advised. These tests help to differentiate common metabolic causes from rarer neoplastic ones. HOMA-IR and HbA1c are especially helpful in detecting IR.[8,11]

- Fasting insulin and glucose
- Homeostatic model assessment of insulin resistance)
- Glycated hemoglobin
- Lipid profile
- Thyroid profile
- Abdominal ultrasound [if obesity or polycystic ovary syndrome (PCOS) is suspected]
- *Malignancy workup:* Indicated if onset is sudden, rapid, and widespread (especially in nonobese adults)

A skin biopsy is rarely necessary unless the diagnosis is unclear. Histopathology may reveal papillomatosis, hyperkeratosis, and minimal dermal inflammation.[9]

■ PATHOPHYSIOLOGY

Understanding the underlying mechanisms highlights the importance of metabolic correction in treatment. AN often serves as a visible sign of systemic imbalance. The main pathway involves hyperinsulinemia, which activates IGF-1 receptors on keratinocytes and fibroblasts, resulting in:

- Epidermal hyperplasia
- Papillomatosis
- Stimulation of melanocytes → hyperpigmentation

In rare cases, paraneoplastic AN occurs due to tumor-secreted growth factors (e.g., TGF-α)[10]

■ DIAGNOSIS

Acanthosis nigricans is diagnosed clinically, based on typical morphology and distribution. Grading aids in

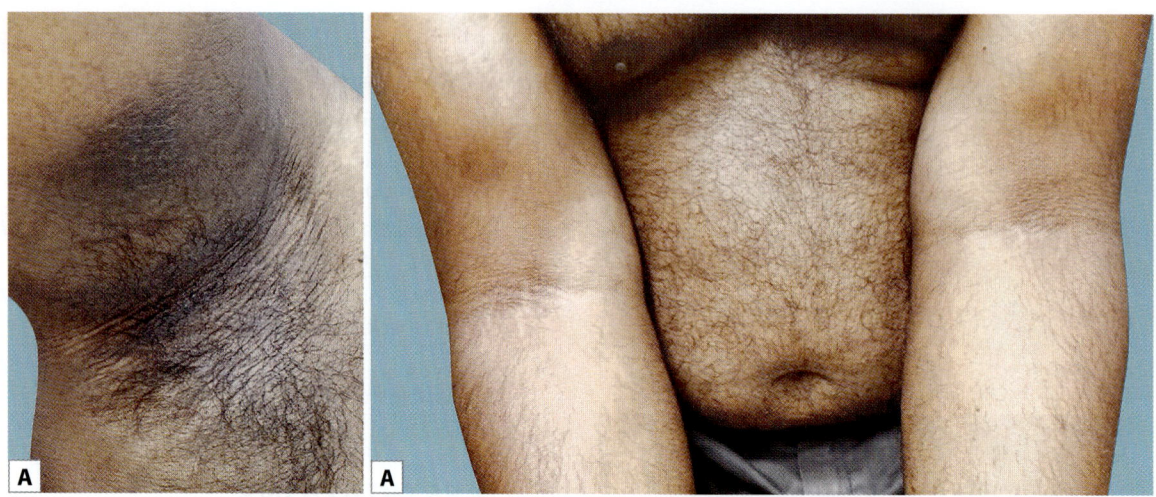

FIGS. 6A AND B: Acanthosis at other areas: Acanthosis nigricans at other areas. (A) Acanthosis nigricans (right axilla); **(B)** Acanthosis nigricans (antecubital fossae).

assessing severity and monitoring progress. Evaluating IR supports confirmation and guides therapy.[7,8]

■ DIFFERENTIAL DIAGNOSIS

The following conditions should be considered in the differential diagnosis. The diagnostic distinction depends on lesion pattern, associated systemic findings, and absence of usual metabolic risk factors.[9]
- Confluent and reticulated papillomatosis
- Hemochromatosis
- Addison disease
- Postinflammatory hyperpigmentation
- Epidermal nevus
- Drug-induced AN (e.g., nicotinic acid, oral contraceptives, and corticosteroids)

■ MANAGEMENT

Dermatologist
- *Topical keratolytics:* Urea, salicylic acid, and retinoic acid
- Topical retinoids (e.g., tretinoin) to reduce skin thickness
- While topical agents enhance appearance, systemic treatment targeting IR offers long-term improvement.[10,11]
- Chemical peels or laser therapy in cosmetically significant cases
- Counseling for aesthetic concerns and regular follow-up

Diabetologist/Physician
- *Weight reduction:* Fundamental to management
- *Addressing IR:* Metformin or pioglitazone
- Glycemic control through dietary changes, physical activity, and medications
- Ongoing screening for metabolic syndrome, PCOS, and NAFLD
- Malignancy screening when clinically indicated[8,12]

Clinical Pearls
- Acanthosis nigricans is a visible indicator of IR and should not be overlooked.[8,9]
- In children, AN may precede type 2 diabetes mellitus by several years.[12]
- Sudden, extensive AN in a nonobese adult warrants evaluation for malignancy.[10]
- The neck is the most commonly affected site—always examine axillae and knuckles as well.
- Grading correlates with insulin levels and BMI.[7]
- Topical therapy offers cosmetic benefits but does not address the underlying metabolic cause.
- Each case of AN is an opportunity to identify and address metabolic disturbances early.[11,12]

Case 3: Acanthosis Nigricans and Multiple Acrochordons (Skin Tags)

■ PRESENTATION

A 65-year-old woman with an 8-year history of type 2 diabetes mellitus presented with a 3–4-year progression of skin darkening and multiple skin tags. Her diabetes is well-controlled (HbA1c 5.13%), but she has elevated triglyceride and cholesterol levels.

- There is no evidence of diabetic retinopathy or nephropathy, and neurological examination is normal. The patient denies any symptoms such as itching, pain, weight loss, or fatigue.
- She has no history of hypertension, and her clinical profile is consistent with features of the metabolic syndrome (central obesity and dyslipidemia).
- Current medications include metformin 1,000 mg twice daily, atorvastatin 20 mg daily, and fenofibrate 160 mg daily, with no insulin or corticosteroid use.
- The skin changes have progressed gradually, with no new medications or rapid changes preceding their onset.

■ EXAMINATION

- Velvety and hyperpigmented plaques were observed on the posterior neck, axillae, and groin **(Fig. 7)**.
- Multiple small, soft, pedunculated papules (acrochordons) were present on the lateral aspects of the neck and upper back **(Fig. 8)**.
- The lesions were asymptomatic and had increased gradually in number and extent over the years.

■ INVESTIGATIONS

- Laboratory results confirmed well-controlled blood glucose (HbA1c 5.13%), along with dyslipidemia marked by elevated triglyceride and cholesterol levels.
- A skin biopsy was not performed, as clinical examination was deemed diagnostic.

■ DIAGNOSIS

The clinical presentation and examination were characteristic of AN and multiple acrochordons (skin tags), well-known cutaneous markers of IR and the metabolic syndrome. The patient's long-standing type 2 diabetes mellitus, dyslipidemia, and central obesity further supported the clinical suspicion. Other systemic causes were excluded by clinical assessment and laboratory evaluation.

Acanthosis nigricans and acrochordons are frequently observed in patients with diabetes, with studies reporting prevalence rates of approximately 16 and 19%, respectively. Their presence highlights the underlying metabolic dysfunction and IR.[13-17]

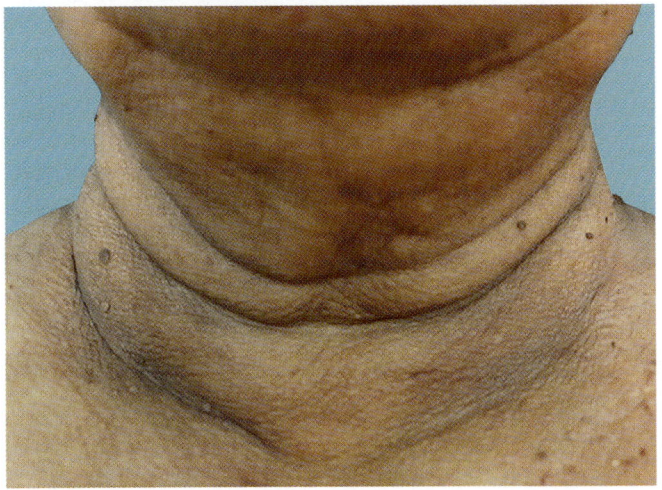

FIG. 7: Velvety, hyperpigmented plaques characteristic of acanthosis nigricans involving the neck.

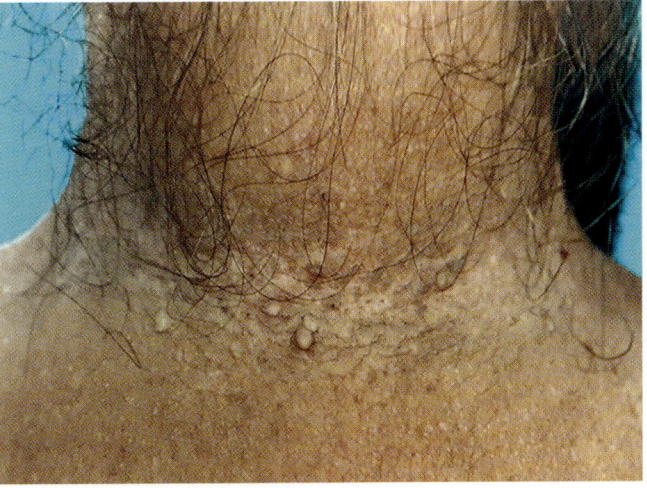

FIG. 8: Multiple soft, pedunculated papules (acrochordons) noted on the lateral neck and upper back.

DIFFERENTIAL DIAGNOSIS

Malignancy-associated Acanthosis Nigricans

Sudden onset of widespread AN, especially with mucosal involvement, may indicate underlying malignancy (commonly gastric cancer). The gradual progression and absence of systemic symptoms in this patient make this unlikely.[13]

Drug-induced Acanthosis Nigricans

Medications such as niacin and glucocorticoids can induce AN-like changes, but the patient has not used these drugs.[13]

Endocrine Disorders

Conditions such as Cushing syndrome or hypothyroidism may cause skin changes, but these typically present with additional systemic features and different skin morphology.[13]

Other Skin Conditions

- Confluent and reticulated papillomatosis presents as hyperpigmented papules but lacks the velvety texture of AN.[13]
- Seborrheic keratoses (Leser–Trélat sign) can mimic skin tags but are keratotic and not associated with diabetes.[13]
- Pedunculated nevi or fibroepithelial polyps may resemble skin tags but are usually fewer in number and not linked to metabolic syndrome.[13]

MANAGEMENT

Dermatological Care

- Educate that AN and skin tags are benign but signal metabolic risk.[13-16]
- Offer removal of bothersome skin tags via cryotherapy or snip excision.[13,15]
- Topical keratolytics or retinoids (e.g., tretinoin) may help to reduce AN thickness.[15]
- Advise friction-reducing strategies (loose clothing and good hygiene).[13]
- Cosmetic procedures (laser and chemical peels) may be considered for resistant plaques.[15,18]

Metabolic and Diabetic Management

- Continue current medications for diabetes and dyslipidemia.[13,17]
- Emphasize lifestyle changes—diet and exercise—to promote weight loss and improve insulin sensitivity, which can lead to regression of AN.[13,14,16,17]
- Regular cancer screening is recommended due to age and metabolic risk factors.[13]
- Maintain optimal glycemic control, as improved insulin sensitivity can reduce skin manifestations.[13,14,17]

PROGNOSIS

Acanthosis nigricans and acrochordons themselves are benign and do not pose a direct health risk. Their improvement is closely tied to metabolic control; weight loss and better insulin sensitivity often lead to gradual fading of AN, though some lesions may persist. Removed skin tags do not recur at the same site, but new ones can develop if IR continues. With well-controlled diabetes, the prognosis is favorable, and skin changes are likely to improve over time.[13,14,16,17]

> **Clinical Pearls**
>
> ▸ Velvety hyperpigmentation in body folds is a hallmark of IR.[13,14]
> ▸ Multiple skin tags clustered on the neck or axillae should prompt evaluation for diabetes and metabolic syndrome.[14,16,17]
> ▸ Both AN and skin tags are cutaneous markers of hyperinsulinemia; aggressive management of metabolic risk factors can improve these lesions.[13,14,16,17]
> ▸ Rapid and extensive AN (especially with mucosal involvement) necessitates evaluation for internal malignancy, but gradual onset with skin tags suggests a benign metabolic cause.[13]

REFERENCES

1. Radu AM, Carsote M, Dumitrascu MC, Sandru F. Acanthosis Nigricans: Pointer of Endocrine Entities. Diagnostics (Basel). 2022;12(10):2519.
2. Sarkar R, Bharati A, Mendiratta V. Facial acanthosis nigricans—a narrative review. Pigment Int. 2023;10(2):80-6.
3. Shah VH, Rambhia KD, Mukhi JI, Singh RP, Kaswan P. Clinico-investigative Study of Facial Acanthosis Nigricans. Indian Dermatol Online J. 2022;13(2):221-8.
4. Kurian B, Kurian SS, George J, Nair PA. Dermoscopic patterns in facial acanthosis nigricans. J Cosmet Dermatol. 2021;20(7):2245-9.

5. Elston D, Ferringer T, Ko C. Acanthosis Nigricans. In: Elston D, Ferringer T, Ko C (Eds). Dermatopathology, 3rd edition. Netherlands: Elsevier; 2019.
6. Agarwal P, Yadav D, Bansal S, Singh RP. Metformin and Acanthosis Nigricans in Insulin Resistance: A Review. J Clin Diagn Res. 2019;13(4):OE01-OE04.
7. Burke JP, Hale DE, Hazuda HP, Stern MP. A quantitative scale of acanthosis nigricans. Diabetes Care. 1999;22(10):1655-9.
8. Stuart CA, Gilkison CR, Smith MM, Bosma AM, Keenan BS, Nagamani M. Acanthosis nigricans as a risk factor for noninsulin dependent diabetes mellitus. Clin Pediatr (Phila). 1998;37(2):73-9.
9. Leung AKC, Lam JM, Barankin B, Leong KF, Hon KL. Acanthosis Nigricans: An Updated Review. Curr Pediatr Rev. 2022;19(1):68-82.
10. HermannsLê T, Scheen A, Piérard GE. Acanthosis nigricans associated with insulin resistance: Pathophysiology and management. Am J Clin Dermatol. 2004;5(3):199-203.
11. Gangwar A, Sharma V, Sharma R. Combinational treatment approaches for acanthosis nigricans: a review. Arch Dermatol Res. 2025;317(1):179.
12. Lopez-Alvarenga JC, Chittoor G, Paul SFD, Puppala S, Farook VS, Fowler SP, et al. Acanthosis nigricans as a composite marker of cardiometabolic risk and its complex association with obesity and insulin resistance in Mexican American children. PLoS One. 2020;15(10):e0240467.
13. Hughes EK, Brady MF, Rawla P. Acanthosis Nigricans. StatPearls [Internet]. 2023.
14. Singh SK, Agrawal N, Vishwakarma AK. Association of acanthosis nigricans and acrochordon with insulin resistance: a cross-sectional study. Indian J Dermatol. 2020;65(2):112-7.
15. Patel NU, Roach C, Alinia H, Huang WW, Feldman SR. Current treatment options for acanthosis nigricans. Clin Cosmet Investig Dermatol. 2018;11:407-13.
16. Tripathy T, Singh BSTP, Kar BR. Association of skin tags with metabolic syndrome: a case–control study. Indian Dermatol Online J. 2019;10(3):284-7.
17. Vâță D, Stanciu D-E, Temelie-Olinici D, et al. Cutaneous manifestations associated with diabetes mellitus: a retrospective study. Diseases. 2023;11(3):106.
18. Zayed AA, Hassan WS, Abdallah K. Trichloroacetic acid peel in acanthosis nigricans: a pilot study. J Dermatolog Treat. 2015;26(4):320-4.

CHAPTER 15

Lichen Planus in a Diabetic Male with Hypothyroidism

Nipul Vara, Vishwa Marvania

■ PRESENTATION

A 57-year-old male, working as an office clerk, presented with a long-standing history of type 2 diabetes mellitus (11 years) and hypothyroidism (7 years), managed with levothyroxine 75 μg daily. He complained of a persistent, intensely pruritic rash over both forearms and wrists, present for the past 6 months.

■ EXAMINATION

- Multiple violaceous, polygonal, flat-topped papules were observed on the flexural surfaces of both wrists and forearms **(Fig. 1)**.
- The lesions displayed fine, white, reticular streaks (Wickham striae) on the surface.

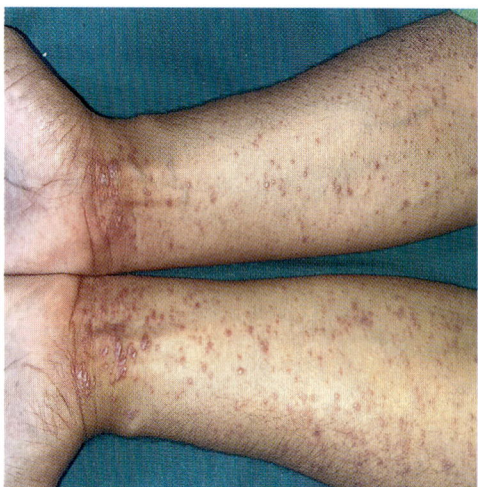

FIG. 1: Multiple violaceous, polygonal, flat-topped papules present on the flexural surfaces of the wrists and forearms, consistent with lichen planus. Several lesions have merged to form plaques, with subtle Wickham striae.

- No evidence of mucosal or nail involvement was observed.

■ INVESTIGATIONS

- Laboratory studies, including fasting glucose and thyroid function tests, confirmed long-standing, well-controlled type 2 diabetes and hypothyroidism.
- No evidence of other autoimmune or systemic disease was found.
- The clinical presentation was highly suggestive of lichen planus (LP), and no further diagnostic biopsy was deemed necessary due to its classic morphology.

■ DIAGNOSIS

Diagnosis is classic LP occurring in a patient with T2DM and hypothyroidism.

■ DIFFERENTIAL DIAGNOSES

- *Lichenoid drug eruption*: Typically symmetrical and less itchy; detailed drug history is crucial; Wickham striae are usually absent.
- *Psoriasis (inverse or guttate):* Characterized by silvery scales and positive Auspitz sign; lesions generally lack polygonal shape
- *Lichen simplex chronicus:* Presents as a single, thickened plaque from chronic scratching; lacks violaceous color
- *Lichen nitidus:* Manifests as tiny, shiny, discrete papules without striae
- *Prurigo nodularis:* Nodular lesions, not flat-topped; pruritus is severe.
- *Graft-versus-host disease (in post-transplant patients):* Requires relevant history; may show lichenoid features.

PATHOPHYSIOLOGY AND ASSOCIATION WITH DIABETES

Lichen planus is a persistent inflammatory disorder affecting the skin and mucous membranes.

PATHOGENESIS

The disease is driven by a T-cell-mediated autoimmune response targeting basal keratinocytes, likely due to altered skin antigens.

LINK WITH DIABETES

- Lichen planus is observed more frequently in individuals with metabolic dysfunctions such as diabetes and thyroid disorders.[1,2]
- The chronic inflammatory state in LP may share pathogenic pathways with insulin resistance and autoimmune thyroiditis.[3]
- Patients with diabetes demonstrate altered immune regulation, predisposing them to autoimmune skin diseases, including LP.[3]

MANAGEMENT

Dermatological Approach

- *Topical therapy:* High-potency corticosteroids (e.g., clobetasol propionate) applied twice daily for 4–6 weeks
- *Steroid-sparing agents:* Topical calcineurin inhibitors (e.g., tacrolimus 0.1%)
- *Symptomatic relief:* Antihistamines such as levocetirizine 5 mg once daily for pruritus
- *Systemic therapy (for extensive or resistant cases):*
  - Oral corticosteroids (prednisolone 0.5 mg/kg, tapered over 4–6 weeks)
  - Low-dose methotrexate or azathioprine for chronic or refractory LP
  - Narrowband ultraviolet B (NB-UVB) phototherapy or psoralen plus ultraviolet A (PUVA) for widespread disease

Diabetology/Physician Considerations

- *Glycemic control:* Emphasize maintaining HbA1c below 7% to reduce disease activity and enhance lesion resolution
- *Steroid-induced hyperglycemia:* Proactively monitor and manage during systemic therapy
- *Thyroid monitoring:* Regular thyroid-stimulating hormone (TSH) assessments and titration of thyroxine as necessary
- *Lifestyle interventions:* Encourage stress management, weight optimization, and avoidance of trauma or irritants at lesion sites

PROGNOSIS

- Lichen planus generally resolves spontaneously within 1–2 years.
- Postinflammatory hyperpigmentation may linger even after lesion resolution.
- Recurrences are not rare, particularly in patients with poorly controlled diabetes or hypothyroidism.
- Aggressive intervention is warranted for nail and mucosal LP due to the risk of scarring.[4,5]

> **Clinical Pearls**
>
> ▶ Wickham's striae (white, lacy lines) are diagnostic for LP.[4]
> ▶ lichen planus is commonly encountered in diabetics with coexistent thyroid dysfunction, reflecting underlying multisystem autoimmune dysregulation.[1,2]
> ▶ Screening for metabolic syndrome and additional autoimmune comorbidities is advisable in LP patients.[1]
> ▶ Oral and genital LP should be excluded, even in the absence of symptoms.[6,7]

REFERENCES

1. Gupta M, Mahajan VK, Mehta KS, Chauhan PS. Lichen Planus and Its Association with Metabolic Syndrome: A Case-Control Study in Indian Patients. Indian J Dermatol. 2018;63(6):490-5.
2. Singh S, Kanwar AJ, Narang T. Lichen Planus and Metabolic Syndrome: Is There a Link? J Dermatol Treat. 2017;28(7):633-6.
3. Teixeira F, Soares-Almeida LM, Filipe P. The Link Between Lichen Planus and Diabetes Mellitus. Acta Med Port. 2019;32(9):628-34.
4. Boyd AS, Neldner KH. Lichen Planus. J Am Acad Dermatol. 1991;25(4):593-619.
5. Samman PD. Lichen Planus. Br J Dermatol. 1961;73:401-16.
6. Kanwar AJ, De D. Lichen Planus in India: An Appraisal of 441 Cases. Int J Dermatol. 2010;49(1):54-60.
7. Lavanya N, Jayanthi P, Rao UK, Ranganathan K. Oral Lichen Planus: An Update on Pathogenesis and Treatment. J Oral Maxillofac Pathol. 2011;15(2):127-32.

CHAPTER 16

Xerosis and Pruritus in Diabetes (Dry Skin and Generalized Itch)

J Thadeus

■ PRESENTATION

A 62-year-old male with a history of type-2 diabetes mellitus for over two decades presented with persistent pruritic dryness of the skin over both lower limbs. Over the preceding year, he experienced recurrent episodes of swelling, discomfort, and ulceration in the same regions.

■ CLINICAL HISTORY

- No recent trauma, infection, or new medications
- Comorbidities included hypertension and established diabetic peripheral neuropathy.
- No prior dermatological interventions or evidence of overt vascular disease.

■ EXAMINATION

- Pronounced xerosis with fine scaling and shallow, transverse fissures on both lower legs (**Figs. 1 and 2**).

A magnified view highlighting the characteristic skin changes—xerosis with fine scaling and shallow transverse fissures—is shown in **Figure 3**.
- Reduced sweating and diminished hair growth were evident over the affected areas.
- The patient reported paresthesia and a sensation of coldness in both feet.
- No active ulceration or secondary infection was present at the time of evaluation.

■ DIAGNOSIS

The diagnosis is asteatotic dermatitis (xerotic eczema) associated with long-standing diabetes mellitus.[1,2]

■ DIFFERENTIAL DIAGNOSES

- *Gravitational (stasis) eczema:* Typically associated with venous insufficiency and hemosiderin deposition[3]

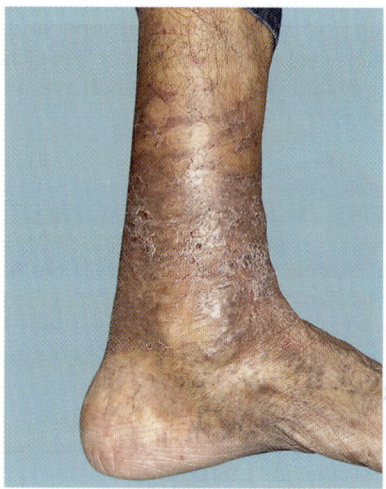

FIG. 1: Pronounced xerosis with fine scaling and shallow, transverse fissures observed on left lower legs.

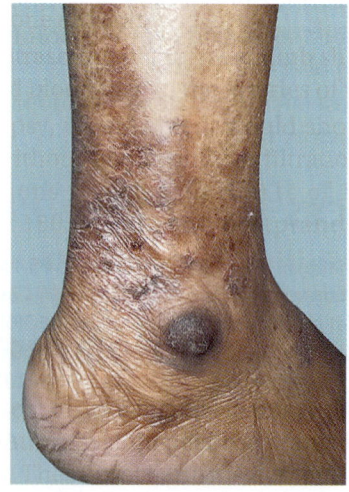

FIG. 2: Pronounced xerosis with fine scaling and shallow, transverse fissures observed on right lower legs.

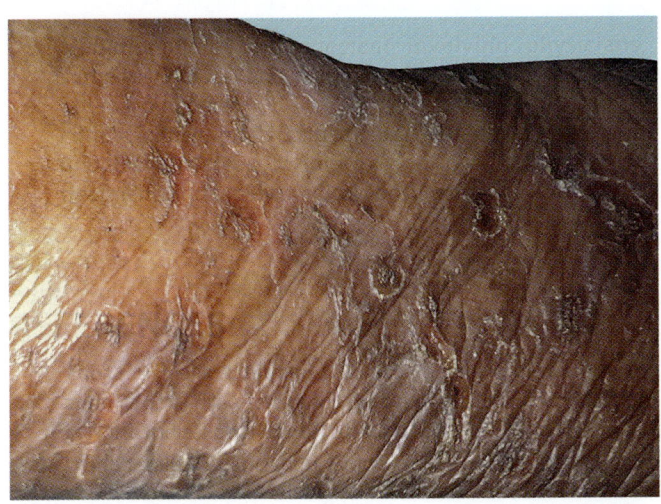

FIG. 3: Magnified view of the lesion demonstrating xerosis with fine scaling and shallow transverse fissures.

- *Diabetic dermopathy:* Characterized by atrophic brown macules without fissuring[4]
- *Ichthyosis vulgaris:* Presents as generalized xerosis from early life[3]
- *Contact dermatitis:* Suggested by a history of exposure to irritants or allergens[3]
- *Psoriasis vulgaris (hypopigmented):* Exhibits sharply demarcated plaques with silvery scales[3]
- *Lichen simplex chronicus:* Features localized lichenification from chronic scratching[3]

■ MANAGEMENT

Dermatological Approach

- *Topical therapy:*
  - Mometasone furoate 0.1% cream applied at night for short-term control of inflammation[3]
  - Liberal use of liquid paraffin emollient in the morning to restore skin moisture[5]
- *Oral medications:*
  - Second-generation antihistamines for relief of pruritus[3]
  - Aspirin 150 mg daily, utilized for its anti-inflammatory and vasodilatory benefits[6]
- *Supportive measures:*
  - Strict avoidance of irritants such as vegetable oils and hot water baths[3]
  - Advice on regular nail trimming and general skin protection
  - Long-term maintenance focused on emollient therapy alone[5]

Diabetology/Physician Management

- Emphasis on optimal glycemic control to mitigate peripheral microvascular complications[2]
- Screening for diabetic neuropathy and other microvascular sequelae:
  - Fundoscopic examination for diabetic retinopathy[4]
  - Urinary albumin-to-creatinine ratio (UACR) to assess nephropathy[4]
- Consideration of α-lipoic acid and methylcobalamin for neuropathic symptoms[4]
- Comprehensive foot care education, including footwear hygiene and prevention of fissure-related infections[7]
- Scheduled follow-up to monitor for secondary infection or recurrence of ulceration[7]

■ PROGNOSIS

Asteatotic dermatitis in individuals with diabetes can serve as a focus for secondary bacterial infections, potentially progressing to cellulitis or diabetic foot ulcers if not addressed promptly. Early institution of emollients and anti-inflammatory agents typically results in rapid symptom improvement and reduces the risk of complications. With diligent skin care and metabolic management, the long-term prognosis is generally favorable.[2,7]

> **Clinical Pearls**
>
> ▶ Asteatotic dermatitis manifests as dry, cracked, and scaly skin, frequently exacerbated by cold weather or excessive bathing.[1,8]
> ▶ Commonly affects the shins and extensor surfaces, especially in elderly or diabetic patients.[2]
> ▶ Peripheral neuropathy and diminished sweating in diabetes contribute to the severity of xerosis.[2]
> ▶ Early and consistent use of emollients is crucial to prevent fissuring and secondary infection.[5]
> ▶ Diabetic microangiopathy leads to impaired dermal perfusion and delayed barrier recovery.[7]

REFERENCES

1. Roupe G. Asteatotic eczema in the elderly. Acta Derm Venereol Suppl (Stockh). 1992;177:61-3.
2. Singh SK, Bansal A, Kaur C. Xerosis in diabetes: common, unrecognized, and under-treated. Indian J Dermatol. 2020;65(3):232-6.
3. Ingram JR. Chapter 39: Eczematous Disorders. In: Barker J, Bleiker TO, Chalmers R, Griffiths CEM, Creamer D (Eds). Rook's Textbook of Dermatology, 9th edition. London: Wiley Blackwell; 2016.
4. Narayanaswamy V, Rajendran S. Diabetic dermopathy and other common skin manifestations in diabetes. J Clin Diagn Res. 2015;9(4):WC01-3.
5. Lodén M. Role of topical emollients and moisturizers in the treatment of dry skin barrier disorders. Am J Clin Dermatol. 2003;4(11):771-88.
6. Stefaniak AA, Chlebicka I, Szepietowski JC. Itch in diabetes: a common underestimated problem. Postepy Dermatol Alergol. 2021;38(2):177-83.
7. Lima AL, Illing T, Schliemann S, Elsner P. Cutaneous manifestations of diabetes mellitus: a review. Am J Clin Dermatol. 2017;18(4):541–53.
8. Williams HC. Atopic dermatitis. N Engl J Med. 2005;352(22):2314-24.

CHAPTER 17

Subacute Eczema with Id Eruption in Metabolic Syndrome and Type 2 Diabetes

Rutul Gokalani, Viral Thakkar

■ PRESENTATION

A 62-year-old male with a 7-year history of type-2 diabetes mellitus (T2DM) presented with progressively worsening erythematous, scaly, and fissured plaques on both hands over several weeks, associated with nail dystrophy and suspected id reaction. He also has a medical history of hypertension and dyslipidemia.

Current medications include:
- *Diabetes*: Glimepiride 0.5 mg, dapagliflozin 10 mg, and metformin 1,000 mg
- *Hypertension*: Telmisartan 40 mg, azelnidipine
- *Dyslipidemia*: Rosuvastatin 20 mg

He denied systemic complaints such as fever or malaise. The clinical picture was highly suggestive of a subacute eczematous reaction associated with long-standing metabolic disturbances.

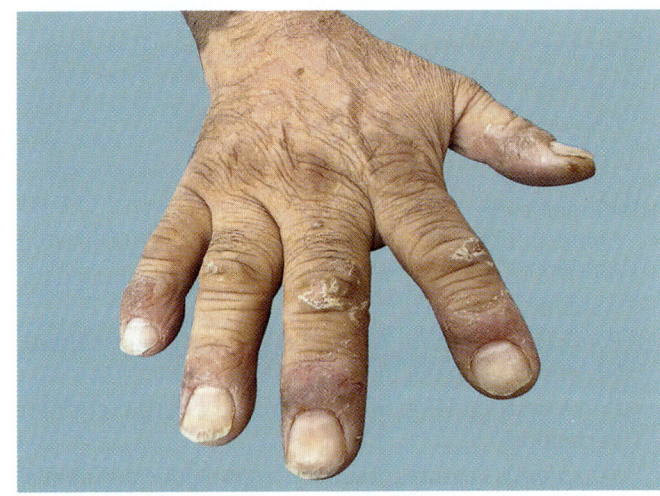

FIG. 1: Well-defined scaly and fissured plaques with mild erythema over the dorsum of the hand, suggestive of an id reaction.

■ EXAMINATION

- Well-defined scaly and fissured plaques with mild erythema were present on both hands, suggesting an id reaction **(Figs. 1 to 3)**.
- Nail examination revealed thickened, discolored, dystrophic nails, with no overt fungal elements.
- No other significant dermatological findings were observed.

■ INVESTIGATIONS

Laboratory parameters:
- *Glycated hemoglobin (HbA1c)*: 7.6%
- *Serum creatinine*: 1.1 mg/dL
- *Serum glutamic pyruvic transaminase (SGPT)*: 33 IU/L
- *Hemoglobin*: 12.8 g/dL

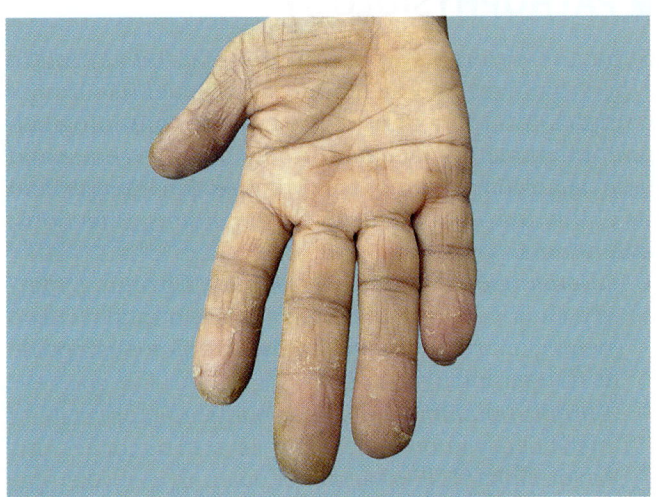

FIG. 2: Involvement of the palm showing erythematous, scaly plaques with superficial fissuring.

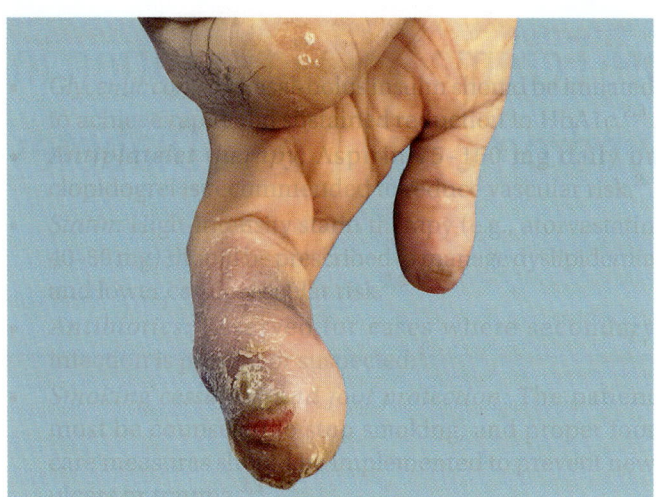

FIG. 3: Fingers displaying scaly plaques and fissures.

- *Low-density lipoprotein (LDL)*: 98 mg/dL
- *Triglyceride*: 187 mg/dL

Additional tests:
- *Complete blood count (CBC), erythrocyte sedimentation rate (ESR), and C-reactive protein (CRP)*: Evaluated for systemic inflammatory status
- *Potassium hydroxide (KOH) mount and fungal culture*: Negative, ruling out tinea
- *Patch testing*: Negative, excluding allergic contact dermatitis
- *Skin biopsy*: Features of subacute spongiotic dermatitis, consistent with eczema
- *Nail microscopy*: No fungal elements detected

PATHOPHYSIOLOGY

Subacute eczema and id eruptions in the setting of type-2 diabetes and metabolic syndrome arise from a complex interplay of microvascular, immunological, and inflammatory factors. Chronic hyperglycemia and associated comorbidities compromise skin integrity and its ability to respond effectively to irritants, infections, and trauma.[1-3]
- *Microangiopathy and neuropathy:* Chronic hyperglycemia leads to impaired skin perfusion and reduced neurogenic response, making the skin more susceptible to trauma and irritants.[1,3,4]
- *Chronic inflammation:* The proinflammatory state of metabolic syndrome, including elevated tumor necrosis factor-alpha (TNF-α) and interleukin-6 (IL-6), disrupts keratinocyte differentiation and compromises stratum corneum integrity.[1,4]
- *Immunosuppression:* Persistent hyperglycemia diminishes the phagocytic activity of neutrophils and macrophages, slowing the resolution of cutaneous inflammation.[5,6]
- *Xerosis from sodium-glucose co-transporter 2 (SGLT2) inhibitors*: Agents such as dapagliflozin may exacerbate skin dryness, intensifying eczematous changes.[5,6]

DIAGNOSIS

The patient is diagnosed with subacute eczema with an id eruption, influenced by a combination of factors associated with long-standing type 2 diabetes and metabolic syndrome.[1,2,4]

Chronic hyperglycemia and dyslipidemia have contributed to skin barrier dysfunction and heightened susceptibility to irritants, while the use of SGLT2 inhibitors may have exacerbated skin dryness, further aggravating the eczematous changes.[3,5,6]

DIFFERENTIAL DIAGNOSIS (RULED OUT)

- *Allergic contact dermatitis:* No relevant allergen exposure, and the patch test was negative.[1,2]
- *Psoriasis*: Absent silvery scale and Auspitz sign[1,2]
- *Tinea manuum:* Negative KOH examination[1,2]
- *Scabies/Norwegian scabies:* No burrows or mite visualization[1,2]
- *Lichen planus/palmoplantar keratoderma:* Not supported by clinical or histopathological findings[1,2]
- *Dyshidrotic eczema:* No vesiculation observed[1,2]

MANAGEMENT

Dermatological Management

- *Topical treatments:*
    - Mometasone (0.1%) cream for its anti-inflammatory action[1,2,4]
    - Tacrolimus (0.1%) ointment for immunomodulation and reducing chronic dermatitis[1,2,4]
    - Regular use of emollients to restore the skin barrier and combat xerosis[1-3]
- *Systemic treatments*:
    - Oral antihistamines to alleviate pruritus[1,2]
    - Careful monitoring of the patient's SGLT2 inhibitor therapy due to its potential role in exacerbating skin dryness[5,6]

Management by a Diabetologist

- Lifestyle counseling focusing on weight loss, balanced nutrition, and increased physical activity to reduce insulin resistance.[1,2,4]
- Continuation of statin therapy for dyslipidemia, addressing lipid-driven vascular and skin complications[1,2,4]
- Optimization of antidiabetic therapy with metformin and dapagliflozin, monitoring for skin changes and xerosis[5,6]
- Glycemic optimization with improved blood glucose control (HbA1c reduced from 7.6 to 6.7%), supporting skin recovery and reducing the risk of complications[1,2]
- Education about hand hygiene, avoidance of irritants, and early detection of skin changes to prevent recurrences

PROGNOSIS

With improved metabolic control and targeted topical therapy, the patient's lesions resolved within 2–3 weeks, with no recurrence observed at the 3-month follow-up.[1,2] The associated nail dystrophy persisted but remained stable and nonprogressive.[1,2]

Clinical Pearls

- Subacute eczema in diabetes can mimic other dermatoses, making biopsy and fungal studies essential for accurate diagnosis.[1-3]
- Dapagliflozin-induced xerosis can exacerbate eczema in predisposed patients, highlighting the need for close monitoring.[5,6]
- Long-standing diabetes, dyslipidemia, and hypertension create a proinflammatory microenvironment that impacts skin health.[1,2,4]
- A collaborative approach between dermatologists and diabetologists improves outcomes in mixed-etiology skin conditions.[1,2,4]
- Reduction in HbA1c is often paralleled by clinical improvement of dermatological lesions.[1-3]

REFERENCES

1. Kim BE, Leung DYM. Significance of skin barrier dysfunction in atopic dermatitis. Allergy Asthma Immunol Res. 2018;10(3):207-15.
2. Edwards E, Yosipovitch G. Skin manifestations of diabetes mellitus. In: Feingold KR, Anawalt B, Boyce A, et al. editors. Endotext [Internet]. South Dartmouth (MA): MDText.com, Inc.; 2025 Mar 21 [cited 2025 Sep 2]. Available from: https://www.ncbi.nlm.nih.gov/books/NBK481900/
3. McAleer MA, Irvine AD. The multifunctional role of filaggrin in allergic skin disease. J Allergy Clin Immunol. 2013;131(2):280-91.
4. Langan SM, Irvine AD, Weidinger S. Atopic dermatitis. Lancet. 2020;396(10247):345-60.
5. Zinman B, Wanner C, Lachin JM, Fitchett D, Bluhmki E, Hantel S, et al.; EMPA-REG OUTCOME Investigators. Empagliflozin, cardiovascular outcomes, and mortality in type 2 diabetes. N Engl J Med. 2015;373(22):2117-28.
6. George NM, Abou-Samra R, Alaaeddine N, Fares Y, El-Zein N. Cutaneous adverse reactions to SGLT2 inhibitors: rare but relevant. J Skin Stem Cell. 2024;11(2):e146625.

SECTION 4

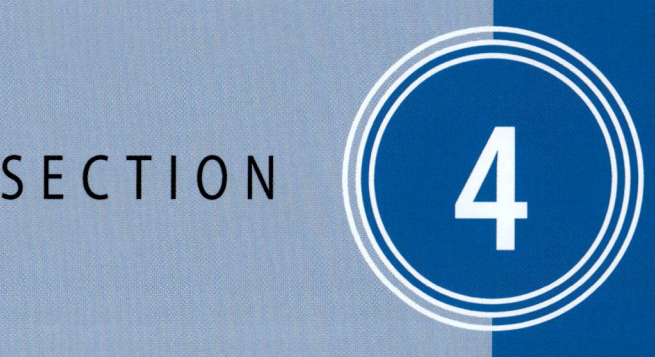

Cutaneous Infections in Diabetes

▶ Section Outline

Chapter 18: Fungal Infections
Arti Muley, Akashkumar N Singh, Yashika Doshi, Bela J Shah, Ashma Surani, Nipul Vara, Dhaivat Joshi, Armaan Mishra, Firdous Shaikh, Avina Jain

Chapter 19: Bacterial Skin Infections in Diabetes
Nipul Vara, Vishwa Marvania, Preya Parag Rana, Hiral Shah, J Thadeus, Aarathy Kannan, Akashkumar N Singh, Ankur Kothari, Suhas Gopal Erande, Anil Patki, Ruchi Shah, Yogesh Marfatia

Chapter 20: Viral Skin Infections in Diabetes: Hemorrhagic Herpes Zoster (Multidermatomal) in an Uncontrolled Diabetic Patient
Bela J Shah

CHAPTER 18

Fungal Infections

Arti Muley, Akashkumar N Singh, Yashika Doshi, Bela J Shah, Ashma Surani, Nipul Vara, Dhaivat Joshi, Armaan Mishra, Firdous Shaikh, Avina Jain

Part A: Dermatophyte Infection in Diabetes (Tinea and Onychomycosis)

Case 1: Onychomycosis in a Type 2 Diabetic Male

■ PRESENTATION

A 48-year-old male painter presented with progressive yellow discoloration and thickening of his fingernails over 6 months. He denied pain, trauma, or systemic symptoms but experienced increasing difficulty with fine motor tasks involving his dominant hand. He had an 8-year history of type 2 diabetes mellitus, managed with metformin 500 mg three times daily. There was no history of paronychia or other systemic illness.

■ EXAMINATION

On examination, the following findings were notable:
- Yellowish discoloration of fingernails
- Subungual hyperkeratosis
- Distal onycholysis with a proximal jagged margin
- Thickened nail plate exhibiting a ruinous pattern on onychoscopy
- Absence of periungual erythema or swelling **(Fig. 1)**
- His BMI was 31.2 kg/m^2.

■ LABORATORY INVESTIGATIONS

Laboratory investigations revealed:
- *Fasting blood glucose*: 120 mg/dL
- *Postprandial blood glucose*: 148 mg/dL
- *Glycated hemoglobin (HbA1c)*: 6.1%
- *Potassium hydroxide (KOH) mount*: Multiple, branching septate hyphae
- *Complete blood count, renal and liver function, thyroid profile, and lipid panel*: All within normal limits

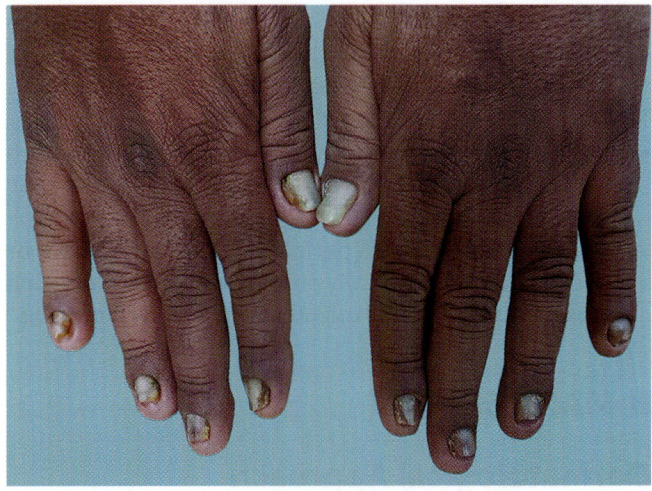

FIG. 1: Yellowish discoloration of the fingernails with subungual hyperkeratosis, distal onycholysis featuring a proximal jagged margin, and a thickened nail.

DIAGNOSIS

Total dystrophic onychomycosis in a patient with well-controlled type-2 diabetes mellitus.

DIFFERENTIAL DIAGNOSIS

- *Nail psoriasis*: Characterized by pitting, oil spots, and subungual debris
- *Candidal paronychia*: Involvement of the proximal nail fold, with erythema and tenderness
- *Eczematous nail changes*: Associated with periungual dermatitis
- *Nail lichen planus*: Longitudinal ridging and pterygium formation

PATHOPHYSIOLOGY

Onychomycosis is a global public health concern, with diabetic patients disproportionately affected.[1"] Onychomycosis is a fungal infection of the nail unit, predominantly caused by dermatophytes, but diabetic individuals are also susceptible to infections by yeasts and nondermatophyte molds.[2-5] Diabetes increases the risk of onychomycosis through several mechanisms:

- Chronic hyperglycemia impairs immune responses, reducing the body's ability to contain fungal proliferation.[3,5]
- Peripheral neuropathy and microvascular disease compromise local immunity and healing capacity.[3,5]
- Poor nail hygiene and increased colonization by *Candida* species and opportunistic molds further contribute to infection risk.[3-5]
- Diabetics are estimated to have a 2.5-fold higher risk of developing onychomycosis compared to nondiabetics, with older men being particularly vulnerable.[3-5]
- The severity of onychomycosis often correlates with the duration of diabetes and is influenced by glycemic control.[3,5]
- Diabetic patients with peripheral vascular disease or neuropathy are especially prone to complications such as secondary bacterial infections and delayed healing.[5]

MANAGEMENT

Dermatological Approach

Systemic Antifungal Therapy

- *Itraconazole pulse regimen*: 200 mg twice daily for 7 days each month, repeated for 3 months[2,6]
- *Alternative*: Terbinafine 250 mg daily for 6 weeks (fingernails)[2,6]

Topical Therapy

- Ciclopirox olamine 8% nail lacquer[2,6]
- For mild cases, amorolfine 5% lacquer applied twice weekly[2,6]

Nail Care Recommendations

- Regular trimming of nails
- Avoidance of occlusive gloves and exposure to solvents or irritants
- Consistent use of emollients for periungual skin

Diabetology/Physician Approach

- Reinforcement of glycemic monitoring and patient education on diabetes management[3,5]
- Continuation of metformin 500 mg TDS
- Screening for diabetic neuropathy and peripheral arterial disease[3,5]
- Counseling on foot and nail care to prevent complications[3,5]
- Recommendation for annual podiatric and dermatological evaluations[3,5]

PROGNOSIS

Onychomycosis in diabetic patients typically follows a chronic, relapsing course and may require extended treatment durations.[3,5,6] Relapse and treatment failure are common, and poor peripheral circulation or neuropathy further elevate the risk of complications such as cellulitis or, in severe cases, amputation.[3,5,6] Vigilant glycemic control and early intervention are crucial to minimize morbidity.[3,5,6]

> **Clinical Pearls**
> - The most prevalent pattern in diabetics is distal and lateral subungual onychomycosis (DLSO).[5,7]
> - Total dystrophic onychomycosis signifies advanced disease with destruction of the nail plate.[5,7]
> - In diabetic patients, KOH positivity should be supplemented with fungal culture or PCR, particularly in nonresponders.[6-8]
> - Diabetic men over 50 years are at the greatest risk.[3-5]
> - Prevention strategies should focus on optimal glycemic control, meticulous nail hygiene, and prompt treatment of early nail changes.[3,5,6]

REFERENCES

1. Tosti A, Hay RJ, Arenas R. Global epidemiology of fungal diseases: what do we know? J Eur Acad Dermatol Venereol. 2020;34 Suppl 1:4-9.
2. Elewski BE, Charif MA. Onychomycosis: current trends in diagnosis and treatment. Am Fam Physician. 1997;55(6):1971-6.
3. Gupta AK, Gupta G, Jain HC. Prevalence and epidemiology of onychomycosis in diabetic patients. Eur J Dermatol. 2000;10(1):19-22.
4. Romano C, Massai L, Asta F. Prevalence of dermatophytes and non-dermatophyte fungi in diabetic and non-diabetic patients. Mycoses. 2001;44(3-4):83-6.
5. Saunte DM, Holgersen JB, Haedersdal M. Onychomycosis in patients with diabetes mellitus. J Eur Acad Dermatol Venereol. 2006;20(7):775-80.
6. Kaur R, Kashyap B, Bhalla P. Onychomycosis: epidemiology, diagnosis and management. Indian J Med Microbiol. 2008;26(2):108-16.
7. Lipner SR, Scher RK. Onychomycosis: clinical overview and diagnosis. J Am Acad Dermatol. 2019;80(4):835-51.
8. Gupta AK, Simpson FC. Diagnosing onychomycosis. Clin Dermatol. 2013;31(5):540-6.

Case 2: Extensive Tinea Corporis in a Diabetic Patient

■ PRESENTATION

A 56-year-old woman presented with multiple itchy, ring-shaped skin lesions over her trunk and extremities for the past year. The patient reported intense pruritus, significantly affecting her daily life and sleep. She had a history of self-medication with ayurvedic formulations and over-the-counter topical steroid-antifungal combinations, used intermittently over the previous 6 months. Such unsupervised and inappropriate topical therapy is a recognized risk factor for chronic and atypical dermatophytosis in India.[1-3]

■ CLINICAL HISTORY

- Known case of type 2 diabetes mellitus for 7 years, on metformin 500 mg BD and vildagliptin 50 mg OD
- No other comorbidities
- No family members reported similar skin complaints

■ EXAMINATION FINDINGS

- Multiple annular plaques, varying in size from 5 × 7 to 10 × 12 cm, with scaly borders and central clearing, symmetrically distributed over the chest **(Fig. 1)**, abdomen **(Fig. 2)**, and lower back.
- No crusting, oozing, or secondary infection was noted.
- KOH mount from active lesions revealed septate hyphae and spores, confirming the diagnosis.[4,5]

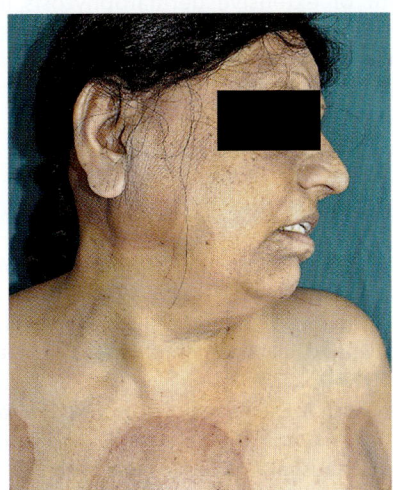

FIG. 1: Annular plaques with scaly borders and central clearing observed over the chest, varying in size and distribution.

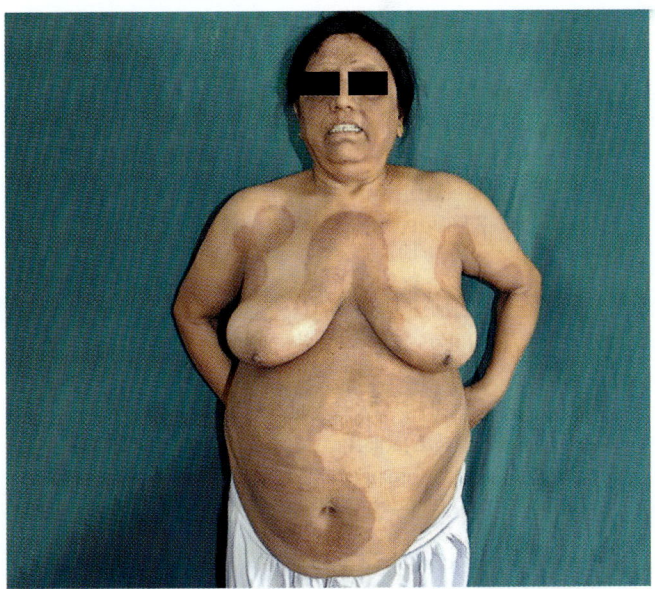

FIG. 2: Similar annular lesions noted on the abdomen, including areas under the breasts, displaying symmetrical involvement.

DIAGNOSIS

The diagnosis is extensive tinea corporis in a patient with type-2 diabetes mellitus and topical steroid misuse.[1,3]

DIFFERENTIAL DIAGNOSES

- *Erythema annulare centrifugum:* Annular plaques but typically without scale and central clearing[4]
- *Granuloma annulare:* Papular annular lesions, nonscaling, often asymptomatic[4]
- *Subacute cutaneous lupus erythematosus*: Photosensitive annular plaques with fine scaling and systemic association[4]

MANAGEMENT

Dermatology Management

- *Oral antifungal therapy:* Super-bioavailable itraconazole 130 mg once daily for 4 weeks, extended as needed based on response[6]
- *Topical antifungal therapy:* Sertaconazole nitrate 2% cream applied twice daily to affected areas[6]
- *Antihistamines*: Levocetirizine 5 mg at night for symptomatic itching relief[6]
- *Patient education*: Advised on strict avoidance of steroid-containing creams and emphasized adherence to the full antifungal course and hygiene practices (such as sun-drying clothes and avoiding synthetic garments)[1,3]

Physician/Diabetologist Management

- Continued metformin and vildagliptin[7]
- Glycemic control reinforced with dietary modifications and self-monitoring of blood glucose (SMBG)[7]
- Recommended routine HbA1c monitoring (initial level assumed >7.5% given delayed healing)[7]
- Advised periodic foot and skin checks to detect recurrence or superinfection early[7]
- *Lifestyle advice*: Regular bathing, weight loss (BMI evaluation not stated), and stress reduction[7]

Other systemic medications that can be used are oral fluconazole, oral terbinafine, and oral griseofulvin, especially in cases of resistance or intolerance to itraconazole.[3,6,8]

PROGNOSIS

With optimized antifungal treatment and improved glycemic control, the lesions resolved completely over 4 months, leaving behind residual hyperpigmentation. Diabetic patients with poor glycemic control or inappropriate steroid use are at increased risk for persistent or recurrent dermatophytosis, often requiring longer or combination therapy.[1,3,7]

Clinical Pearls

- Large, annular scaly plaques with central clearing are hallmarks of tinea corporis[4,5]
- Involves multiple body areas, including the trunk, limbs, and intertriginous regions.[1,5]
- Intense itching, aggravated by heat and sweating[1,5]
- Lesions may persist or worsen despite antifungal therapy, especially due to nonadherence and poorly controlled diabetes.[3,7]
- Common in individuals with diabetes, obesity, or immunocompromised status[1,7]
- Increased sweating due to hot/humid climate or tight clothing[1,5]
- Positive KOH test showing septate hyphae, confirmed by fungal culture[4,5]
- Steroid-modified tinea (tinea incognito) is increasingly common in India due to irrational fixed-dose combinations.[1-3]
- Recurrent or extensive dermatophytosis in diabetics requires systemic antifungal therapy and assessment of underlying metabolic derangements.[3,7]

REFERENCES

1. Verma SB, Panda S. The great Indian epidemic of superficial dermatophytosis: an appraisal. Indian J Dermatol. 2017;62(3):227-36.
2. Bishnoi A, Vinay K, Dogra S. Emergence of recalcitrant dermatophytosis in India. BMJ. 2018;361:k1614.
3. Narang T, Batta A, Kumaran MS. Antifungal resistance and topical steroid abuse: A dangerous alliance in India. Clin Dermatol Rev. 2020;4(1):1-6.
4. Hay RJ. Tinea corporis. In: Barker J, Bleiker TO, Chalmers R, Griffiths CEM, Creamer D (Eds). Rook's Textbook of Dermatology, 9th edition. London: Wiley-Blackwell; 2016.
5. Durdu M, Ilkit M. First steps in the dermatophyte world: Diagnosis and treatment. J Fungi. 2021;7(3):169.
6. Singal A, Khanna D. Superficial fungal infections: Clinical perspective and management. Indian J Dermatol Venereol Leprol. 2011;77(6):628-32.
7. Ghosh S, Ghosh A. Extensive tinea corporis: Clinical implications in diabetics. J Assoc Physicians India. 2020;68(7):45-8.
8. Pathania S, Kaushal A, Kaur S. Current trends in antifungal resistance among dermatophytes. J Infect Dev Ctries. 2022;16(4):561-7.

Case 3: Onychomycosis in a Diabetic Daily Wage Laborer

PRESENTATION

Mr RK, a 63-year-old male manual laborer working at construction sites, presented with progressive yellow discoloration and thickening of all fingernails for the past 2 years. He complained of increasing difficulty in trimming the nails, occasional pain during manual work, and social embarrassment due to the unsightly appearance. The nail changes initially began in the right thumb and gradually spread to involve all fingernails bilaterally. He reported nail brittleness, subungual debris, and discomfort while grasping tools. There was no history of recent trauma, systemic illness, or chemical exposure. His occupation involves frequent exposure to moisture and dust, and he seldom uses protective gloves, often working with wet hands.

He has a 13-year history of type 2 diabetes mellitus with poor glycemic control (HbA1c 9.1%). He is on irregular oral hypoglycemic therapy (metformin and glimepiride) and is not on insulin. There is no history of peripheral vascular disease or immunosuppressive disorders. He belongs to a low socioeconomic group, with poor hygiene practices and inadequate hand and foot protection.

EXAMINATION

- *Nails*: All fingernails were involved. The nails appeared thickened, dystrophic, and discolored (yellowish–brown). Subungual debris and distal onycholysis were noted. Surface changes included longitudinal ridging and irregular texture, consistent with onychomycosis **(Figs. 1 and 2)**.
- *Skin*: Mild xerosis (dryness) was observed over the hands and forearms, likely related to chronic moisture exposure.
- *Feet*: The feet were intact, with no signs of fungal involvement such as tinea pedis or intertrigo.
- *Neurological examination*: There was mild peripheral sensory loss detected on monofilament testing, suggesting early diabetic neuropathy.
- *Vitals*: Blood pressure and other vital signs were stable at presentation.

INVESTIGATIONS

Laboratory investigations revealed:
- *Glycemic profile*: Poor diabetes control was confirmed with an HbA1c of 9.1%. Fasting blood glucose was 176 mg/dL and postprandial blood sugar was 242 mg/dL.
- *Mycological testing*:
  - KOH mount of nail clippings demonstrated septate fungal hyphae.
  - Fungal culture identified *Trichophyton rubrum*, a common dermatophyte associated with onychomycosis.
- *Baseline safety profile*: Liver function tests (LFTs) were within normal limits, indicating suitability for systemic

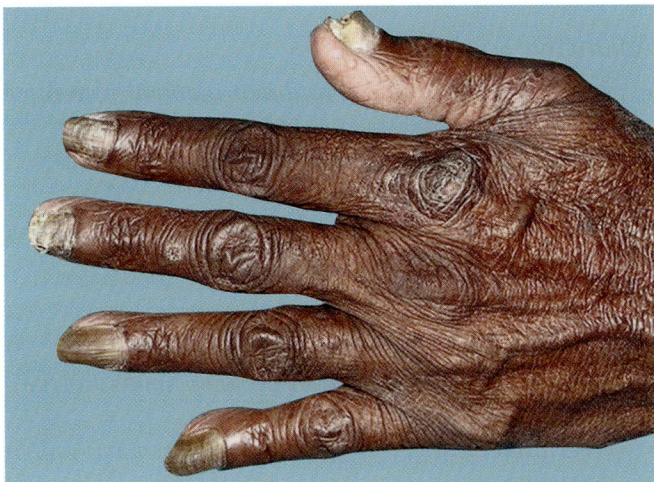

FIG. 1: All fingernails appear thickened, dystrophic, and yellowish–brown in color, with subungual debris, distal onycholysis, longitudinal ridging, and irregular surface texture.

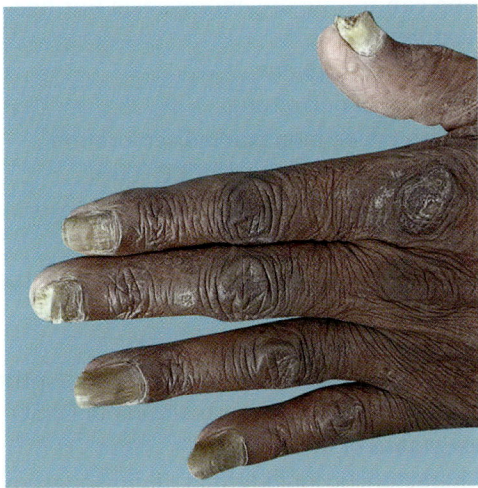

FIG. 2: A closer view of the same hand reveals pronounced nail dystrophy, subungual debris, distal onycholysis, and surface irregularities consistent with onychomycosis.

antifungal treatment. Complete blood count (CBC) and renal function tests (RFTs) were also normal.

PATHOPHYSIOLOGY AND ASSOCIATION WITH DIABETES

Onychomycosis is more prevalent and severe in individuals with diabetes due to multiple factors:
- *Peripheral neuropathy* leads to unnoticed trauma and altered nail growth.
- *Impaired immunity* at the skin/nail interface enhances fungal colonization.
- *Hyperglycemia* facilitates fungal proliferation through increased glucose in skin tissue and reduced neutrophil function.[1,2]
- Studies show prevalence of onychomycosis in diabetics ranges from 22 to 35%, with *T. rubrum* being the predominant pathogen.[3,4]

DIAGNOSIS

- Distal and lateral subungual onychomycosis (DLSO)
- The patient is diagnosed with DLSO, a common fungal nail infection, and has poorly controlled type 2 diabetes mellitus, which may contribute to increased susceptibility and delayed healing.

DIFFERENTIAL DIAGNOSIS

The classification and diagnostic criteria for onychomycosis have been well established in standard mycology texts.[5] When evaluating a case of suspected DLSO, several differential diagnoses must be considered. Each of these conditions can mimic onychomycosis but has distinct clinical features:
- *Psoriatic nail dystrophy:*
  - Presence of nail pitting
  - Oil drop or salmon patch discoloration
  - Negative fungal culture or KOH test
  - Often associated with skin lesions of psoriasis
- *Traumatic nail dystrophy:*
  - History of repetitive or acute localized trauma to the nail
  - No evidence of fungal infection
  - Nail plate may show discoloration, splitting, or subungual hyperkeratosis similar to DLSO
- *Lichen planus of the nails:*
  - Characteristic longitudinal ridging or grooving
  - Possible dorsal pterygium formation (adhesion of proximal nail fold to the nail bed)
  - May be accompanied by violaceous papules on the skin or mucosa
- *Chronic paronychia:*
  - Involves inflammation and swelling of the proximal nail fold
  - Associated with frequent exposure to water or irritants
  - Can cause nail dystrophy, but usually has signs of persistent periungual inflammation
- *Yellow nail syndrome:*
  - Nails are uniformly yellow, thickened, and may lack a cuticle
  - Often associated with systemic conditions such as lymphedema and chronic respiratory disorders
  - Typically involves multiple nails without evidence of fungal infection

MANAGEMENT

Dermatological Management

Management of onychomycosis involves a combination of systemic and topical antifungal strategies, along with preventive care to reduce recurrence.

Systemic Antifungal Therapy

- *Oral terbinafine* 250 mg once daily for 6 weeks (for fingernail involvement)
- *Monitoring:* Liver function tests should be performed prior to initiation and repeated every 4 weeks during treatment

Adjunctive Local Therapy

- Regular *nail trimming and debridement* to reduce fungal load
- Application of *topical antifungal lacquers*, such as:
  - *Amorolfine 5%* or
  - *Ciclopirox 8%*—applied once or twice weekly as per product instructions

Patient Education and Preventive Measures

- Avoid prolonged water exposure; keep hands and nails dry
- Wear protective *gloves while handling cement, soil, or detergents*

- Maintain *nail hygiene*: Keep nails short, clean, and filed
- Do not share personal items such as nail cutters or gloves
- Manage comorbid conditions such as *diabetes and immunosuppression*

Physician/Diabetologist Management

A multidisciplinary approach is essential to optimize glycemic control and minimize the risk of infection-related complications in diabetic patients.

Optimized Glycemic Control

Transitioned to a regimen of *basal insulin* combined with *metformin* for improved and sustained glycemic management

Patient Counseling and Education

- Emphasis on *daily foot and hand care*, including inspection for cuts, blisters, or discoloration
- Strong recommendation to *avoid walking barefoot*, especially outdoors or on wet surfaces
- Education on recognizing *early signs of infection*, such as:
  - Redness, warmth, or swelling around nails or skin folds
  - Unusual pain, discharge, or foul odor
  - Changes in skin color or texture

Preventive Guidance

- Encourage regular follow-up with a diabetologist and a podiatrist
- Reinforce adherence to glycemic targets and medication compliance
- Promote general hygiene and early reporting of minor injuries

PROGNOSIS

- Good prognosis if treated early with systemic antifungals and lifestyle correction
- Recurrence is common without glycemic control and personal hygiene reinforcement
- Nail appearance may take 6–9 months to improve, especially in diabetics.

> **Clinical Pearls**
> - Always suspect *onychomycosis in chronic nail dystrophy* in diabetics
> - *Combined systemic + topical therapy* offers better outcomes
> - Check for *tinea pedis*, which often co-exists (the "two feet-one hand" syndrome)
> - Recurrence is *higher in diabetics*, stressing the need for *foot and nail surveillance*
> - *KOH microscopy + fungal culture* remains the gold standard for diagnosis

REFERENCES

1. Gupta AK, Konnikov N, MacDonald P, Rich P, Rodger NW, Edmonds MW, et al. Epidemiology and prevalence of onychomycosis in diabetic patients: A systematic review. J Eur Acad Dermatol Venereol. 2017;31(10):1532-41.
2. Navarro-Pérez D, Tardáguila-García A, García-Oreja S, Álvaro-Afonso FJ, López-Moral M, Lázaro-Martínez JL. Treatment of onychomycosis and the drug–drug interactions in patients with diabetes mellitus and diabetic foot syndrome: A systematic review. Infect Dis Rep. 2025;17(1):4.
3. Rajagopalan M, Inamadar A, Mittal A, Miskeen AK, Srinivas CR, Sardana K, et al. Expert consensus on the management of dermatophytosis in India (ECTODERM India). BMC Dermatol. 2018;18(1):6.
4. Hay RJ, Baran R. Onychomycosis: A proposed revision of the clinical classification. J Am Acad Dermatol. 2011;65(6):1219-27.
5. Chander J. Textbook of Medical Mycology, 4th edition. New Delhi: Jaypee Brothers Medical Publisher; 2018.

Part B: Candidiasis and Other Yeast Infections in Diabetes

Case 1: Candidal Intertrigo in a Diabetic Patient

■ PRESENTATION

A 45-year-old woman, a homemaker, with a 6-year history of type 2 diabetes mellitus, presented with complaints of pruritus and mild burning over the groin for the past 20 days. She reported multiple recurrences of similar lesions over the preceding 6 months. Her diabetes was managed with metformin 500 mg once daily and glimepiride 1 mg once daily. She denied any other systemic symptoms.

■ EXAMINATION

- Physical examination revealed confluent erythematous plaques with peripheral satellite pustules in the groin folds **(Figs. 1 and 2)**.
- Wood's lamp examination was negative for fluorescence.
- The patient was obese, with a body mass index (BMI) of 32 kg/m².

■ INVESTIGATIONS

- Potassium hydroxide (KOH) mount of the skin scraping demonstrated pseudohyphae, consistent with *Candida albicans*.
- *Fasting blood glucose*: 288 mg/dL
- *Postprandial glucose*: 308 mg/dL
- *HbA1c*: 8.1%
- *Total cholesterol*: 302 mg/dL
- *Triglycerides*: 252 mg/dL
- *Liver, renal, and thyroid profiles*: Normal
- *Viral markers*: Negative

■ DIAGNOSIS

The diagnosis is Candidal intertrigo in the setting of poorly controlled type-2 diabetes mellitus and dyslipidemia.[1]

■ DIFFERENTIAL DIAGNOSES

- Irritant or frictional intertrigo
- Tinea cruris
- Erythrasma
- Inverse psoriasis
- Seborrheic dermatitis
- Hailey–Hailey disease
- Darier's disease
- Systemic contact dermatitis[1,4]

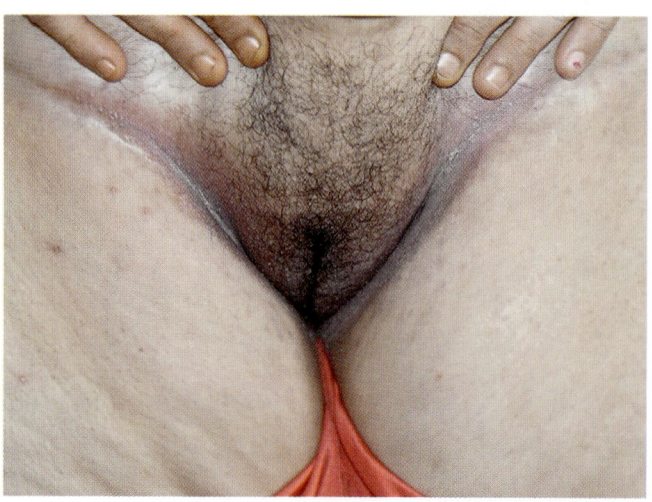

FIG. 1: Physical examination revealed confluent erythematous plaques with peripheral satellite pustules in the groin folds.

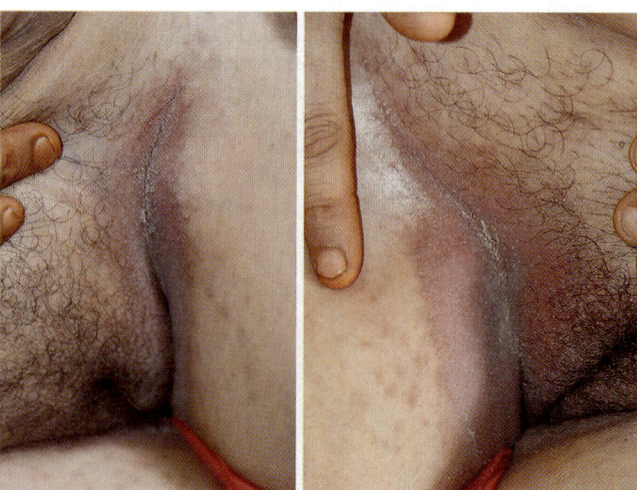

FIG. 2: Closer view of the left and right groin fold showing erythematous plaque with distinct satellite pustules along the periphery.

MANAGEMENT

Dermatology Management

- *Topical antifungal therapy*: Clotrimazole 1% cream applied twice daily for 15 days is recommended as first-line treatment for candidal intertrigo.[2,3]
- *Systemic antifungal therapy*: For extensive, severe, or recurrent cases, fluconazole 100 mg orally once daily for 10 days may be used. In resistant cases, itraconazole 200 mg/day or fluconazole 50–100 mg/day for 2–6 weeks can be considered.[2,3]
- *Adjunctive measures*: Patients should be advised to keep the affected skin folds dry, wear loose and breathable clothing, and regularly clean and pat-dry the area. In cases of persistent moisture, astringent solutions such as Burow's solution or zinc oxide ointment may be helpful.[2-6]
- *Alternative topical agents*: Nystatin or ketoconazole creams can be alternated in resistant cases. Castellani's paint or vinegar-water solutions may be used for acute lesions, especially in cases involving interdigital spaces.[2,7]
- *Combination therapy*: In cases with significant inflammation or pruritus, topical antifungal-corticosteroid combinations (e.g., hydrocortisone) may be added for short-term use.[2]

Diabetology/Physician Management

- *Glycemic and lipid control*: Referral to a diabetologist is essential for optimizing metabolic parameters. The antidiabetic regimen was intensified to metformin 500 mg twice daily and glimepiride 1 mg once daily, and atorvastatin 40 mg at bedtime was initiated for dyslipidemia.[1]
- *Monitoring*: Regular monitoring of fasting and postprandial blood glucose every 2 weeks, and reassessment of HbA1c and lipid profile after 3 months, is advised.[1]
- *Lifestyle interventions*: A calorie-restricted diabetic diet, weight reduction, and daily physical activity are crucial for long-term control and prevention of recurrences.[1,8]

PROGNOSIS

Candidal intertrigo generally responds well to appropriate topical and/or systemic antifungal therapy in immunocompetent individuals. However, in patients with uncontrolled diabetes or obesity, the disease tends to be more severe, recurrent, and may require prolonged systemic therapy. Early recognition and correction of underlying risk factors are vital for preventing recurrence.[2,8]

> **Clinical Pearls**
>
> ▶ Candidal intertrigo typically affects large intertriginous areas such as the groin, inframammary, axillary, and gluteal folds.[2,4]
> ▶ The hallmark features include pruritic, erythematous, and macerated patches with characteristic satellite vesicopustules. These pustules rupture easily, forming collarette scaling.[2]
> ▶ Diabetes mellitus and obesity are the most significant predisposing factors.[2,8]
> ▶ Diagnosis is supported by lack of fluorescence on Wood's lamp and demonstration of pseudohyphae on KOH mount.[1,4]
> ▶ Prevention of recurrence requires a multifaceted approach, including topical therapy, metabolic control, and lifestyle modification.[2,8]

REFERENCES

1. Sobel JD. Vulvovaginal candidosis. Lancet. 2007;369(9577):1961-71.
2. Metin A, Dilek N, Bilgili SG. Recurrent candidal intertrigo: challenges and solutions. Clin Cosmet Investig Dermatol. 2018;11:175-85.
3. Scheinfeld N. Candidal intertrigo. Drugs of Today. 2005;41(10):661-67.
4. Weitzman I, Summerbell RC. The dermatophytes. Clin Microbiol Rev. 1995;8(2):240-59.
5. Gupta AK, Cooper EA, Feldman SR. Candidiasis. In: Kang S, Amagai M, Bruckner AL, Enk AH, Margolis DJ, McMichael AJ, Orringer JS (Eds). Fitzpatrick's Dermatology, 9th edition. New York: McGraw Hill; 2019.
6. Korting HC, Braun-Falco O. The effect of the environment on the skin and its microflora. Zentralbl Hyg Umweltmed. 1995;197(5):423-34.
7. Sundaram SV, Srinivas CR, Thirumurthy M. Candidal intertrigo: Treatment with filter paper soaked in Castellani's paint. Indian J Dermatol Venereol Leprol. 2006;72:386-7.
8. Medscape. Practice Essentials, Pathophysiology, Etiology of Intertrigo. New York: Medscape; 2024.

Case 2: Candidal Balanoposthitis with Phimosis in an Undiagnosed Diabetic

■ PRESENTATION

A 45-year-old married man, working as a school teacher, presented with a 3-day history of difficulty retracting the foreskin (phimosis). He denied any prior episodes, genital discharge, or ulcers. His wife was asymptomatic.

■ EXAMINATION

- The inner surface of the prepuce was erythematous with fissuring, and the foreskin was tight and non-retractable **(Fig. 1)**.
- No inguinal lymphadenopathy or mucosal involvement elsewhere was noted.

■ INVESTIGATIONS

- Complete blood count, liver and renal profiles, fasting lipid panel, thyroid function, rapid plasma reagin (RPR), and viral markers were within normal limits.
- Random blood glucose was 250 mg/dL, and urine analysis showed glycosuria without ketonuria.
- KOH mount of preputial discharge revealed budding yeast and pseudohyphae.
- Culture on Sabouraud dextrose agar confirmed *Candida albicans*.

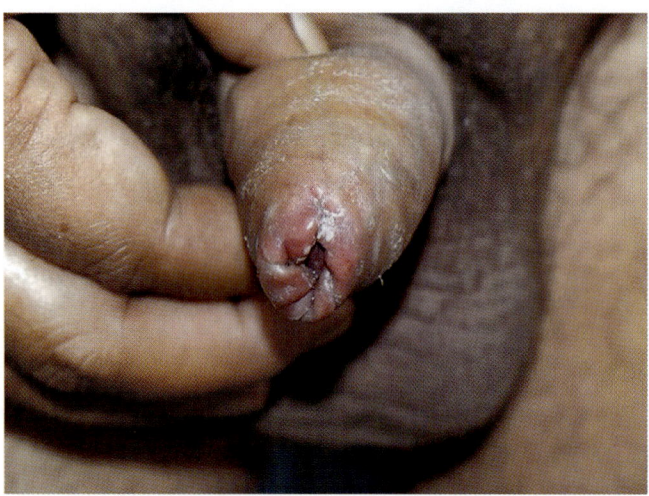

FIG. 1: Erythema and fissuring observed on the inner surface of the prepuce, with a tight, nonretractable foreskin suggestive of balanoposthitis with phimosis.

■ DIAGNOSIS

The diagnosis is Candidal balanoposthitis with phimosis in a previously undiagnosed diabetic male.[1,2]

■ DIFFERENTIAL DIAGNOSES

- *Sexually transmitted infections (STIs)*: Herpes genitalis and chancroid may present with painful ulcers or vesicles.[3]
- *Poor genital hygiene:* Particularly relevant in uncircumcised men, leading to smegma accumulation and secondary inflammation[4]
- *Lichen sclerosus (balanitis xerotica obliterans):* Characterized by atrophic white plaques and fibrosis.
- *Psoriasis or eczema of the glans:* Considered in cases with chronic, noninfectious plaques or fissures.
- *Zoon's balanitis:* Presents as persistent, reddish-orange moist patches on the glans, typically in middle-aged uncircumcised men[2,4]

■ MANAGEMENT

Dermatology/Urology Management

- *Systemic antifungal therapy:* Fluconazole 100 mg orally once daily for 10 days
- *Topical antifungal:* Application of 2% miconazole cream twice daily to the glans and inner foreskin
- *Hygiene measures:* Advise gentle cleansing with lukewarm water and avoidance of irritants. Instruction on proper foreskin hygiene after recovery is essential.
- *Assessment for circumcision:* Consider surgical intervention only if phimosis persists after inflammation resolves.[5]

Diabetology/Physician Management

- The patient was newly diagnosed with diabetes mellitus and started on metformin 500 mg twice daily, along with dietary modifications.
- Counseling focused on the importance of glycemic control to prevent the recurrence of infections.
- Regular follow-up was planned, including monitoring fasting blood glucose, HbA1c, and urine microalbumin over the next 3 months.

- Education was provided regarding foot care, sexual hygiene, and awareness of infection risks.[1,2]

PROGNOSIS

The patient experienced marked improvement within 5 days of initiating therapy, with complete resolution of both inflammation and phimosis by the end of 1 week. With diligent glycemic control and maintenance of local hygiene, the prognosis is excellent, and surgical intervention can often be avoided.[1,2]

> **Clinical Pearls**
>
> - Balanoposthitis and phimosis may be initial clinical indicators of undiagnosed diabetes, especially in middle-aged uncircumcised men.[1,2]
> - *Candida albicans* is the predominant pathogen in diabetic patients, attributed to glycosuria and impaired local immunity.[1]
> - Preputial fissures and vertical splitting are linked to the accumulation of advanced glycation end-products (AGEs) in chronically hyperglycemic skin. Repeated trauma from intercourse or urination can exacerbate these fissures, leading to reversible phimosis.[2]
> - Early recognition and appropriate management can prevent unnecessary surgical procedures such as circumcision.[4-6]

REFERENCES

1. Achkar JM, Fries BC. Candida infections of the genitourinary tract. Clin Microbiol Rev. 2010;23(2):253-73.
2. Donders GG. Balanitis and balanoposthitis: a neglected problem in men. Expert Opin Pharmacother. 2010;11(4):629-35.
3. Workowski KA, Bachmann LH, Chan PA, Johnston CM, Muzny CA, Park I, et al. Sexually Transmitted Infections Treatment Guidelines, 2021. MMWR Recomm Rep. 2021;70(4):1-187.
4. Edwards S. Balanitis and balanoposthitis: A review. Genitourin Med. 1996;72(3):155-59.
5. Lee YJ, Park SC. Foreskin problems in children and adults. Korean J Urol. 2012;53(7):481-6.
6. Vasudevan B, Verma R, Suri J. Balanitis and balanoposthitis: A clinicomycological study. Indian J Sex Transm Dis AIDS. 2010;31(2):91-4.

Case 3 — Candidal Vulvovaginitis in Type 2 Diabetes Mellitus

PRESENTATION

A 38-year-old woman, homemaker, with a 4-year history of type-2 diabetes mellitus, presented with complaints of vaginal discharge and pruritus persisting for 15–20 days. She reported experiencing recurrent episodes of similar symptoms over the preceding year. There was no history of systemic symptoms or urinary tract infections. Her antidiabetic regimen included metformin 500 mg twice daily for the past 6 years. Her BMI was 28.9 kg/m².

EXAMINATION

- On per speculum examination, there was thick, white, curdy vaginal discharge and mild vulvar edema, without any foul odor, ulcers, or trauma **(Fig. 1)**.
- Microscopic evaluation of the discharge using 10% KOH preparation revealed pseudohyphae, indicating *Candida albicans* infection.
- Wet mount and Gram stain showed no significant findings.

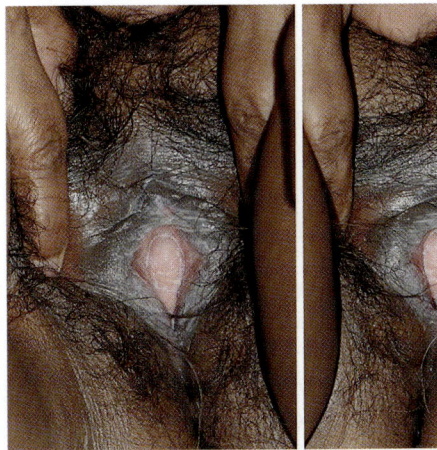

FIG. 1: Examination reveals thick, white, curdy vaginal discharge with mild vulvar edema; no foul odor, ulcers, or signs of trauma observed.

INVESTIGATIONS

- Laboratory investigations revealed fasting blood sugar of 234 mg/dL, postprandial blood sugar of 298 mg/dL,

- HbA1c of 7.8%, serum cholesterol of 290 mg/dL, and serum triglycerides of 252 mg/dL.
- Viral markers were negative, and other hematological, hepatic, renal, and thyroid parameters were within normal ranges.

PATHOPHYSIOLOGY AND RISK FACTORS

Diabetes mellitus predisposes to vulvovaginal candidiasis (VVC) through multiple mechanisms, including hyperglycemia-induced impairment of neutrophil function, increased glucose availability in vaginal secretions, and enhanced adhesion of Candida to vaginal epithelial cells.[1-3] Poor glycemic control is directly correlated with increased frequency and severity of VVC episodes.[1-3] Sodium–glucose transport protein 2 (SGLT2) inhibitors, by increasing urinary glucose excretion, further elevate the risk of genital mycotic infections.[1]

EPIDEMIOLOGICAL INSIGHTS

Studies indicate that women with type 2 diabetes are at significantly higher risk for both symptomatic and recurrent VVC, with *C. albicans* being the most common isolate, though nonalbicans species are more prevalent in this population.[2,3] The incidence of VVC may also serve as an early indicator for undiagnosed diabetes, especially in women over 55 years of age.[4,5]

DIAGNOSIS

The diagnosis is recurrent Candidal vulvovaginitis in a patient with uncontrolled type-2 diabetes mellitus and dyslipidemia.[2,6]

DIFFERENTIAL DIAGNOSES

- *Bacterial vaginosis:* Characterized by fishy odor, thin homogeneous discharge, and presence of clue cells on microscopy[2]
- *Trichomoniasis:* Presents with frothy greenish discharge and motile trichomonads on wet mount[2]
- *Atrophic vaginitis:* Typically seen in postmenopausal women, with dry, thin vaginal mucosa and dyspareunia[2]
- *Irritant or allergic contact vaginitis*: History of exposure to irritants, with erythema but usually no discharge[2]
- *Inflammatory vaginitis*: Usually idiopathic, associated with elevated vaginal pH and increased leukocytes[2]

MANAGEMENT

Dermatology/Gynecology Management

- *Oral antifungal*: Fluconazole 100 mg daily for 14 days[1,6]
- *Topical therapy*: 1% Clotrimazole cream applied twice daily to the vulvovaginal area for 14 days[6,7]
- Emphasized genital hygiene, avoidance of irritants, and use of breathable undergarments[7]
- For recurrent vulvovaginal candidiasis (VVC) (>4 episodes/year), maintenance therapy with weekly fluconazole for 6 months is advised.[7,8]
- Adjunctive use of probiotics to support vaginal microbiota may be considered.[1]

Diabetology/Physician Management

- The patient was referred for metabolic optimization. Her diabetes regimen was intensified by adding glimepiride 1 mg once daily to ongoing metformin.[6]
- Atorvastatin 40 mg at bedtime was initiated for dyslipidemia.[6]
- SGLT2 inhibitors such as dapagliflozin were avoided due to their association with increased risk of genital mycotic infections.[1]
- Lifestyle advice included a calorie-restricted diabetic diet, weight management, and stress reduction.
- Regular follow-up with quarterly HbA1c, lipid profile, and infection surveillance was recommended.[1]

PROGNOSIS

Uncomplicated VVC generally has an excellent prognosis with appropriate therapy. However, in diabetic patients, recurrent and complicated VVC is common due to impaired immunity and glycosuria, necessitating prolonged antifungal regimens and strict glycemic control. With optimal management, long-term symptom resolution and prevention of recurrences are achievable.[1,6]

> **Clinical Pearls**
>
> ▶ Candidal Vulvovaginitis typically presents with thick, curdy white vaginal discharge, vulvar pruritus, and mild erythema or edema.[7]
> ▶ *Candida albicans* is the predominant pathogen, but nonalbicans species such as *C. glabrata* and *C. krusei* are increasingly observed in diabetic women and may require prolonged or alternative antifungal regimens due to reduced susceptibility to azoles.[1,2,8]

- Recurrent infections (>4 per year) are more likely in women with poor glycemic control, obesity, or recent use of broad-spectrum antibiotics.[7,8]
- Extended antifungal therapy and suppression protocols are often necessary in diabetic women.[8] In cases of recurrent or atypical presentation, vaginal culture and antifungal sensitivity testing are beneficial.[8]
- Fluconazole remains the first-line therapy for VVC, with topical azoles as effective alternatives.[1,7]
- In cases of recurrent or complicated VVC, extended or maintenance regimens are required, and nonalbicans Candida infections may necessitate alternative antifungals due to variable azole susceptibility.[1,8]
- Patient education and adherence to therapy are crucial for successful management.[8]

REFERENCES

1. Marchaim D, Lemanek L, Bheemreddy S, Kaye KS, Sobel JD. Fluconazole-resistant *Candida albicans* vulvovaginitis. Obstet Gynecol. 2012;120(6):1407-14.
2. Spence D, Melville C. Vaginal discharge. BMJ. 2007;335(7630): 1147-51.
3. Mondragón Rosas E, González Flores JE, Zamudio Carías AD, García Martínez N, Díaz Salcedo EX, Navarro López PE, et al. Pathogenesis and Clinical Management of Vulvovaginal Candidiasis in Mexican Diabetic Patients: A Literature Review. Cureus. 2025;17(6):e86012.
4. Workowski KA, Bachmann LH, Chan PA, Johnston CM, Muzny CA, Park I, et al. Sexually Transmitted Infections Treatment Guidelines, 2021. MMWR Recomm Rep. 2021;70(4):1-187.
5. Achkar JM, Fries BC. Candida infections of the genitourinary tract. Clin Microbiol Rev. 2010;23(2):253-73.
6. Sobel JD. Vulvovaginal candidosis. Lancet. 2007;369(9577): 1961-71.
7. Zeng X, Liu H, Zhang L, Leaman D, Nyirjesy P, Weitz MV, et al. Risk factors of recurrent vulvovaginal candidiasis in females: a meta-analysis. Front Microbiol. 2021;12:697211.
8. Patel DA, Gillespie B, Sobel JD, Leaman D, Nyirjesy P, Weitz MV, et al. Risk factors for recurrent vulvovaginal candidiasis in women receiving maintenance antifungal therapy: results of a prospective cohort study. Am J Obstet Gynecol. 2004;190(3):644-53.

Case 4: Candidal Balanoposthitis in Undiagnosed Type 2 Diabetes Mellitus

■ PRESENTATION

A 52-year-old male farmer reported persistent pruritus and fissuring affecting the glans penis and foreskin for 3 months. He also experienced increased smegma accumulation and progressive difficulty in retracting the prepuce. Over the preceding 2 weeks, the patient developed dysuria and painful micturition, which prompted him to seek medical evaluation. He denied any prior history of diabetes, hypertension, or medication use. Laboratory investigations revealed an HbA1c of 12% and urine glucose of 3+, confirming previously undiagnosed diabetes mellitus. There were no systemic symptoms such as fever or malaise.

■ EXAMINATION

Physical examination demonstrated fissures over the prepuce, mild erythema of the glans, and adherent white patches, without purulent discharge or lymphadenopathy. His sexual partner remained asymptomatic **(Fig. 1)**.

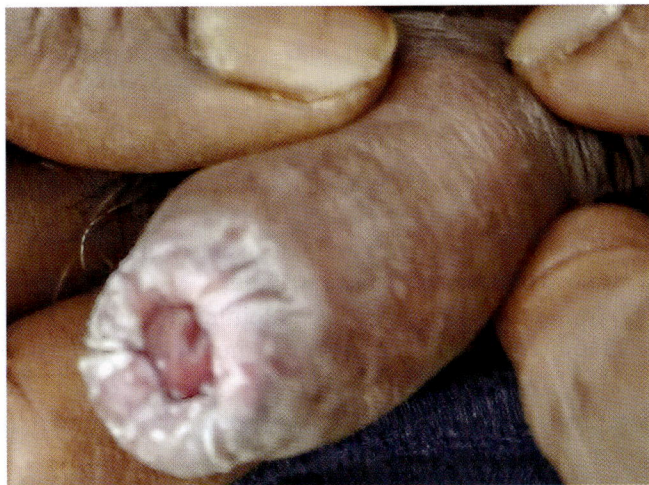

FIG. 1: Fissures over the prepuce with mild erythema of the glans and adherent white patches, without purulent discharge or lymphadenopathy.

DIAGNOSIS

The diagnosis is Candidal balanoposthitis associated with newly diagnosed type-2 diabetes mellitus.[1,2]

DIFFERENTIAL DIAGNOSIS

Infective causes

- *Bacterial balanitis:* Typically presents with confluent erosions over the glans and prepuce, often accompanied by purulent subpreputial discharge.[1]
- *Herpetic balanitis:* Characterized by painful, superficial, irregular erosions, sometimes with systemic symptoms.[1]

NONINFECTIVE CAUSES

- *Irritant contact dermatitis:* Manifests as patchy, dry erythema and is often linked to recent exposure to topical agents or medications[1]
- *Lichen sclerosus:* Presents with atrophic white plaques and may progress to phimosis[1]
- *Psoriatic balanitis*: Features well-demarcated, erythematous plaques with silvery scales[1]

MANAGEMENT

Dermatology/Urology Management

- *Topical antifungal therapy*: Clotrimazole 1% cream applied locally twice daily for 7–10 days is recommended as first-line therapy. Miconazole 2% cream serves as an alternative.[1,3]
- *Systemic antifungal therapy*: For moderate-to-severe or refractory cases, oral fluconazole 150 mg as a single dose, repeated after 3 days if necessary, is indicated.[3,4]
- *Local hygiene*: Advise gentle cleansing with warm water and avoidance of soaps or irritants[1]
- *Sexual partner management*: Routine treatment is not required unless the partner is symptomatic.[5]
- *Follow-up:* Suggested for persistent or recurrent cases; circumcision may be considered in refractory situations.[1,4]

Diabetology/Physician Management

- *Newly diagnosed diabetes:* Initiate oral antidiabetic therapy (e.g., metformin 500 mg twice daily)[2]
- *Patient education*: Emphasize the importance of genital hygiene, optimal glycemic control, and early recognition of infections[1,2]
- *Monitoring*: Plan quarterly assessment of HbA1c, fasting and postprandial blood glucose, renal function, and urine microalbumin to optimize diabetes management and reduce recurrence risk.[2]

PROGNOSIS

With appropriate antifungal therapy, candidal balanoposthitis generally resolves favorably. However, the risk of recurrence is increased in individuals with poor genital hygiene or inadequate glycemic control. Early diagnosis and effective management of diabetes facilitate symptom resolution and decrease recurrence rates.[1,2]

> **Clinical Pearls**
> - Classic findings include fissuring of the prepuce and smegma accumulation.
> - *Candida* species proliferate in warm, moist, glucose-rich environments, making poorly controlled diabetes a significant predisposing factor.[2,3,6,7]
> - The accumulation of advanced glycation end products in the skin and microvascular dysfunction in diabetic patients may contribute to preputial fissuring.[2]
> - The presence of candidal balanoposthitis in an otherwise healthy male should prompt evaluation for underlying diabetes, as it may serve as a cutaneous marker of the disease.[1,2]

REFERENCES

1. Edwards S. Balanitis and balanoposthitis: a review. Genitourin Med. 1996;72(3):155-59.
2. Verma SB, Wollina U. Looking through the cracks of diabetic candidal balanoposthitis! Int J Gen Med. 2011;4:511-3.
3. Achkar JM, Fries BC. Candida infections of the genitourinary tract. Clin Microbiol Rev. 2010;23(2):253-73.
4. Donders GG. Balanitis and balanoposthitis: a neglected problem in men. Expert Opin Pharmacother. 2010;11(4):629-35.
5. Workowski KA, Bachmann LH, Chan PA, Johnston CM, Muzny CA, Park I, et al. Sexually Transmitted Infections Treatment Guidelines, 2021. MMWR Recomm Rep. 2021;70(4):1-187.
6. Sobel JD. Recurrent vulvovaginal candidiasis. Am J Obstet Gynecol. 2016;214(1):15-21.
7. Bjekić M, Šipetić-Grujičić S, Marinković J. Risk factors for development of balanitis in uncircumcised men. Srp Arh Celok Lek. 2016;144(1-2):79-84.

Case 5: Type-2 Diabetes Mellitus with Cutaneous Candidiasis

PRESENTATION

A 54-year-old woman with type 2 diabetes presented with a 2-week history of pruritus, erythema, and maceration in the groin and vaginal folds. The lesions worsened gradually. Random blood glucose was 400 mg/dL. She was on dapagliflozin 10 mg once daily and sitagliptin–metformin (50/500 mg) twice daily. No systemic symptoms were reported.

EXAMINATION

Well-defined erythematous patches with maceration and mild pruritus were observed in the groin and vaginal folds **(Fig. 1)**.

INVESTIGATIONS

- KOH mount of skin scrapings revealed pseudohyphae and yeast forms of *Candida*.
- No other laboratory or clinical evidence of systemic infection was found.

DIAGNOSIS

The diagnosis is type-2 diabetes mellitus with cutaneous candidiasis.

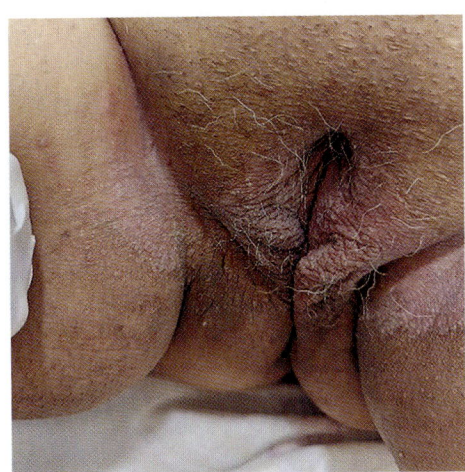

FIG. 1: Well-defined erythematous patches with maceration and mild pruritus observed in the groin and vaginal folds.

DIFFERENTIAL DIAGNOSES

- Noninfectious intertrigo
- Tinea cruris (dermatophyte infection)
- Inverse psoriasis
- Contact dermatitis

MANAGEMENT

Dermatological Approach

- *Oral antifungal*: Fluconazole 200 mg once daily for 4 days
- *Topical antifungal*: Clotrimazole cream applied twice daily for 2 weeks
- *Hygiene*: Advised to maintain cleanliness, dryness, and ventilation of affected sites. Recommended use of loose-fitting cotton undergarments and avoidance of occlusive attire.

Diabetology/Physician Management

- The patient was initially referred for diabetes evaluation, with no baseline laboratory results available.
- Dapagliflozin was discontinued due to its association with an increased risk of genital fungal infections, particularly in women and those with a prior history of such infections.[1,2]
- Initiated therapy with gliclazide 60 mg plus metformin 500 mg twice daily
- *Advised follow-up investigations*: HbA1c, fasting and postprandial glucose, serum creatinine, urinary albumin-to-creatinine ratio (UACR), and urine routine with microscopy.

Follow-up Findings (after 1 week)

- *HbA1c*: 8.1%
- *Fasting blood sugar*: 180 mg/dL
- *Postprandial blood sugar*: 250 mg/dL
- *Serum creatinine*: 1.1 mg/dL
- *Urine routine and microscopy*: Yeast ++
- Other parameters were within normal limits

Revised Management

- Continued gliclazide plus metformin regimen.
- Added sitagliptin 50 mg plus metformin 500 mg once daily.
- Reinforced the importance of lifestyle modification and regular glycemic monitoring.
- Scheduled follow-up in 3 months with repeat HbA1c and glucose profiles.

■ PROGNOSIS

Cutaneous candidiasis, although superficial, can substantially diminish quality of life due to persistent itching and risk of secondary excoriations. With targeted antifungal therapy and optimization of glycemic control, lesions typically resolve within 1–2 weeks. Long-term prevention hinges on sustained glycemic management and strict hygiene.[2,3]

Clinical Pearls

- Cutaneous candidiasis is a prevalent but often under-recognized complication in individuals with poorly controlled diabetes, especially in moist, intertriginous areas.[4-7]
- SGLT2 inhibitors such as dapagliflozin, while effective for glycemic control, are linked to an elevated risk of genital mycotic infections, particularly in women.[1]
- The initial manifestation of candidiasis may serve as an early indicator of undiagnosed or inadequately managed diabetes mellitus.[6,7]
- Prompt recognition and coordinated care between dermatology and diabetology are essential to prevent complications and recurrences.

REFERENCES

1. Bennett JE, Dolin R, Blaser MJ. Mandell, Douglas, and Bennett's Principles and Practice of Infectious Diseases, 9th edition. Philadelphia: Elsevier; 2020.
2. Seufert J, Laimer M. SGLT2 inhibitors and risk of genital infections: current understanding and clinical guidance. Ther Adv Endocrinol Metab. 2021;12:20420188211012877.
3. Nampoothiri S, Vellappally S, John J. Mucocutaneous manifestations in diabetes mellitus. J Assoc Physicians India. 2020;68(6):48-52.
4. Sobel JD. Genital candidiasis: a common infection with serious consequences. J Womens Health (Larchmt). 2006;15(6):529-39.
5. Geerlings SE. Urinary tract infections in patients with diabetes mellitus: epidemiology, pathogenesis and treatment. Int J Antimicrob Agents. 2008;31(Suppl 1):S54-7.
6. Katsambas A, Antoniou C. Candidiasis (cutaneous). In: Bolognia JL, Jorizzo JL, Schaffer JV (Eds). Dermatology, 3rd edition. Philadelphia: Elsevier Saunders; 2012. pp. 1190-6.
7. Goldenberg RL, Thompson C. Infections and diabetes: an overview. Clin Infect Dis. 1996;22(Suppl 2):S1-S3.

CHAPTER 19

Bacterial Skin Infections in Diabetes

*Nipul Vara, Vishwa Marvania, Preya Parag Rana, Hiral Shah,
J Thadeus, Aarathy Kannan, Akashkumar N Singh, Ankur Kothari,
Suhas Gopal Erande, Anil Patki, Ruchi Shah, Yogesh Marfatia*

Part A: Acute Paronychia in a Diabetic Male

PRESENTATION

A 47-year-old male with a 7-year history of type 2 diabetes mellitus, currently managed with metformin and glimepiride, presented with a sudden onset of swelling and severe throbbing pain localized to the lateral margin of his right great toenail, persisting for the past 3 days. There was no preceding trauma or ingrown nail reported, and no prior similar episodes.

EXAMINATION

- On examination, there was localized erythema, swelling, and tenderness along the lateral nail fold, with yellowish pus pointing at the edge **(Fig. 1)**.
- The patient was afebrile, had stable vital signs, and showed no other nail changes or foot ulcers.

DIAGNOSIS

Acute paronychia involving the right great toe, most likely of bacterial origin (*Staphylococcus aureus* or *Streptococcus species*).[1,2]

DIFFERENTIAL DIAGNOSES

- *Ingrown toenail with secondary infection*—commonly presents with similar swelling and tenderness[3]
- *Chronic paronychia*—slower onset, multiple recurrences, often candidal[1]
- *Felon*—deeper pulp space infection of the fingertip or toe
- *Herpetic whitlow*—grouped vesicles, more common on fingers, burning pain
- *Diabetic foot abscess*—deeper infection, systemic signs are more common[4]

PATHOPHYSIOLOGY AND DIABETES LINK

- High glucose levels impair neutrophil function and promote bacterial growth.[4,5]

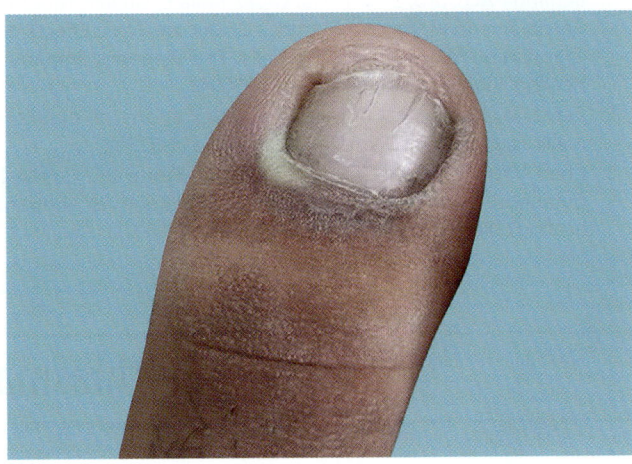

FIG. 1: inflamed, swollen lateral nail fold with a yellowish, pointed pustule and surrounding erythema at the right great toe nail—classic of acute paronychia.

- Diabetic patients often have compromised microcirculation and skin barrier function.[5]
- Increased risk of minor trauma from trimming toenails or footwear pressure can precipitate infection.[3,5]
- Poor wound healing in diabetes can delay resolution and complicate even minor infections.[4,5]

MANAGEMENT

Dermatology/Surgical Management

- *Incision and drainage (I and D)*: Standard treatment once pus is localized and fluctuance appears.[2]
- *Topical care*:
  - Daily dressing with antiseptic solution (e.g., povidone–iodine or chlorhexidine)
  - Mupirocin or fusidic acid if topical therapy alone is initiated early.[2]
- *Culture and sensitivity*: Swab may be sent for microbiological testing if recurrence occurs or systemic antibiotics fail.[1]

Physician/Diabetology Management

- *Antibiotic therapy*:
  - Oral antibiotics covering gram-positive cocci (e.g., amoxicillin–clavulanic acid or cephalexin)
  - Clindamycin or linezolid in methicillin-resistant *Staphylococcus aureus* (MRSA)-prone settings[2,3]
- *Glycemic optimization:* Reinforce blood sugar monitoring and adjustment of oral medications or insulin if needed[4]
- *Foot care education:*
  - Avoid trauma from improper nail cutting
  - Footwear counseling and regular foot examinations[3,5]

PROGNOSIS

- Excellent with early drainage and appropriate antibiotics[1,2]
- Delay in intervention may result in:
  - Cellulitis
  - Osteomyelitis in diabetics[4]
  - Chronic paronychia or nail dystrophy
- Healing may be prolonged in uncontrolled diabetes.[5]

> **Clinical Pearls**
> - Paronychia is a common soft tissue infection in diabetics and must be promptly treated.[1,5]
> - Always assess for deeper spread (e.g., tracking cellulitis or abscess extension)[3]
> - Reinforce diabetic foot hygiene and footwear education.
> - Surgical intervention (I and D) is often curative when done early.[2]

REFERENCES

1. Berlanga-Acosta J, Schultz GS, López-Mola E, Guillen-Nieto G, García-Siverio M, Herrera-Martínez L. Glucose Toxic Effects on Granulation Tissue Productive Cells: The Diabetics' Impaired Healing. BioMed Res Int. 2013;2013:256043.
2. Pérez M, Kohn SR. Cutaneous manifestations of diabetes mellitus. J Am Acad Dermatol. 1994;30(4):519-31.
3. Chen VY, Siegfried LG, Tomic-Canic M, Stone RC, Pastar I. Cutaneous changes in diabetic patients: Primed for aberrant healing? Wound Repair Regen. 2023;31(5):700-12.
4. Ferguson MWJ, Herrick SE, Spencer M, Shaw JE, Boulton AJM, Sloan P. The Histology of Diabetic Foot Ulcers. Diabetic Med. 1996;13:S30-3.
5. Levin ME; American Diabetes Association. Classification of Diabetic Foot Wounds. Diabetes Care. 1998;21(5):681.

Part B: Erythrasma in a Diabetic Patient

PRESENTATION

A 50-year-old female with poorly controlled type 2 diabetes mellitus (random blood sugar: 200 mg/dL) presented with asymptomatic erythematous to hyperpigmented patches localized to the groin and both axillae for 1 month. She reported no pruritus, systemic complaints, or fever. Her medical history was notable for long-standing diabetes with suboptimal glycemic control, a common risk factor for cutaneous infections such as erythrasma.

EXAMINATION

On examination, well-defined erythematous to hyperpigmented patches were observed in the axillae (**Fig. 1**), under the breasts and over the upper abdomen (**Fig. 2**), and in the groin region (**Fig. 3**). The patient had no associated signs of systemic illness.

INVESTIGATIONS

- Direct microscopic examination with potassium hydroxide (KOH) preparation was negative, excluding dermatophytosis.
- Under Wood's lamp examination, the lesions exhibited a characteristic coral-red fluorescence, attributed to coproporphyrin III produced by *Corynebacterium minutissimum*, the causative organism. This fluorescence is a hallmark feature, aiding in the rapid bedside diagnosis of erythrasma.

DIAGNOSIS

The diagnosis of erythrasma was established based on clinical and laboratory findings.

DIFFERENTIAL DIAGNOSIS

The clinical presentation necessitated differentiation from several other intertriginous dermatoses:
- *Tinea cruris*: Excluded by negative KOH mount.[1]
- *Intertrigo*: Typically presents as macerated, inflamed plaques, often with secondary infection.[2]
- *Inverse psoriasis:* Characterized by sharply demarcated erythematous plaques, usually lacking the brownish hue seen in erythrasma[3]
- *Candidiasis:* Distinguished by satellite pustules and positive KOH findings[4]
- *Pityriasis versicolor*: Occurs in different anatomical locations and demonstrates yellowish, rather than coral-red, fluorescence under Wood's lamp[5]

PATHOPHYSIOLOGY

Erythrasma is caused by *Corynebacterium minutissimum*, a Gram-positive bacillus that thrives in moist, occluded skin folds. Diabetic patients are particularly susceptible due to:
- Increased moisture retention in intertriginous areas[6]

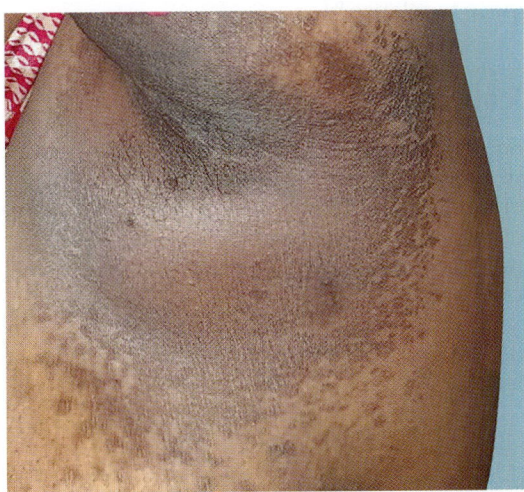

FIG. 1: Well-defined, erythematous to hyperpigmented patches in the axillary region.

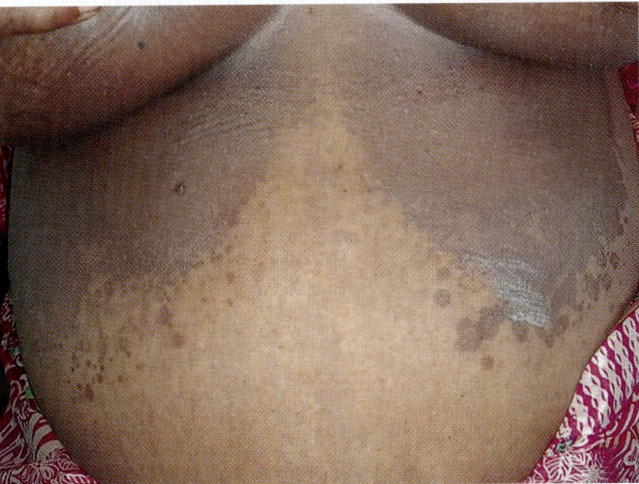

FIG. 2: Erythematous to hyperpigmented lesions with maceration observed under the breasts and over the upper abdomen.

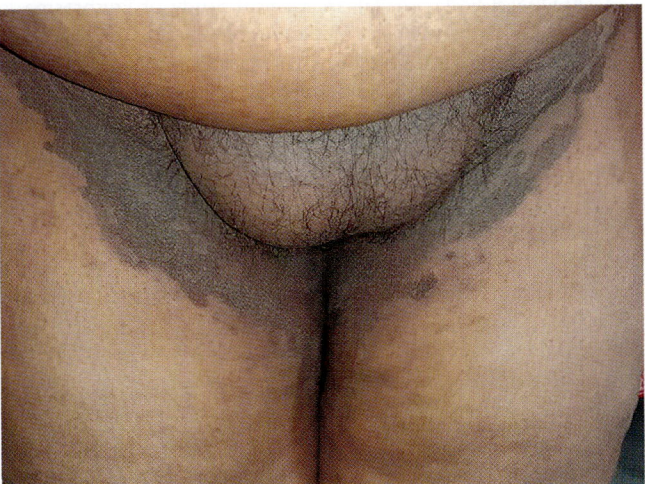

FIG. 3: Hyperpigmented patches involving the groin folds with mild erythema.

- Hyperglycemia-mediated impairment of local immune defenses[7]
- Altered skin surface pH, which promotes bacterial overgrowth[7]

The pathognomonic coral-red fluorescence under Wood's lamp is due to the accumulation of porphyrins, specifically coproporphyrin III, produced by the organism.[5,6]

■ MANAGEMENT

Dermatology Management

First-line therapy for localized erythrasma involves topical agents:

- Fusidic acid 2% cream applied twice daily for 2 weeks[5]
- Clindamycin 1% solution or Whitfield's ointment as alternatives[7]
- For extensive or refractory cases, systemic antibiotics are indicated:
  - Erythromycin 500 mg orally four times daily for 7 days (as used in this case)[5,7]
  - Alternatives include clarithromycin or doxycycline[7]

Adjunctive measures may include:

- Benzoyl peroxide wash to reduce bacterial load[3]
- Photodynamic therapy for recalcitrant or recurrent lesions[2]

Diabetology/Physician Management

Effective management extends beyond antimicrobial therapy and requires addressing underlying risk factors:

- Achieve optimal glycemic control (target HbA1c <7%)[6]
- Maintain meticulous hygiene in intertriginous zones[7]
- Encourage weight reduction in overweight or obese individuals[7]
- Educate patients on early recognition and reporting of suspicious skin lesions[6]
- Advise against tight clothing and practices that promote excessive moisture retention[6]

■ PROGNOSIS

With appropriate therapy, erythrasma lesions typically resolve within 1–2 weeks. Recurrence is uncommon when predisposing factors, particularly glycemic control and obesity, are adequately managed. However, persistent hyperglycemia or failure to address local risk factors may predispose to relapse.[6,7]

> **Clinical Pearls**
>
> ▶ Consider erythrasma in any diabetic patient presenting with brown, scaly patches in body folds.[6]
> ▶ Coral-red fluorescence under Wood's lamp is a rapid, noninvasive diagnostic clue.[7]
> ▶ Always exclude co-existing tinea or candidiasis with KOH examination.[1,4]
> ▶ Erythrasma is frequently misdiagnosed as a fungal infection but responds promptly to appropriate antibacterial therapy.[5,7]

REFERENCES

1. Al-Obaidi RMD, Khallaf SA. Clinical Study of Erythrasma in Diabetic Patients. Prensa Médica Argentina. 2021;107(2):1-3.
2. Medscape. (2024). Erythrasma: Practice Essentials, Pathophysiology, & Epidemiology. [online] Available from https://emedicine.medscape.com/article/1052532-overview. [Last accessed August, 2025]
3. Groves JB, Nassereddin A, Freeman AM. (2024). Erythrasma. [online] Available from https://www.ncbi.nlm.nih.gov/books/NBK513352/. [Last accessed August, 2025]
4. MDedge – The Hospitalist. (2022). Erythrasma: Clinical Presentation and Epidemiology. [online] Available from https://community.the-hospitalist.org/content/erythrasma. [Last accessed August, 2025]
5. Janeczek M, Kozel Z, Bhasin R, Tao J, Eilers D, Swan J. High Prevalence of Erythrasma in Patients with Inverse Psoriasis: A Cross-sectional Study. J Clin Aesthet Dermatol. 2020;13(3):12-14.
6. Rajkumar V. Erythrasma: A Superficial Cutaneous Bacterial Infection Overlooked in Clinical Practice. Rev Bact Fungal Infect. 2023;2(1):19-25.
7. Martínez-Ortega JI, Franco González S. Erythrasma Revisited: Diagnosis, Differential Diagnoses, and Comprehensive Review of Treatment. Cureus. 2024;16(8):e10733.

Part C: Furunculosis in Diabetic Patients

Case 1 — Furunculosis with Carbuncles: A Staphylococcal Infection of the Hair Follicle

■ PRESENTATION

A 45-year-old male presented with multiple painful, ulcerated nodules discharging pus over the body for 14 days. The lesions began as tender, erythematous papules, progressed to fluctuant nodules (furuncles), and coalesced into a large carbuncle with draining sinuses on the left leg. The patient had no prior medical consultation and was newly diagnosed with diabetes mellitus.

■ EXAMINATION

- Multiple furuncles with central necrosis and purulent discharge were observed on the beard region, neck, and upper chest **(Figs. 1 and 2)** and limbs **(Fig. 3)**.
- A large carbuncle with multiple sinus openings was present on the left leg **(Fig. 3)**.
- there were no systemic signs such as fever or lymphadenopathy.

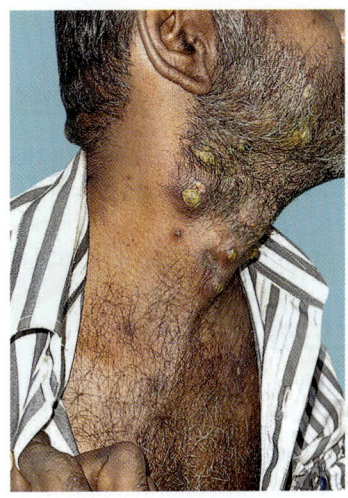

FIG. 2: Multiple furuncles with central necrosis and purulent discharge involving the right side of the bearded region, extending to the adjacent neck and hairy areas of the upper chest.

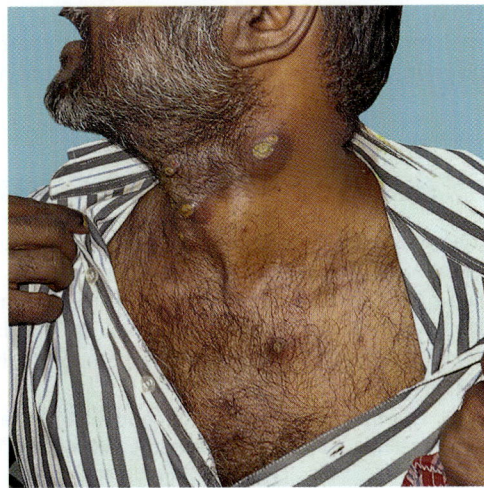

FIG. 1: Multiple furuncles with central necrosis and purulent discharge involving the left side of the bearded region, extending to the adjacent neck and hairy areas of the upper chest.

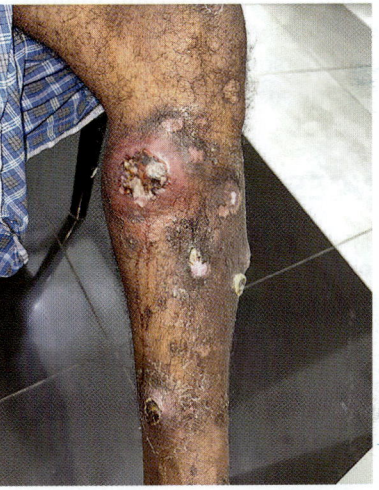

FIG. 3: Multiple furuncles with central necrosis and purulent discharge on the leg, along with a large carbuncle on the left leg exhibiting multiple sinus openings and surrounding inflammation.

INVESTIGATIONS

- On initial assessment, he was found to have newly diagnosed diabetes mellitus.
- no other significant laboratory or clinical abnormalities were noted.

DIAGNOSIS

Furunculosis with carbuncle: *Staphylococcus aureus* infection of hair follicles in a background of previously undiagnosed type 2 diabetes mellitus.

DIFFERENTIAL DIAGNOSES

- *Multiple bacterial abscesses*: Generally deeper and more fluctuant than furuncles or carbuncles.
- *Cold abscess (tubercular)*: Characterized by chronic, nontender swellings that lack overt inflammatory signs.[1]

MANAGEMENT

Dermatology Management

- Oral cephalexin 500 mg four times daily for 10 days, targeting methicillin-sensitive *Staphylococcus aureus* (MSSA).[1]
- Topical mupirocin to reduce local bacterial load in superficial pustules.[2]
- Analgesics and anti-inflammatory agents for pain control.
- Warm compresses and incision-drainage for fluctuant or nonresolving lesions.
- Guidance on personal hygiene, including daily cleansing with antiseptic soap and wearing clean clothing.[1,2]

Diabetology/Physician Management

- Diabetes mellitus was newly diagnosed during admission; random blood sugar was >200 mg/dL.
- Initiation of oral antidiabetic therapy (e.g., metformin) and dietary counseling
- Education on foot care and strategies to prevent further infections
- Regular monitoring of fasting and postprandial blood glucose, HbA1c, and screening for other diabetes complications
- Scheduled follow-up to evaluate glycemic control and monitor for recurrence of skin infections[3-5]

PROGNOSIS

With prompt initiation of systemic antibiotics and optimization of glycemic control, the patient's condition improved rapidly, and all lesions resolved within 10 days, leaving only post-inflammatory pigmentation. If not managed appropriately, furunculosis may progress to systemic infection or become chronic and recurrent, especially in diabetic individuals.[2,3,5]

> **Clinical Pearls**
>
> ▶ Furunculosis and carbuncles are cutaneous indicators of immunosuppression, most commonly due to diabetes mellitus.[3,4]
> ▶ Staphylococcal skin infections are prone to recur in those with poor glycemic control.
> ▶ All patients presenting with multiple boils or carbuncles should be evaluated for undiagnosed diabetes.
> ▶ Maintaining good hygiene, effective glycemic control, and regular skin surveillance are vital to prevent recurrence.[4-7]

REFERENCES

1. Dryden MS. Skin and soft tissue infection: microbiology and epidemiology. Int J Antimicrob Agents. 2009;34(Suppl 1):S2-S7.
2. Simonart T. Cutaneous staphylococcal infections. Clin Dermatol. 2008;26(2):193-201.
3. Rayner BL, Abdullah MS. Carbuncle—a marker for diabetes mellitus. S Afr Med J. 1997;87(3):352.
4. Yosipovitch G, Hodak E, Vardi P, Shraga I, Karp M. The prevalence of cutaneous manifestations in IDDM patients and their association with diabetes risk factors and microvascular complications. Diabetes Care. 1998;21(4):506-9.
5. Mahajan BB, Kaur S, Singh A. Diabetic dermatoses and their correlation with diabetic status. Int J Dermatol. 2003;42(7):498-500.
6. Foster TJ. The *Staphylococcus aureus* "superbug." J Clin Invest. 2004;114(12):1693-6.
7. Bhat YJ, Gupta V, Kudyar RP. Cutaneous manifestations of diabetes mellitus. Int J Diabetes Dev Ctries. 2006;26(4):152-55.

Case 2: Furunculosis with Carbuncle in an Uncontrolled Diabetic Male: Neglected Skin Infection Leading to MRSA Abscess

■ PRESENTATION

Mr AR (pseudonym), a 42-year-old male auto mechanic residing in an urban slum with poor sanitation, presented with a 1-week history of a painful, red swelling over the mid-upper back. He has been a known case of type 2 diabetes mellitus for the past 8 years, with poor glycemic control. The swelling gradually increased in size, became more painful, and eventually developed central necrosis with pus drainage and multiple sinus tracts—features typical of a carbuncle. He also reported associated symptoms of fever and malaise, with a noted delay in seeking medical attention due to socioeconomic limitations.

■ EXAMINATION

- On examination, the lesion presented as a classic carbuncle, characterized by a necrotic central core, surrounding induration, marked erythema, and purulent discharge **(Fig. 1)**.
- Such skin and soft tissue infections are commonly observed in poorly controlled diabetic patients and are often associated with furunculosis and impaired wound healing.

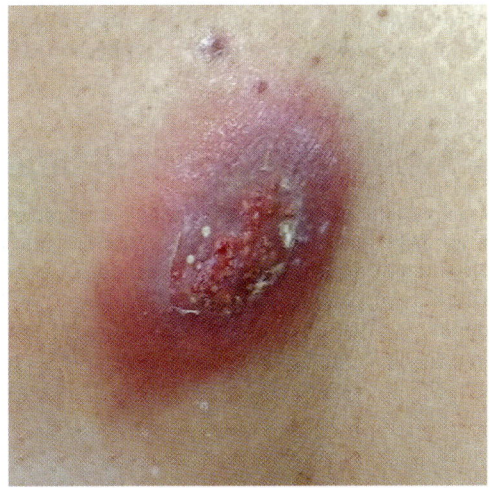

FIG. 1: Carbuncle on the upper back showing a necrotic center, surrounding erythema, pus discharge, and slough.
Source: Case image from RSSDI Atlas (with consent)

■ INVESTIGATIONS

- Random blood sugar (RBS) is 286 mg/dL, which is markedly elevated. This indicates poor short-term glycemic control and suggests the patient is currently hyperglycemic.
- HbA1c is 9.4%, which reflects chronic poor blood sugar control over the past 2–3 months. This level is significantly above the recommended target (usually <7%) and increases the risk of diabetes-related complications, especially infections and delayed wound healing.
- Total leukocyte count is 14,200/mm^3, which indicates leukocytosis. The pattern is neutrophilic, suggesting a bacterial infection.
- C-reactive protein (CRP) is elevated, which supports the presence of active inflammation or infection in the body.
- Pus culture has isolated MRSA (methicillin-resistant *Staphylococcus aureus*). This confirms a serious bacterial infection that requires targeted antibiotic treatment with drugs effective against MRSA, such as vancomycin or linezolid.
- HIV, HBsAg, and HCV tests are nonreactive, indicating there is no evidence of viral immunosuppression. This is a favorable finding for recovery and treatment response.
- Liver function tests (LFTs) and renal function tests (RFTs) are normal, indicating that there is no liver or kidney dysfunction at this time. This is important for the safe administration of antibiotics and other medications.

■ DIAGNOSIS

- *Confirmed*: Carbuncle arising from underlying furunculosis
- *Underlying comorbidity*: Uncontrolled type 2 diabetes mellitus

■ DIFFERENTIAL DIAGNOSIS

- Cutaneous abscess
- Infected epidermoid cyst
- Infected hidradenitis suppurativa

MANAGEMENT

Medical Management

- *Initial empiric intravenous antibiotics*:
  - Amoxicillin–clavulanic acid 1.2 g TID
  - Metronidazole 500 mg TID
- *After MRSA was identified on culture:* Switched to intravenous linezolid as per sensitivity
- *Glycemic management*:
  - Started on a basal-bolus insulin regimen
  - Frequent blood glucose checks
  - Endocrinology referral for optimization

Surgical and Local Wound Care

- Prompt incision and drainage by the surgical team
- Daily sterile wound dressings
- Application of topical antimicrobials (mupirocin or iodine gauze)

Education and Lifestyle Modification

- Counseling on the necessity of stringent diabetes control to avoid recurrence
- Emphasis on hygiene to prevent further infections
- Education regarding early signs of skin infection

FOLLOW-UP AND PROGNOSIS

The wound began to heal within 7–10 days after surgical drainage and linezolid therapy. Glycemic control improved with insulin; repeat HbA1c testing was scheduled for 3 months later. The patient was advised to perform regular skin checks and continue follow-up care.

Clinical Pearls

- Carbuncles are deep-seated abscesses resulting from the coalescence of adjacent furuncles and are most commonly seen in immunocompromised individuals, especially those with poorly controlled diabetes.[1,2]
- Chronic hyperglycemia in diabetes impairs neutrophil function, including chemotaxis and phagocytosis, thereby reducing microbial clearance and increasing susceptibility to skin infections.[1,2]
- *Staphylococcus aureus*, including methicillin-resistant strains (MRSA), is the most frequently isolated organism in furuncles and carbuncles.[3,4]
- Key risk factors for furunculosis and carbuncle formation in diabetic individuals include persistent hyperglycemia, inadequate hygiene, malnutrition, and delayed medical attention.[3,4]
- The rising incidence of MRSA in community-acquired skin infections necessitates early microbiological diagnosis and targeted antimicrobial therapy to ensure effective treatment.[5,6]
- Surgical drainage remains the cornerstone of carbuncle management, supported by systemic antibiotics and strict blood glucose control to facilitate healing and prevent complications.[5]
- Delayed treatment in diabetic patients can result in serious outcomes such as cellulitis, bacteremia, or sepsis. Prompt recognition, appropriate antibiotic coverage, and glycemic optimization are vital.[1,5]
- Empirical MRSA coverage should be considered in cases with delayed presentation or frank pus discharge, especially in diabetic individuals.[5]
- Always send pus for culture and sensitivity testing in diabetic patients with skin abscesses to guide definitive antimicrobial therapy.[6]
- Patient education on personal hygiene, wound care, early signs of infection, and routine skin/foot inspection is essential to prevent recurrence and complications.[4]

REFERENCES

1. Delamaire M, Maugendre D, Moreno M, Le Goff MC, Allannic H, Genetet B. Impaired leucocyte functions in diabetic patients. Diabet Med. 1997;14(1):29-34.
2. Dryden M. Skin and soft tissue infection: microbiology and epidemiology. Int J Antimicrob Agents. 2009;34:S2-7.
3. Joshi N, Caputo GM, Weitekamp MR, Karchmer AW. Infections in patients with diabetes mellitus. N Engl J Med. 1999;341(25):1906-12.
4. Lipsky BA. Infections in diabetes: pathogenesis and management. Clin Infect Dis. 2001;33(9):1535-41.
5. Abrahamian FM, Snyder EW. Community-associated methicillin-resistant *Staphylococcus aureus*: incidence, clinical presentation, and treatment decisions. Current Infectious Disease Reports. 2007;9(5):391-7.
6. Gadepalli R, Dhawan B, Sreenivas V, Kapil A, Ammini AC, Chaudhry R. A clinico-microbiological study of diabetic foot ulcers in an Indian tertiary care hospital. Diabetes Care. 2006;29(8):1727-32.

Part D: Fournier's Gangrene in an Undiagnosed Diabetic Male

■ PRESENTATION

A 35-year-old male presented with purulent discharge, pain, and black discoloration over the right side of the scrotum for 1 week. He denied any preceding trauma, insect bite, or systemic symptoms such as fever, nausea, or vomiting.

No significant past medical history, including diabetes, hypertension, tuberculosis, or asthma, was reported.

■ EXAMINATION

- Local examination revealed a raw, ulcerated area (~4 × 3 cm) with purulent discharge and adjacent skin necrosis on the right scrotum **(Figs. 1 and 2)**.
- Systemic examination was unremarkable, with a soft, nontender abdomen, normal bowel sounds, and no abnormalities detected in respiratory, cardiovascular, or neurological systems.

■ INVESTIGATIONS

- Random blood glucose was 151 mg/dL on admission.
- Due to the necrotizing nature of the lesion and the clinical context, a diagnosis of Fournier's Gangrene was established.
- further metabolic assessment revealed previously undiagnosed type 2 diabetes mellitus, likely a contributing factor to the severity of the infection.

■ DIAGNOSIS

The diagnosis is Fournier's gangrene (necrotizing fasciitis of the perineum and genitalia) in a patient with newly diagnosed type 2 diabetes mellitus and poor genital hygiene.[1,2]

■ DIFFERENTIAL DIAGNOSIS

- *Necrotizing fasciitis (non-Fournier)*: Generally affects the limbs or trunk rather than the genitalia[3]
- *Scrotal cellulitis*: Characterized by superficial inflammation without deep tissue necrosis
- *Scrotal abscess*: Localized collection, typically without fascial involvement
- *Hidradenitis suppurativa*: Chronic, with nodules and sinus tract formation
- *Traumatic scrotal ulcer*: Associated with a clear history of injury
- *Tubercular epididymo-orchitis*: Insidious onset, often with constitutional symptoms
- *Scrotal carcinoma*: Rare, presents as a chronic nonhealing ulcer[4]

■ PATHOPHYSIOLOGY

Fournier's gangrene is a rapidly advancing, polymicrobial necrotizing fasciitis of the perineal, scrotal, and genital regions.[2]

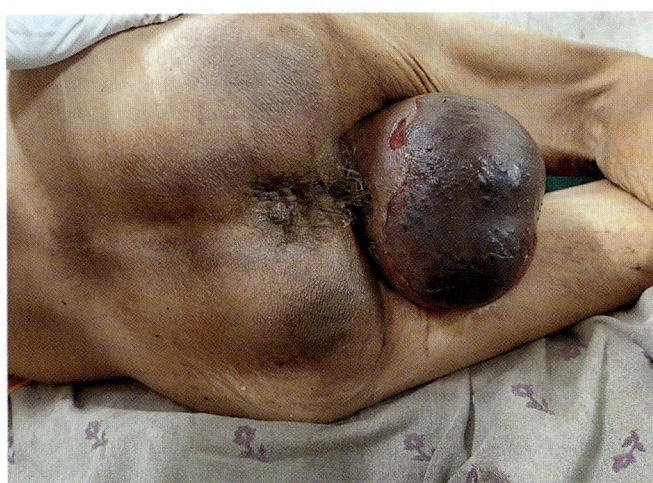

FIG. 1: Raw, ulcerated area (~4 × 3 cm) with purulent discharge and surrounding skin necrosis observed on the right scrotum back view.

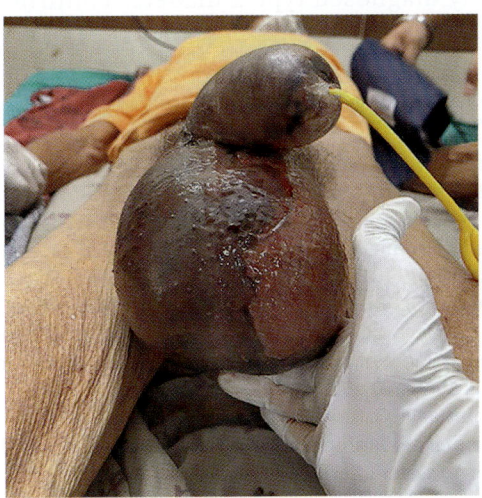

FIG. 2: Raw, ulcerated area (~4 × 3 cm) with purulent discharge and surrounding skin necrosis observed on the right scrotum front view.

- *Polymicrobial synergy*: Both aerobic and anaerobic organisms (e.g., *E. coli*, *Bacteroides*, *Streptococcus*, and *Klebsiella*) collaborate to induce tissue necrosis.[2]
- *Microvascular thrombosis and enzymatic tissue destruction:* Facilitate swift spread of infection[2]
- *Role of diabetes mellitus*:
  - Impaired immune response
  - Defective neutrophil chemotaxis
  - Reduced tissue perfusion
  - Glucosuria, which fosters local microbial growth[5]
- *Common entry points:* Periurethral glands, hair follicles, trauma, or inadequate genital hygiene[2]

MANAGEMENT

Surgical and Wound Care

- Immediate surgical debridement of necrotic tissue is essential.[6]
- Daily wound care with povidone–iodine, hydrogen peroxide, or saline dressings.
- Empiric broad-spectrum intravenous antibiotics, such as:
  - Piperacillin-tazobactam
  - Clindamycin
  - Metronidazole
  - Adjusted according to culture and sensitivity results[3]
- Obtain wound swab and blood cultures at admission.
- Extensive cases may require secondary closure, skin grafting, or testicular transposition.[6]

Diabetes and Medical Management

- Newly diagnosed type 2 diabetes confirmed after admission.[7]
- Initial glycemic management with intravenous insulin infusion, targeting blood glucose of 140–180 mg/dL[7]
- Transition to basal-bolus insulin regimen after stabilization
- Oral hypoglycemic agents (e.g., metformin and glimepiride) introduced post-acute phase
- Sodium-glucose transport protein 2 (SGLT-2) inhibitors should be avoided in this context.[5]
- Monitor for diabetic ketoacidosis, renal complications, and sepsis
- Patient education on genital hygiene, diabetic foot and skin care, and the importance of sustained glycemic control[7]

PROGNOSIS

Outcome is strongly dependent on prompt diagnosis, urgent surgical intervention, and adequate glycemic control.[8]

Mortality rates can reach 20–40% in cases with delayed or inadequate treatment.[2]

In this patient, timely debridement and metabolic correction resulted in favorable recovery without systemic complications.[8]

> **Clinical Pearls**
>
> - Fournier's gangrene should be considered in diabetics with rapidly progressing genital skin necrosis, particularly if accompanied by pus discharge or crepitus.[3]
> - Disproportionate pain, skin discoloration, and systemic decline are warning signs.[2]
> - SGLT2 inhibitor-induced glycosuria increases genital infection risk; caution is advised in patients with poor hygiene or infection history.[5]
> - Imaging (CT/MRI) may be helpful to delineate the extent of fascial involvement if diagnosis is uncertain.[3]

REFERENCES

1. Sorensen MD, Krieger JN, Rivara FP, Broghammer JA, Klein MB, Mack CD, et al. Fournier's Gangrene: Population Based Epidemiology and Outcomes. J Urol. 2009;181(5):2120-6.
2. Eke N. Fournier's gangrene: a review of 1726 cases. Br J Surg. 2000;87(6):718-28.
3. Stevens DL, Bisno AL, Chambers HF, Dellinger EP, Goldstein EJ, Gorbach SL, et al. Practice Guidelines for Diagnosis and Management of Skin and Soft Tissue Infections. Clin Infect Dis. 2014;59(2):e10-e52.
4. Yilmazlar T, Ozturk E, Ozguc H, Ercan I, Vuruskan H, Oktay B. Fournier's gangrene: an analysis of 80 patients and a novel scoring system. Tech Coloproctol. 2010;14(3):217-23.
5. Bersoff-Matcha SJ, Chamberlain C, Cao C, Kortepeter C, Chong WH. Fournier gangrene associated with sodium-glucose cotransporter-2 inhibitors: a review of spontaneous postmarketing cases. Ann Intern Med. 2019;170(11):764-9.
6. Shyam DC, Rapsang AG. Fournier's gangrene. Surgeon. 2013;11(4):222-32.
7. American Diabetes Association. Standards of Medical Care in Diabetes—2023. Diabetes Care. 2023;46(Suppl_1):S1–S291.
8. Yanar H, Taviloglu K, Ertekin C, Guloglu R, Zorba U, Cabioglu N, et al. Fournier's Gangrene: Risk Factors and Strategies for Management. World J Emerg Surg. 2006;1:16.

Part E: Carbuncle in a Diabetic Female

■ PRESENTATION

A 58-year-old female, known case of poorly controlled type 2 diabetes mellitus, presented with recurrent painful skin swellings associated with pus discharge. She reported repeated episodes over several months. The current episode involved a painful swelling over the nape of the neck with multiple openings and pus discharge lasting 5–7 days. She also experienced mild fever and malaise. The patient is a homemaker. A carbuncle is defined as a deep-seated pyogenic infection consisting of a cluster of interconnected furuncles, characterized by multiple pustular openings and extensive inflammation. A classic sign is pus discharge from multiple sinuses producing a "sieve-like" appearance.

■ EXAMINATION

- On physical examination, a tender, erythematous, swollen mass approximately 5 cm in diameter was observed over the nape of the neck. Multiple pustular openings and sinus tracts were noted, exuding purulent discharge. The surrounding skin was warm, inflamed, and indurated **(Fig. 1)**.
- Regional lymphadenopathy was present.
- No signs of systemic toxicity, such as hypotension or altered consciousness, were observed.

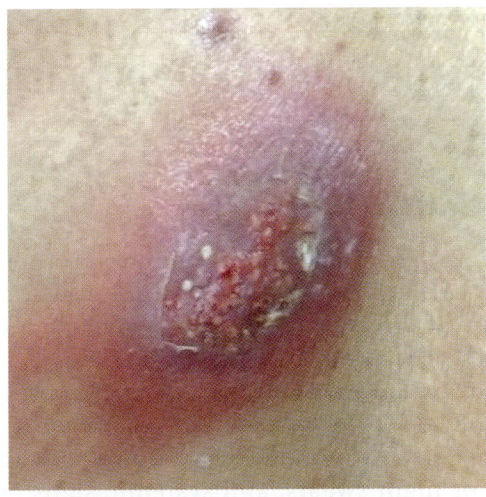

FIG. 1: Tender, erythematous, swollen mass over the nape of the neck (~5 cm in diameter) with multiple pustular openings and sinus tracts exuding purulent discharge; surrounding skin appears warm, inflamed, and indurated.

■ INVESTIGATION

- Complete blood count showed leukocytosis consistent with infection.
- Blood glucose and HbA1c levels were elevated, confirming poor glycemic control.
- Pus culture and sensitivity identified (e.g., *Staphylococcus aureus*) as the causative organism.
- Ultrasound of the lesion revealed a complex abscess with multiple interconnected loculations consistent with a carbuncle.

■ DIAGNOSIS

- Carbuncle
- The diagnosis of carbuncle was established based on the clinical presentation of a painful, swollen mass with multiple pustular openings and purulent discharge, supported by examination findings and investigations.[1]

■ DIFFERENTIAL DIAGNOSIS

- *Furuncle:* Single inflamed follicular nodule with central pus point
- *Hidradenitis suppurativa:* Recurrent nodules in apocrine-rich areas; chronic relapsing course
- *Cutaneous abscess:* Localized pus collection without multiple draining points
- *Necrotizing fasciitis:* Rapidly progressive with systemic toxicity and subcutaneous emphysema
- *Epidermoid cyst with secondary infection:* Central punctum with cheesy discharge; lacks sieve-like discharge[1,2]

■ PATHOPHYSIOLOGY

Diabetes impairs neutrophil function, microvascular perfusion, and skin barrier integrity.[3] *Staphylococcus aureus* is the most common causative organism; Methicillin-resistant Staphylococcus aureus (MRSA) may be involved.[3-5] Carbuncles often begin as furuncles and expand due to deep dermal and subcutaneous tissue involvement.[2-4]

MANAGEMENT

Dermatology Management

- *Local care*: Warm compresses, incision and drainage (I and D), and topical antibiotics like mupirocin or fusidic acid[1,2,6]
- *Wound care*: Daily dressing and decolonization (especially in MRSA cases)[5,6]

Diabetology/Physician Management

- *Antibiotics*: Start empiric therapy; adjust based on culture results[1,3,4]
- *Glycemic optimization*: Intensify anti-diabetic therapy and monitor blood sugar levels[3,4,6]
- *Education*: Emphasize skin hygiene and regular glucose control to prevent recurrence[6]

PROGNOSIS

Carbuncles generally heal within 10–14 days with proper antibiotics and wound care. However, poor glycemic control may increase the risk of complications such as cellulitis, sepsis, or recurrence.[3,4]

> **Clinical Pearls**
> - Sieve-like pus discharge is characteristic of a carbuncle.[2,4]
> - Always screen for diabetes or immunosuppression in recurrent skin infections.[1,2,5]
> - Early intervention prevents complications.[3,5]
> - Reinforce foot and skin hygiene in diabetic patients.[1,6]

REFERENCES

1. Jain AKC, Nisha ST, Viswanath S. Carbuncle in Diabetics – Our Experience. Sch J Appl Med Sci. 2013;1(5):493-5.
2. Troxell T, Hall CA. (2023). Carbuncle. [online] Available from https://www.ncbi.nlm.nih.gov/books/NBK554459/. [Last accessed August, 2025]
3. Sahin A, Aydına F, Kellecia Y, Canturk MT. Massive carbuncle in a patient with diabetes mellitus. J Exp Clin Med. 2019;36(1):31-3.
4. Venkatesan R, Baskaran R, Asirvatham AR, Mahadevan S. 'Carbuncle in diabetes': a problem even today! BMJ Case Rep. 2017;2017:bcr2017220628.
5. Wang X, Zhu F, Tang H, Xiao S, Hu X. Treatment for Giant Nape Carbuncle Complicated by Diabetic Ketoacidosis and Sepsis: A Case Report and Literature Review. Open Access Emerg Med. 2021;13:619.
6. Jain AKC. "Carbuncle Is an Uncle of Furuncle" – A Case Report. EAS J Med Surg. 2019;6(1):175-6.

Part F: Cutaneous Nontuberculous Mycobacterium Infections in Diabetes

PRESENTATION

A 42-year-old male laborer with an 18-year history of type 2 diabetes mellitus, on Mixtard and plain insulin for 2.5 years, presented with low-grade fever, painful swelling, and pus discharge from insulin injection sites. The lesions had persisted for 1 month. Clinical examination revealed nonhealing nodules and plaques, abscesses, and draining sinuses at the injection sites. Chronic ulcerated or granulomatous lesions were observed, often mimicking cellulitis or panniculitis. These lesions were notably refractory to conventional antibiotics.

EXAMINATION

- On examination, multiple tender, erythematous nodules, and plaques were noted at the insulin injection sites, with discharging sinuses and evidence of abscess formation **(Fig. 1)**.
- Chronic, nonhealing ulcers with features of granulomatous inflammation were present.
- There were no constitutional symptoms such as weight loss or night sweats, and systemic signs of acute infection were absent.

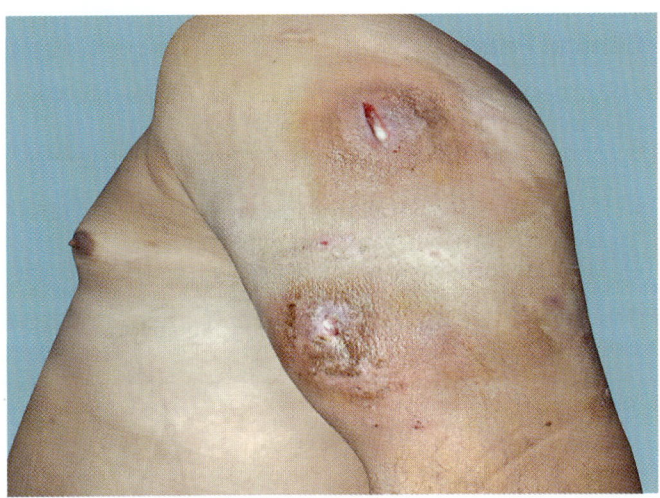

FIG. 1: Multiple tender, erythematous nodules and plaques at insulin injection sites, with discharging sinuses and abscess formation.

INVESTIGATIONS

- *Histopathology:* Biopsy from two different sites showed suppurative granulomatous inflammation, with or without necrosis.
- *Microbiology:* Mycobacterial culture on Lowenstein–Jensen medium or automated BACTEC systems confirmed the organism. Polymerase chain reaction (PCR) was used for species-level confirmation.
- *Immunological tests:* Both interferon-gamma release assay (IGRA) and Mantoux tests were negative.
- *Imaging:* Ultrasonography or MRI was performed when deeper or poorly resolving lesions were suspected.

PATHOPHYSIOLOGY

Cutaneous nontuberculous mycobacterium (NTM) infections are caused by environmental mycobacteria such as *Mycobacterium fortuitum*, *Mycobacteroides abscessus*, *Mycobacteroides chelonae*, and *Mycobacterium marinum*. Transmission typically occurs through direct skin inoculation, including injections, trauma, or surgery, and can also result from contaminated medical equipment. Diabetes increases susceptibility due to immune dysfunction (impaired neutrophil and macrophage function), chronic inflammation, and poor wound healing with compromised skin integrity.[1-3] The incidence of cutaneous NTM infections has been rising globally, with regional epidemiological data from Alberta, Canada, highlighting a growing burden, particularly among immunocompromised individuals such as diabetics.[4]

DIAGNOSIS

- The final diagnosis was cutaneous nontuberculous mycobacterial infection at insulin injection sites.
- This was confirmed by histopathological evidence of granulomatous inflammation, along with positive mycobacterial culture and PCR for species identification.[1,2,5]

DIFFERENTIAL DIAGNOSIS

- *Bacterial abscess:* Usually presents with acute onset, more pronounced inflammation, and rapid progression. Commonly caused by *Staphylococcus* or *Streptococcus* species.[1,5]
- *Fungal infections:* Conditions such as sporotrichosis or blastomycosis may present similarly but often have a history of trauma and distinct morphological features.[1,5]
- *Cutaneous tuberculosis:* Typically shows slower progression, may be associated with constitutional symptoms, and is usually positive for IGRA or Mantoux tests.[1,5]
- *Actinomycosis:* Characterized by sinus tracts and the presence of sulfur granules.[1,5]
- *Pyoderma gangrenosum:* Presents as painful, undermined ulcers and is often associated with systemic disease.[1,5]

MANAGEMENT

Dermatology Management

Antibiotic therapy is tailored to the specific NTM species:
- For *M. abscessus* and MAC, at least three drugs are used for 6–12 months.[1,2,6]
- For *M. chelonae* and *M. fortuitum*, at least two drugs are administered for a minimum of 4 months.[1,2,6]
- For *M. marinum*, therapy lasts 3–4 months or until 1–2 months after symptom resolution.[1,2,6]
- Newer agents such as bedaquiline, omadacycline, tedizolid, and linezolid may be considered for resistant cases.[1,2,6]

Surgical intervention is indicated for deep necrotic lesions, persistent sinuses, or when medical therapy fails. Procedures include incision and drainage, debridement, or excision.[1,2,6,7]

Diabetology/Physician Management

- Optimizing glycemic control is essential, involving tailored insulin regimens and frequent glucose

monitoring, which supports healing and prevents recurrence.
- Patients should be educated on injection hygiene—using clean sites, changing needles, rotating injection sites, and avoiding reuse of syringes or needles. Monitoring for systemic spread is crucial, especially in immunosuppressed individuals.[1,3,7,8]

■ PROGNOSIS

With early diagnosis and targeted therapy, the prognosis is generally good. Delayed or misdiagnosed cases can lead to chronic discharging sinuses and deeper tissue involvement. Recurrence is possible if glycemic control or injection practices remain suboptimal.[1,3,5]

> **Clinical Pearls**
> - Suspect cutaneous NTM in diabetics with nonhealing injection site nodules or abscesses.[1,3,5]
> - Always biopsy persistent, nonresponsive lesions in diabetic patients.[1,3,5]
> - Chronic granulomas with negative Mantoux and IGRA suggest NTM rather than tuberculosis.[1,3,5]
> - Strict aseptic technique and optimal glycemic control are crucial for prevention.[1,3]
> - Employ species-directed multidrug therapy to prevent resistance and recurrence.[1,2,6]

REFERENCES

1. Lamb RC, Dawn G. Cutaneous nontuberculous mycobacterial infections: a review. Int J Dermatol. 2014;53(10):1197-204.
2. Bridson T, Govan B, Ketheesan N, Norton R. Overrepresentation of Diabetes in Soft Tissue Nontuberculous Mycobacterial Infections. Am J Trop Med Hygiene. 2016;95(3):528-30.
3. Jeon DS, Kim S, Kim MA, Chong YP, Shim TS, Jung CH, et al. Type 2 Diabetes Mellitus- and Complication-Related Risk of Nontuberculous Mycobacterial Disease in a South Korean Cohort. Microbiol Spectr. 2023;11(2):e0451122.
4. Sander MA, Isaac-Renton JL, Tyrrell GJ. Cutaneous Nontuberculous Mycobacterial Infections in Alberta, Canada: An Epidemiologic Study and Review. J Cutan Med Surq. 2018;22(5):479-83.
5. Li JJ, Beresford R, Fyfe JAM, Henderson C. Clinical and histopathological features of cutaneous nontuberculous mycobacterial infection: a review of 13 cases. J Cutan Pathol. 2017;44(5):433-43.
6. Wang JY, Lin HC, Lin HA, Chung CH, Chen LC, Huang KY, et al. Associations between Diabetes Mellitus and Nontuberculous Mycobacterium-Caused Diseases in Taiwan: A Nationwide Cohort Study. Am J Trop Med Hyg. 2021;105(6):1672-9.
7. Chung J, Ince D, Ford BA, Wanat KA. Mycobacterium: Recognition and Management. Am J Clin Dermatol. 2018;19:867-78.

Part G: Necrotizing Skin and Soft Tissue Infections in Uncontrolled Diabetes

■ PRESENTATION

A 52-year-old female with a 10-year history of poorly controlled type-2 diabetes mellitus presented with multiple painful, necrotic ulcers and purulent discharge on both lower legs for 3 weeks. The lesions were progressively enlarging, associated with low-grade fever, malaise, and a foul smell. No history of trauma was elicited. The patient had a background of hypertension (4 years) and was irregular with medications (metformin, glimepiride). She led a sedentary lifestyle, and her BMI was 30.2 kg/m².

■ EXAMINATION

Inspection

Multiple punched-out ulcers with necrotic slough and purulent discharge on the right leg, smaller necrotic papulonodular lesions on the left leg, perilesional induration, signs of cellulitis, hyperpigmentation, and ecchymosis **(Fig. 1)**. Healing scars were observed on the medial ankle.

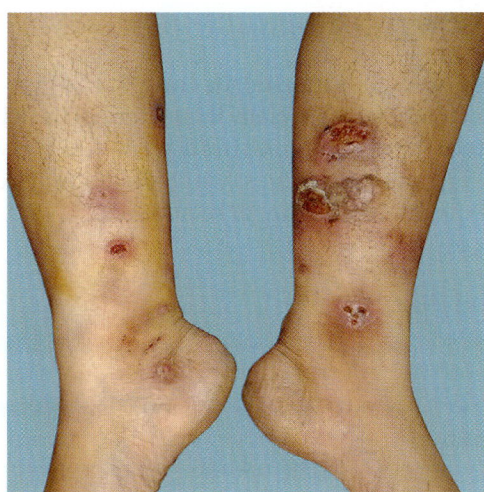

FIG. 1: Multiple punched-out ulcers with necrotic slough and purulent discharge on the right leg, along with smaller necrotic papulonodular lesions on the left leg.

Palpation

Areas were warm and tender with firm induration, no crepitus or fluctuant areas.

■ INVESTIGATIONS

Laboratory Results

- *Glycated hemoglobin (HbA1c)*: 10.6%
- *Random blood sugar (RBS)*: 328 mg/dL
- *White blood cell (WBC)*: 17,800/mm³ (neutrophilic leukocytosis)
- *C-reactive protein (CRP)*: 168 mg/L; erythrocyte sedimentation rate (ESR): 72 mm/h; Procalcitonin: Elevated
- *Renal function*: Mild uremia

Microbiology

Pus culture and sensitivity revealed polymicrobial growth (*Escherichia coli*, *Klebsiella*, and anaerobes). Blood cultures were negative.

Imaging

- *X-ray*: No evidence of osteomyelitis
- *Doppler*: Mild atherosclerosis, normal venous flow
- *Magnetic resonance imaging (MRI)*: Features of fasciitis, no evidence of gas or abscess

■ PATHOPHYSIOLOGY

- Chronic hyperglycemia compromises the host defense and tissue integrity, leading to necrotizing infections.[1,2]
- Microvascular ischemia reduces tissue perfusion and causes hypoxia, making the area susceptible to infection.[1,3]
- Sensory neuropathy diminishes pain perception, allowing trauma and wounds to go unnoticed and untreated.[4]
- Hyperglycemia promotes bacterial growth and polymicrobial invasion.[4]
- Together, these factors facilitate the progression of minor wounds into severe necrotizing soft tissue infections (NSTIs).[1,2,4]

■ DIAGNOSIS

- *Primary diagnosis*: Diabetic neuroischemic skin ulcers with superimposed NSTI[1,4]
- *Probable type*: Nonclostridial polymicrobial necrotizing fasciitis/ecthyma gangrenosum-like lesions[2,3]

■ DIFFERENTIAL DIAGNOSIS

- *Pyoderma gangrenosum*: A neutrophilic dermatosis presenting as painful, rapidly progressing ulcers with violaceous borders, usually associated with systemic disease[3]
- *Ecthyma gangrenosum*: Caused by *Pseudomonas aeruginosa*, presenting as necrotic, crater-like ulcers with a black eschar[1]
- *Cellulitis*: A superficial soft tissue infection presenting with erythema, warmth, and tenderness, typically without deep necrosis[5]
- *Cutaneous mucormycosis*: A deep fungal infection presenting as black, necrotic eschars due to angioinvasion and tissue infarction[4]
- *Vasculitic ulcers*: Ulcers caused by small or medium vessel vasculitis, often associated with purpura and systemic signs of vasculitis[3]

■ MANAGEMENT

Surgical/Wound Care

- Immediate and thorough surgical debridement of all necrotic tissue is essential.[1,5,6]

- Dressings with hydrogel or alginate help maintain a moist environment, while negative pressure wound therapy (NPWT) can be added later to support granulation.[7,8] Skin grafting may be required for defect closure.[8]

Antibiotic Therapy

- Start broad-spectrum IV therapy (piperacillin-tazobactam, clindamycin, and metronidazole) and adjust based on culture results[1,5,6]
- Typically, a 2–3-week IV course is followed by an oral step-down regimen.[4,5]

Diabetologist's Role

- Initiation of a basal–bolus insulin regimen and intensive glucose monitoring every 4–6 hours are vital for optimizing blood glucose control.[4,7]
- Supportive fluid and electrolyte replacement, along with nutrition optimization, aid recovery and prevent complications.[7]

PROGNOSIS

The prognosis is guarded in long-standing, poorly controlled diabetes, especially if intervention is delayed.[1,4] Early debridement combined with tight glycemic control improves outcomes, while delays may result in disfigurement, amputation, or recurrence.[5,8]

Clinical Pearls

- Always suspect NSTI in any rapidly spreading diabetic ulcer.[2,5]
- Ensure anaerobic coverage when treating diabetic foot infections.[4,6]
- Do not delay surgical debridement for confirmatory imaging.[1,5,6]
- Early and intensive insulin therapy improves wound healing.[4,7]
- Chronic or atypical skin ulcers may be a sign of deeper systemic disease.[3,4]

REFERENCES

1. Stevens DL, Bryant AE. Necrotizing Soft-Tissue Infections. N Engl J Med. 2017;377(23):2253-65.
2. Das DK, Baker MG, Venugopal K. Necrotizing fasciitis: Diagnostic challenges and current practices. Infect Dis Health. 2020;25(3):182-8.
3. Anaya DA, Dellinger EP. Necrotizing soft-tissue infection: Diagnosis and management. Clin Infect Dis. 2007;44(5):705-10.
4. Boulton AJM, Armstrong DG, Albert S, Frykberg RG, Hellman R, Kirkman MS, et al. Comprehensive foot examination and risk assessment: a report of the task force of the foot care interest group of the American Diabetes Association, with endorsement by the American Association of Clinical Endocrinologists. Diabetes Care. 2008;31(8):1679-85.
5. Bonne SL, Kadri SS. Evaluation and management of necrotizing soft tissue infections. Infect Dis Clin North Am. 2017;31(3):497-511.
6. Sartelli M, Guirao X, Hardcastle TC, Kluger Y, Ansaloni L, Baiocchi G, et al. 2018 WSES consensus conference: guidelines for the management of skin and soft tissue infections. World J Emerg Surg. 2018;13:58.
7. Chishti S, Ghosh A, Singh AK. Management of diabetic foot ulcers: Current concepts and future directions. Curr Diabetes Rev. 2022;18(3):e030421196637.
8. Elraiyah T, Prutsky G, Domecq JP, Tsapas A, Nabhan M, Frykberg RG, et al. A systematic review and meta-analysis of débridement methods for chronic diabetic foot ulcers. J Vasc Surg. 2016;63(2 Suppl):37S-45S.e2.

CHAPTER 20

Viral Skin Infections in Diabetes: Hemorrhagic Herpes Zoster (Multidermatomal) in an Uncontrolled Diabetic Patient

Bela J Shah

■ PRESENTATION

A 46-year-old woman, a homemaker by occupation, presented with a 2-day history of painful, fluid-filled lesions over the left thigh. The lesions were associated with mild burning and pain. She had a 14-year history of type-2 diabetes mellitus and dyslipidemia, managed with metformin (500 mg) twice daily, glimepiride (1 mg) once daily, and atorvastatin (40 mg) at bedtime. There were no systemic symptoms such as fever or malaise.

■ EXAMINATION FINDINGS

On examination, multiple grouped hemorrhagic vesicles and bullae were observed on an ecchymotic base, involving both dorsal (**Fig. 1**) and ventral aspects (**Fig. 2**) of the left thigh, indicating multidermatomal involvement (**Figs. 1 and 2**). The patient was obese (BMI: 32.1 kg/m²). Tzanck smear from a blister revealed a few acantholytic cells. There was no lymphadenopathy or evidence of systemic involvement.

Laboratory Investigations

- *Fasting blood glucose*: 258 mg/dL
- *Postprandial blood glucose*: 307 mg/dL
- *glycated hemoglobin (HbA1c)*: 10.3%
- *Viral markers (HBsAg, HCV, HIV)*: Nonreactive
- *Complete blood count, liver and renal function tests, thyroid profile*: Within normal limits

■ DIAGNOSIS

The diagnosis is multidermatomal hemorrhagic herpes zoster in a patient with uncontrolled diabetes mellitus.[1-3]

■ DIFFERENTIAL DIAGNOSES

- *Purpura fulminans:* Rapidly progressive purpuric rash with systemic toxicity
- *Contact dermatitis:* Pruritic, often bilateral, not following a dermatomal pattern

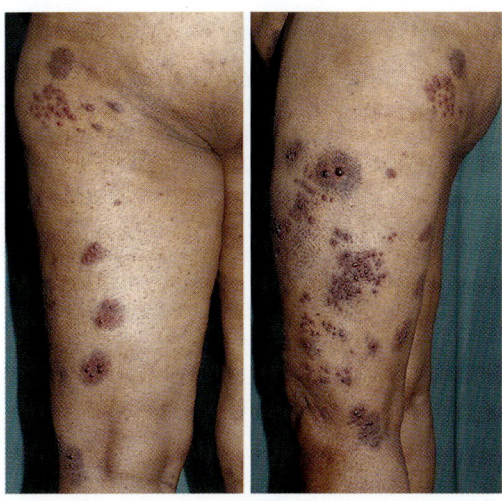

FIG. 1: Grouped hemorrhagic vesicles and bullae on an ecchymotic base involving the dorsal aspect of the left thigh.

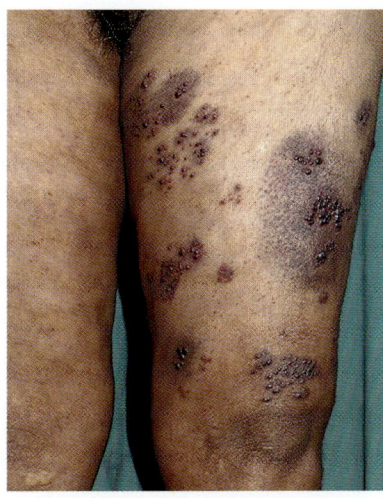

FIG. 2: Grouped hemorrhagic vesicles and bullae with surrounding ecchymosis involving the ventral aspect of the left thigh.

- *Herpes simplex virus infection*: May mimic but typically localized and not dermatomal
- *Bullous impetigo*: More common in children, with honey-colored crusts
- *Insect bite hypersensitivity*: Localized, edematous, and nondermatomal
- *Fixed drug eruption*: Recurrent, sharply demarcated plaques, often at the same site
- *Anticoagulant-induced cutaneous necrosis (warfarin, heparin):* Necrotic lesions after starting anticoagulant therapy[1,4]

MANAGEMENT

Dermatology/Infectious Disease Management

- *Oral antiviral therapy:* Acyclovir 800 mg five times daily for 7–10 days[4,5]
- *Topical antibiotic:* Fusidic acid 2% cream, applied twice daily over ruptured lesions to prevent secondary infection[4]
- *Pain management:* Paracetamol for mild pain; oral pregabalin may be considered for persistent pain or burning sensation
- *Monitoring:* Watch for signs of secondary bacterial infection or dissemination, especially in immunocompromised patients[3,4]

Diabetology/Physician Management

- *Glycemic control:* Intensified diabetes regimen with metformin 500 mg three times daily and glimepiride 1 mg once daily; atorvastatin 40 mg at bedtime continued[2]
- *Lifestyle modification:* Dietary advice, regular self-monitoring of blood glucose, and patient education on infection risk[2]
- *Complication screening:* Referral for evaluation of diabetic retinopathy, nephropathy, and neuropathy[2]

PROGNOSIS

Herpes zoster generally has a favorable outcome in immunocompetent individuals.[6] However, in patients with diabetes, especially those with poor glycemic control, the disease may present with more extensive, multidermatomal, and hemorrhagic lesions, and a prolonged course. The risk of developing postherpetic neuralgia (PHN) is higher in diabetic patients, particularly with severe or delayed presentations. Early initiation of antiviral therapy within 72 hours of rash onset reduces the risk of complications and speeds recovery.[4,5]

Clinical Pearls

- Herpes zoster results from reactivation of latent varicella zoster virus (VZV) in sensory ganglia.[1,4]
- The classic rash consists of grouped vesicles on an erythematous base, typically following a dermatomal distribution.
- Diabetic patients are at increased risk for atypical presentations, including multidermatomal and hemorrhagic forms, due to impaired immunity.[2,7]
- Poor glycemic control is associated with more severe disease and a higher likelihood of PHN, defined as pain persisting for more than 3 months after rash resolution.[2,4]
- Hemorrhagic vesicles in a zosteriform pattern are uncommon and may indicate underlying vascular fragility or immune dysfunction, often related to diabetes.[1-3]

REFERENCES

1. Oxman MN. Herpes zoster pathogenesis and cell-mediated immunity and immunosenescence. J Am Osteopath Assoc. 2009;109(6 Suppl 2):S13-7.
2. Schmader K, Dworkin RH. The epidemiology and natural history of herpes zoster and postherpetic neuralgia. Herpes. 2008;15(Suppl 2):3A-7A.
3. Cohen JI. Herpes zoster. N Engl J Med. 2013;369(3):255-63.
4. Johnson RW, Rice AS. Clinical practice: Postherpetic neuralgia. N Engl J Med. 2014;371(16):1526-33.
5. Ke CC, Lai HC, Lin CH, Hung CJ, Chen DY, Sheu WHH, et al. Increased risk of herpes zoster in diabetic patients comorbid with coronary artery disease and microvascular disorders: a population-based study in Taiwan. PLoS One. 2016;11(1):e0146750.
6. Schmader KE. Herpes zoster in older adults. Clin Infect Dis. 2001;32(10):1481-6.
7. Kawai K, Gebremeskel BG, Acosta CJ. Systematic review of incidence and complications of herpes zoster: towards a global perspective. BMJ Open. 2014;4(6):e004833.

SECTION 5

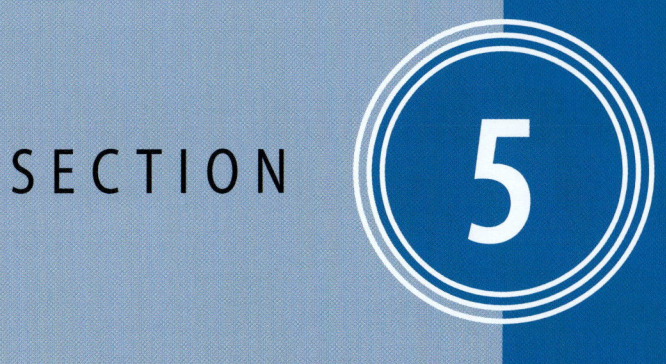

Rare Dermatological Manifestations of Diabetes (Musculoskeletal and Connective Tissue Manifestations in Diabetes)

▶ Section Outline

- **Chapter 21: Diabetic Cheiroarthropathy (Diabetic Hand Syndrome/Stiff Skin Syndrome) in Long-standing Diabetes**
  Suhas Gopal Erande, Anil Patki
- **Chapter 22: Scleredema Diabeticorum (Diabetic Scleroderma)**
  Suhas Gopal Erande
- **Chapter 23: Granuloma Annulare in Diabetes**
  Firdous Shaikh, Avina Jain, Bela J Shah, Akashkumar N Singh, Anuradha Kapoor, Ruchi Shah, Yogesh Marfatia
- **Chapter 24: Eruptive Xanthomas in Uncontrolled Diabetes Mellitus**
  NK Singh, Akashkumar N Singh, Anuradha Kapoor
- **Chapter 25: Abdominal Pseudohernia due to Diabetic Truncal Neuropathy**
  Santosh B
- **Chapter 26: Porphyria Cutanea Tarda in Patients with Type 2 Diabetes Mellitus**
  Suhas Gopal Erande, Anil Patki

CHAPTER 21

Diabetic Cheiroarthropathy (Diabetic Hand Syndrome/Stiff Skin Syndrome) in Long-standing Diabetes

Suhas Gopal Erande, Anil Patki

■ PRESENTATION

A 55-year-old man with a 16-year history of type 2 diabetes mellitus (T2DM) presented with progressive stiffness and reduced mobility of his fingers over the past year. He reported difficulty in fully extending or opposing his fingers but denied any pain, swelling, or prior trauma. There was no history suggestive of arthritis. His medical history included diabetic neuropathy. He was on irregular insulin along with metformin and glimepiride.

■ EXAMINATION

On inspection and palpation of the hands, the following features were noted:
- Waxy thickening of the skin over the dorsum of left hand **(Fig. 1)**.

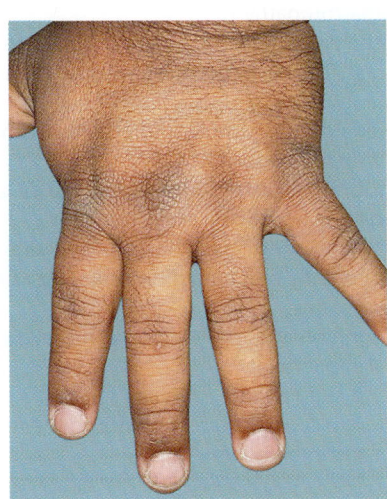

FIG. 1: Waxy thickening of the skin over the dorsum of left hand with prominent skin creases over the proximal interphalangeal (PIP) joints.

- Prominent skin creases over the proximal interphalangeal (PIP) joints.
- No evidence of swelling, inflammation, or joint tenderness.
- Findings suggestive of limited joint mobility (LJM), consistent with diabetic cheiroarthropathy.

■ INVESTIGATION

Relevant laboratory tests, imaging, and clinical assessments were performed to support the diagnosis and rule out other causes:

Laboratory Tests
- *Glycated hemoglobin (HbA1c)*: 9.8% (poor glycemic control)
- *Fasting blood glucose*: 164 mg/dL
- *Postprandial blood glucose*: 289 mg/dL
- *Erythrocyte sedimentation rate (ESR) and C-reactive protein (CRP)*: Normal
- *Antinuclear antibody (ANA) and rheumatoid factor*: Negative
- *Thyroid stimulating hormone (TSH)*: Normal

Imaging
X-ray: No joint er show thickened tendon sheaths

Clinical Tests
Positive prayer sign or tabletop sign (if performed), supporting the diagnosis of LJM

PATHOPHYSIOLOGY

In diabetic cheiroarthropathy, chronic hyperglycemia results in nonenzymatic glycation of collagen, leading to cross-linking and increased stiffness of dermal and periarticular collagen. This process causes thickening of tendon sheaths, reduced skin extensibility, and restricted joint mobility. The condition is estimated to affect approximately 30% of individuals with long-standing diabetes mellitus.[1-4]

DIAGNOSIS

Diabetic cheiroarthropathy (also known as LJM or stiff hand syndrome).

The patient's clinical presentation of waxy skin thickening, prominent finger creases, and restricted joint mobility, along with supportive findings on laboratory tests and imaging, is consistent with diabetic cheiroarthropathy (also known as LJM or stiff hand syndrome).[1,2,5]

This condition, sometimes referred to as diabetic scleredema or diabetic hand syndrome, is a well-recognized musculoskeletal complication of long-standing diabetes mellitus.[1-4]

DIFFERENTIAL DIAGNOSIS

Several conditions can mimic the clinical features of diabetic cheiroarthropathy and should be considered during evaluation:
- *Scleroderma:* Raynaud's phenomenon, positive ANA.
- *Rheumatoid arthritis (RA):* Swelling of metacarpal phalangeal (MCP) and proximal interphalangeal (PIP) joints and morning stiffness.
- *Dupuytren's contracture:* Palmar cord thickening.
- *Hypothyroidism:* Puffy hands and elevated TSH.
- *Tenosynovitis:* Localized swelling and tenderness of the tendon sheath.[1-3,5]

MANAGEMENT

Management of diabetic cheiroarthropathy requires a multidisciplinary approach involving dermatologists, orthopedicians, and diabetologists to improve joint function and metabolic control.[1-3,5]

Dermatologist/Orthopedician Management

- Physiotherapy, including stretching exercises and wax bath therapy, to improve joint mobility.[1-3,5]
- Topical emollients to manage associated dry skin and maintain skin integrity.[1-3]

Diabetologist/Physician Management

- Optimize glycemic control through appropriate adjustments in therapy, including consideration of insulin or glucagon-like peptide-1 (GLP-1) receptor agonists.[1-3]
- Regular monitoring for other microvascular complications, such as retinopathy and nephropathy.

PROGNOSIS

- The prognosis of diabetic cheiroarthropathy is generally favorable if identified early.[1-3]
- Nonprogressive if detected and managed in the early stages.[1-3]
- Partial improvement is achievable with good glycemic control and regular physiotherapy.
- While not life-threatening, the condition can significantly impair hand function if left untreated.[1-3]

Clinical Pearls

Key points to remember in the evaluation and management of diabetic cheiroarthropathy"
- ▶ Always check for LJM in patients with long-standing diabetes, as it may signal the presence of other microvascular complications.[1-3,5]
- ▶ The prayer sign is a simple and effective clinical tool to detect LJM at the bedside.[2,3,5]
- ▶ The condition is often misdiagnosed as arthritis or attributed to aging.[1-3]
- ▶ There is a strong association between diabetic cheiroarthropathy and complications such as retinopathy and nephropathy.[1-3]
- ▶ Early recognition and intervention can prevent significant functional impairment.[5]
- ▶ Studies also suggest that LJM may serve as a predictor for diabetic foot ulcers, further emphasizing the need for early detection and intervention.[6]

REFERENCES

1. Rosenbloom AL. Limited joint mobility in diabetes mellitus. J Diabetes Complications. 2011;25(1):17-21.
2. Arkkila PE, Gautier JF. Musculoskeletal disorders in diabetes mellitus: an update. Best Pract Res Clin Rheumatol. 2003;17(6):945-70.
3. Smith LL, Burnet SP, McNeil JD. Musculoskeletal manifestations of diabetes mellitus. Br J Sports Med. 2003;37(1):30-35.
4. Gerrits EG, Landman GW, Nijenhuis-Rosien L, Bilo HJ. Limited joint mobility syndrome in diabetes mellitus: A minireview. World J Diabetes. 2015;6(9):1108-12.
5. Sugrue D, McEvoy M, Dempsey J, Fitzgerald G, Drury MI. Diabetic stiff hand syndrome. Ir J Med Sci. 1983;152(4):152-6.
6. Delbridge L, Perry P, Marr S, Arnold N, Yue DK, Turtle JR, Reeve TS. Limited joint mobility in the diabetic foot: relationship to neuropathic ulceration. Diabet Med. 1988;5(4):333-7.

CHAPTER 22

Scleredema Diabeticorum (Diabetic Scleroderma)

Suhas Gopal Erande

■ PRESENTATION

A 48-year-old woman with type 2 diabetes mellitus for approximately 18 years presented with a gradual onset of woody and nonpitting induration over her upper back and posterior neck. The affected skin had a "peau d'orange" (orange peel) texture with reduced pliability and limitation of neck and shoulder movements. The skin changes were mildly erythematous but asymptomatic, with no associated pain or itching.

- She had a history of obesity [body mass index (BMI) = 31 kg/m²] and poor glycemic control [glycated hemoglobin (HbA1c) ~9.0%].
- There was no history of preceding infections or monoclonal gammopathy.
- The patient also had diabetic peripheral neuropathy and mild diabetic retinopathy.

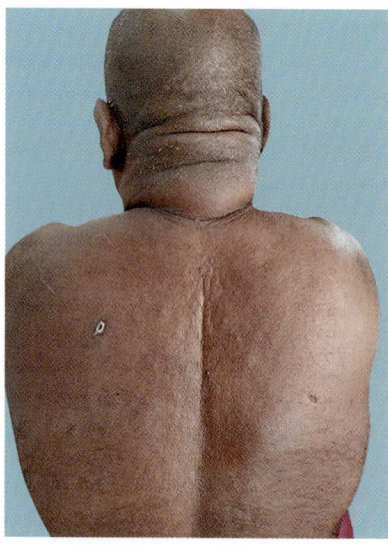

FIG. 1: Symmetrical, ill-defined, and firm plaques noted over the upper back and posterior neck on physical examination.

■ EXAMINATION

- On physical examination, there were symmetrical, ill-defined, firm plaques involving the upper back and posterior neck **(Fig. 1)**.
- The skin could not be pinched, and the induration extended bilaterally across the shoulders.
- There was no evidence of sclerodactyly or Raynaud's phenomenon, helping to rule out systemic sclerosis.

■ INVESTIGATIONS

- *The laboratory and supportive investigations showed:* HbA1c was elevated at 9.2%, indicating poor glycemic control.
- *Renal function tests* were within normal limits.
- *Serum protein electrophoresis* revealed no monoclonal protein bands, ruling out associated gammopathies.
- *Autoimmune screening* showed ANA negativity.
- *Further testing included:*
    - *Chest X-ray and spirometry,* both of which were normal.
    - *Skin biopsy* demonstrated marked dermal thickening with mucin deposition (Alcian blue-positive staining) and thickened collagen bundles without significant inflammation.

■ PATHOPHYSIOLOGY

Chronic hyperglycemia leads to nonenzymatic glycation of collagen, reducing collagenase activity and causing excessive accumulation of dermal collagen.[1]

Diabetic microangiopathy contributes through microvascular changes and tissue hypoxia, which stimulate fibroblast activation and mucopolysaccharide (mucin) deposition in the dermis.[1]

This condition is most commonly associated with long-standing, poorly controlled diabetes, obesity, and male gender, although it can also occur in females, as in this case.[1] Prevalence estimates suggest that approximately 2.5–14% of diabetic patients may develop this condition, particularly those on insulin or with diabetic complications.[1] Importantly, tight glycemic control typically does not reverse the established skin changes.[1,2]

DIAGNOSIS

This condition represents type 3 scleredema, which is strongly associated with long-standing, poorly controlled diabetes.[1]

Differential Diagnosis

- *Systemic sclerosis:* Characterized by sclerodactyly, Raynaud's phenomenon, and the presence of specific autoantibodies.[1]
- *Nephrogenic systemic fibrosis:* Typically seen after exposure to gadolinium-based contrast agents.[1]
- *Scleromyxedema:* Distinguished by systemic involvement, an associated monoclonal gammopathy, and mucin deposition predominantly in the upper dermis.[1]
- *Thyroid dermopathy:* Usually localized to the pretibial area and shows a different pattern of mucin deposition on histology.[1]

MANAGEMENT

Dermatologist Management

- Physical therapy to maintain musculoskeletal mobility and prevent joint contractures.[1-3]
- Topical or intralesional steroids provide limited benefit and rarely lead to significant improvement in symptoms.[1-3]
- Systemic therapy
- *Methotrexate:* Mixed outcomes with partial improvement in some cases.[1,2]
- *Tranilast (antifibrotic agent):* Successful use reported in small case series.[1,4]
- *Phototherapy [ultraviolet A1 (UVA-1)],* intravenous immunoglobulin, or radiotherapy [volumetric modulated arc therapy (VMAT)] may be considered for refractory cases, with some reported functional gains.[1-3,5,8]

Diabetologist/Physician Management

Maintain optimized glycemic control, aiming for a target HbA1c of <7%.[1,2]

Manage comorbidities such as hypertension, dyslipidemia, and obesity.[1,2]

Screen annually for monoclonal gammopathies, particularly if the condition shows atypical progression.[1,7]

PROGNOSIS

The condition is generally benign but chronic and permanent; while inflammatory signs may subside, the induration usually persists.[1,7]

Functional limitations can occur, especially involving neck and shoulder mobility, and in rare cases, restricted breathing.[1,7]

Relapse is common, so regular physical therapy is essential to preserve range of motion.[1-3]

> ### Clinical Pearls
>
> ▶ Suspect scleredema when symmetric, woody hardening of the skin develops over the upper back and neck in long-standing diabetic patients.[1,8]
> ▶ A skin biopsy helps to confirm the diagnosis by showing collagenous and mucinous dermal thickening, while serologic testing is useful to exclude mimics.[1,8]
> ▶ Glycemic improvement alone typically does not reverse sclerosis; a multimodal therapeutic approach is required.[1,2]
> ▶ Successful management integrates physical therapy, systemic agents such as methotrexate or tranilast, and advanced options like UVA-1 phototherapy or radiotherapy in select cases.[1-6]

REFERENCES

1. Fang C, et al. Scleredema diabeticorum – under-recognized complication? Practical Diabetology International. 2009;26(5):142-5.
2. Ranabahu M, Karunarathna W, Asanthi J, Dassanayake D, Senanayake H. Scleredema Diabeticorum: A rare metabolic connective tissue manifestation of type 2 diabetes mellitus causing external restrictive lung disease. Cureus. 2024;16(5):e60374.
3. Adachi M, et al. Scleredema diabeticorum in a patient with Type 2 Diabetes Mellitus. Case Reports in Medicine. 2012;2012:560273. doi:10.1155/2012/560273 [PMC] (pmc.ncbi.nlm.nih.gov)
4. McPherson T, Gru1mph JD. Scleredema diabeticorum partially treated with low-dose methotrexate. J Eur Acad Dermatol Venereol. 2014;28(7):928-32.

5. Sun M, Yang F, Hou M. Tranilast treatment: Successful Treatment of Scleredema Diabeticorum With Tranilast. Diabetes Care. 2018;41(4):e40-1.
6. Gracie JR, Whitaker R. Treatment-Refractory Scleredema Diabeticorum Managed With Radiation. Cureus. 2024;16(9):e69279.
7. Rongioletti F, Kaiser F, Cinotti E, Metze D, Battistella M, Calzavara-Pinton PG, et al. Scleredema: A multicentre study of characteristics, comorbidities, course and therapy in 44 patients. J Eur Acad Dermatol Venereol. 2015;29(12):2399-404.
8. eMedicine Medscape. (2024). Scleredema Treatment and Management. [online] Available from emedicine.medscape.com. [Last accessed August, 2025].

CHAPTER 23

Granuloma Annulare in Diabetes

Firdous Shaikh, Avina Jain, Bela J Shah, Akashkumar N Singh, Anuradha Kapoor, Ruchi Shah, Yogesh Marfatia

Case 1: Granuloma Annulare (Interstitial Type) Associated with Type 2 Diabetes Mellitus

■ PRESENTATION

A 40-year-old male schoolteacher presented with a 6-month history of mildly pruritic papules on both forearms. The lesions were persistent, unrelated to trauma or seasonal changes, and unresponsive to over-the-counter antihistamines and emollients.

There was no history of insect bites, photosensitivity, or systemic complaints such as fever or joint discomfort.

The patient had hypothyroidism for 10 years (on levothyroxine 75 µg daily) and was recently diagnosed with type 2 diabetes mellitus during routine screening.

■ EXAMINATION

Multiple flesh-colored to reddish papules were observed, merging to form annular plaques on both forearms **(Figs. 1A and B)**. The lesions showed no evidence of scaling, ulceration, or systemic involvement.

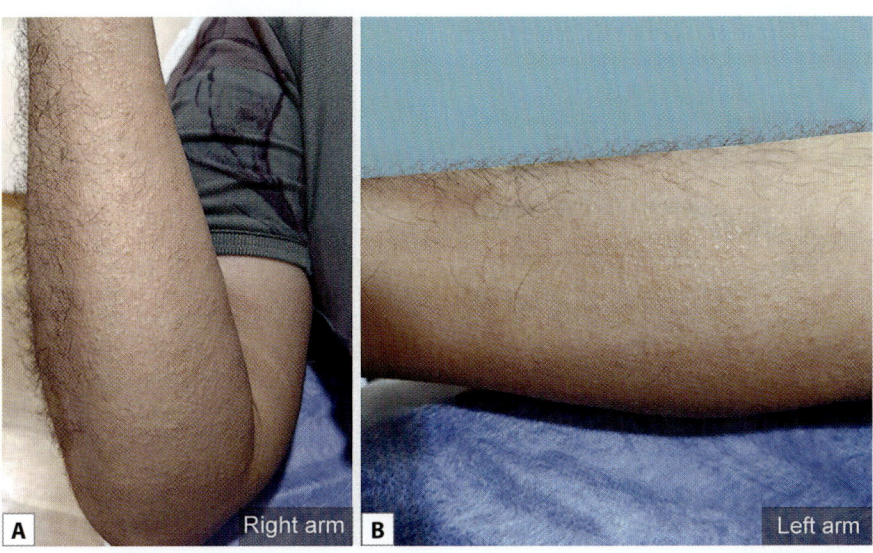

FIGS. 1A AND B: Multiple flesh-colored to reddish papules coalescing to form annular plaques on both forearms.

INVESTIGATIONS

- Type 2 diabetes mellitus was recently identified during routine screening.
- A skin biopsy was performed to confirm the clinical suspicion and exclude other conditions. Histopathology showed features characteristic of the interstitial variant of granuloma annulare (GA), including interstitial histiocytic infiltrates, mucin accumulation, and collagen breakdown.

DIAGNOSIS

Granuloma annulare (interstitial type) associated with type 2 diabetes mellitus. The diagnosis was confirmed by skin biopsy, which revealed interstitial histiocytic infiltrates, mucin accumulation, and collagen breakdown.[1-4]

DIFFERENTIAL DIAGNOSIS

- *Polymorphic light eruption:* Ruled out due to the lack of photosensitivity and localized distribution.
- *Papular urticaria:* Excluded as there was no history of insect exposure or recurrent episodes.
- *Lichen nitidus:* Not considered due to the absence of shiny, flat-topped, and pinpoint papules.

MANAGEMENT

Management by a Dermatologist

- Initiated topical corticosteroids to reduce inflammation and control pruritus.[2,5]
- For persistent lesions, oral isotretinoin 10 mg/day was prescribed under monitoring.[2,6]
- Emphasized that improved glycemic control may aid resolution of skin findings.[7]

Management by a diabetologist or physician. Patient referred after dermatological diagnosis.

- Initiated metformin SR 500 mg once daily [glycated hemoglobin (HbA1c) = 6.2% and serum creatinine = 0.9].
- *Advised lifestyle modification:* Diet, exercise, and weight control.
- Scheduled follow-up with HbA1c, lipid profile, liver function test (LFT), and thyroid function tests at 3 months.

PROGNOSIS

Granuloma annulare is often self-limiting.[1,3] In this case, partial remission was observed over 1–2 years, likely due to improved blood sugar control and the natural disease course.[7] Chronic or recurring cases may persist but generally remain localized and nondestructive.[5,6]

Clinical Pearls

- Interstitial GA is an uncommon skin condition, sometimes linked to diabetes and hypothyroidism.[4,7]
- Typically appears as itchy, ring-shaped papules on the limbs, and can be mistaken for eczema or urticaria.[3,5]
- Biopsy is essential for accurate diagnosis.[1,4] Systemic associations may include diabetes, autoimmune thyroid disease, and sometimes lipid disorders.[4,7]
- Skin lesions may resolve on their own or with improved metabolic control and anti-inflammatory therapy.[2,6]

REFERENCES

1. Dabski K, Winkelmann RK. Generalized granuloma annulare: clinical and laboratory findings in 100 patients. J Am Acad Dermatol. 1989;20(1):39-47.
2. Lukács J, Schliemann S, Elsner P. Treatment of generalized granuloma annulare - a systematic review. J Eur Acad Dermatol Venereol. 2015;29(8):1467-80.
3. Khalifa ES, Thamir AK, Inas KS. Granuloma annulare as a leading mimicking granulomatous disease: Clinical and histopathological study in a series of 47 cases. Journal of Pakistan Association of Dermatologists. JPAD. 2024;34(4):938-46.
4. Piette EW, Rosenbach M. Granuloma annulare: Pathogenesis, disease associations and triggers, and therapeutic options. J Am Acad Dermatol. 2016;75(3):467-9.
5. Keimig EL. Granuloma Annulare. Dermatol Clin. 2015;33(3):315-29.
6. Joshi TP, Duvic M. Granuloma Annulare: An Updated Review of Epidemiology, Pathogenesis, and Treatment Options. Am J Clin Dermatol. 2022;23(1):37-50.
7. Barbieri JS, Rosenbach M, Rodriguez O, Margolis DJ. Association of Granuloma Annulare With Type 2 Diabetes, Hyperlipidemia, Autoimmune Disorders, and Hematologic Malignant Neoplasms. JAMA Dermatol. 2021;157(7):817-23.

Case 2: Granuloma Annulare in a Diabetic Male Associated with Glycemic Control

■ PRESENTATION

A 34-year-old male businessman came with a 4-month history of pruritic, red skin lesions that had developed over his forehead, neck, trunk, back, and both upper and lower limbs. The number and size of these lesions had progressively increased. He did not report systemic symptoms such as fever, weight loss, or joint pain. His medical background included type 2 diabetes mellitus, for which he was taking metformin 500 mg twice daily for the last 2 years.[1]

■ EXAMINATION

- On examination, there were multiple annular papules and plaques, some discrete and others merging, with elevated borders, present over the forehead (**Fig. 2**), trunk (**Fig. 3**), neck (**Fig. 4**), back (**Fig. 5**), and extremities.
- No mucosal surfaces were involved.
- Lesions appeared erythematous and were pruritic.[1]

Laboratory Findings

- *Fasting blood glucose:* 156 mg/dL
- *Postprandial blood glucose:* 285 mg/dL
- *Glycated hemoglobin (HbA1c):* 8.1%, reflecting poor glycemic control
- *Complete blood count, liver and renal function tests, and lipid profile:* Within normal range
- *Serological tests for hepatitis B, hepatitis C, and HIV:* Negative.[1]

■ HISTOPATHOLOGY

A 4-mm punch biopsy from a lesion on the back revealed palisaded granulomas with central mucinous necrobiotic collagen, surrounded by lymphocytes, histiocytes, and multinucleated giant cells. These findings confirmed the diagnosis of GA.[1]

■ DIAGNOSIS

Disseminated GA associated with uncontrolled type 2 diabetes mellitus.[1,2]

■ DIFFERENTIAL DIAGNOSIS

- Tinea corporis
- Erythema annulare centrifugum
- Annular lichen planus

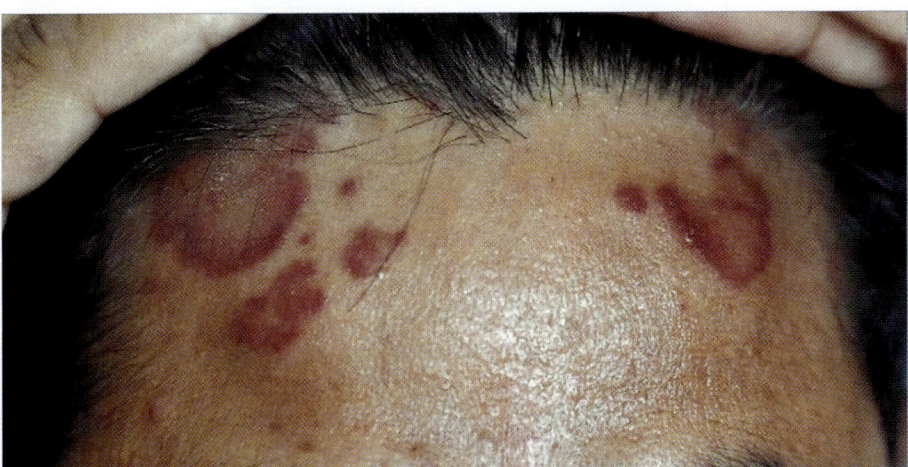

FIG. 2: Multiple annular papules and plaques with elevated borders over the forehead.

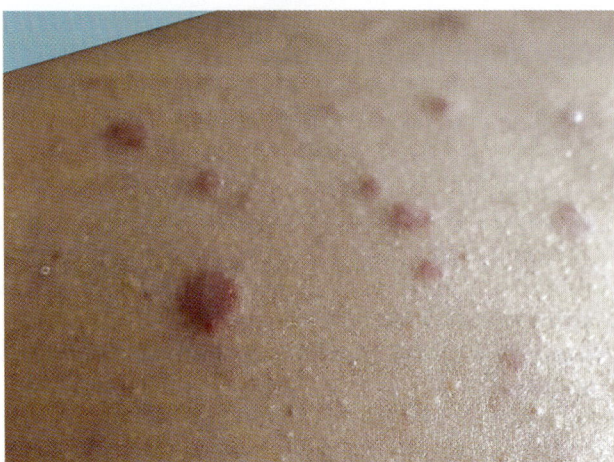

FIG. 3: Similar lesions involving the trunk.

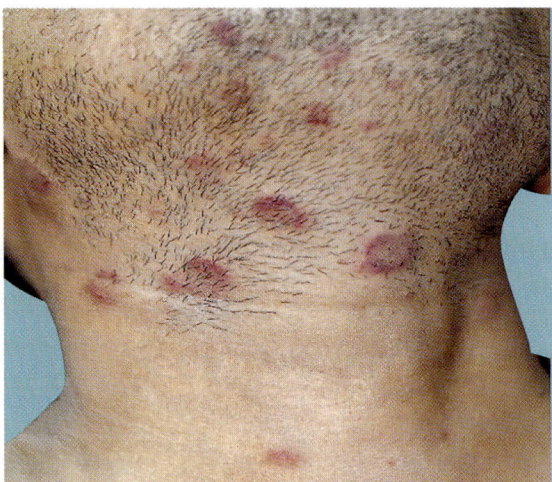

FIG. 4: Annular papules and plaques with coalescence noted over the neck.

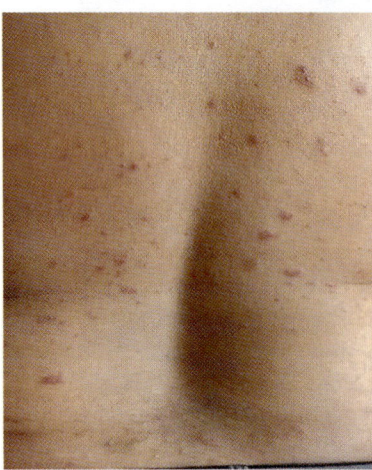

FIG. 5: Discrete and merging annular lesions seen over the back.

- Porokeratosis
- Secondary syphilis
- Erythema multiforme
- Annular elastolytic giant cell granuloma
- Cutaneous sarcoidosis[1,3]

MANAGEMENT

- *Dermatologic therapy:* Isotretinoin was started at 0.1 mg/kg/day for 3 months, with regular monitoring of liver function and lipid profile.[4,5]
- *Diabetes care:* The antidiabetic regimen was intensified to metformin 500 mg three times daily and glimepiride 1 mg once daily, in consultation with a physician.[6]
- *Supportive care:* Emollients were prescribed to maintain skin hydration and reduce pruritus.[1]
- *Monitoring:* The patient was reviewed monthly to assess response to treatment and monitor for adverse effects.[4,5]
- The management plan was guided by the treatment algorithm for GA described by Pathave et al. (Turk J Dermatol, 2020).[6]

PROGNOSIS

With better glycemic control and systemic therapy, the patient's skin lesions resolved fully within 3 months, leaving only mild postinflammatory hyperpigmentation. Laboratory values normalized, and no recurrence was observed during follow-up.[6]

Clinical Pearls

▶ Granuloma annulare is a benign, necrobiotic granulomatous condition, most often seen in a localized form.
▶ The disseminated or generalized type is defined by the presence of at least 10 lesions and usually affects adults.[3,7]
▶ Disseminated GA tends to be chronic, is less likely to resolve on its own, and often requires systemic treatment.[4,7]
▶ Diabetes mellitus is linked to GA in up to 20% of cases, possibly due to microangiopathic changes or collagen damage from chronic hyperglycemia.[2,3]
▶ Compared to localized GA, the disseminated form appears later in life, involves a wider distribution, is more pruritic, and has a lower rate of spontaneous remission.[3,7]
▶ Several reports have shown that GA lesions may regress with improved glycemic control, highlighting the importance of addressing metabolic abnormalities in management.[2,6]

REFERENCES

1. Agrawal P, Pursnani N, Jose R, Farooqui M. Granuloma annulare: A rare dermatological manifestation of diabetes mellitus. J Family Med Prim Care. 2019;8(10):3419-21.
2. Barbieri JS, Rosenbach M, Rodriguez O, Margolis DJ. Association of Granuloma Annulare With Type 2 Diabetes, Hyperlipidemia, Autoimmune Disorders, and Hematologic Malignant Neoplasms. JAMA Dermatol. 2021;157(7):817-23.
3. Dabski K, Winkelmann RK. Generalized granuloma annulare: clinical and laboratory findings in 100 patients. J Am Acad Dermatol. 1989;20(1):39-47.
4. Lukács J, Schliemann S, Elsner P. Treatment of generalized granuloma annulare - a systematic review. J Eur Acad Dermatol Venereol. 2015;29(8):1467-80.
5. Wang J, Khachemoune A. Granuloma Annulare: A Focused Review of Therapeutic Options. Am J Clin Dermatol. 2018;19(3):333-344.
6. Pathave H, Barve V, Gadade H, Nayak C. A case of generalized granuloma annulare with diabetes mellitus: regressed with antidiabetic therapy. Turk J Dermatol. 2020;14(3):79-81.
7. Joshi TP, Duvic M. Granuloma Annulare: An Updated Review of Epidemiology, Pathogenesis, and Treatment Options. Am J Clin Dermatol. 2022;23(1):37-50.

Case 3: Disseminated Granuloma Annulare

■ PRESENTATION

A 54-year-old patient with an 8-year history of type 2 diabetes mellitus presents with numerous, small, elevated papules and plaques, typically annular or arcuate in shape. The lesions are skin-colored, erythematous, or yellowish, distributed symmetrically over the trunk, arms, legs, and occasionally the neck and face. Most lesions are asymptomatic, though mild pruritus may be reported. The clinical course is chronic, with a tendency for persistence and recurrence, especially in adults and those with associated metabolic disturbances. In this patient, long-standing diabetes and suboptimal glycemic control were evident, along with common associated features such as obesity, acanthosis nigricans (AN), skin tags, and other diabetic dermopathies.[1-5]

■ EXAMINATION

Well-defined annular or arcuate plaques and papules were observed across the trunk **(Fig. 6)** and extremities **(Figs. 7 and 8)**. The lesions varied in color from skin-toned to erythematous or yellowish. Mucosal involvement was rare, and the lesions were generally nontender.

■ INVESTIGATIONS

Laboratory Findings

- Blood glucose measurement to assess diabetic status
- Liver and kidney function tests as part of the systemic work-up
- Viral serology (hepatitis B, hepatitis C, and HIV) in selected cases

Histopathology

- Skin biopsy is recommended for confirmation and to exclude other conditions.
- The hallmark finding is a palisaded granulomatous infiltrate with central necrobiotic collagen, surrounded by lymphocytes, histiocytes, and occasional multi-nucleated giant cells.

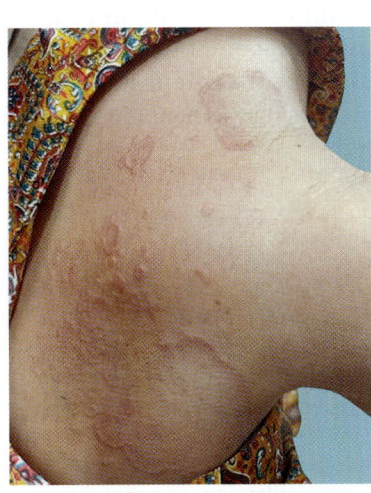

FIG. 6: Well-defined annular and arcuate plaques observed over the trunk.

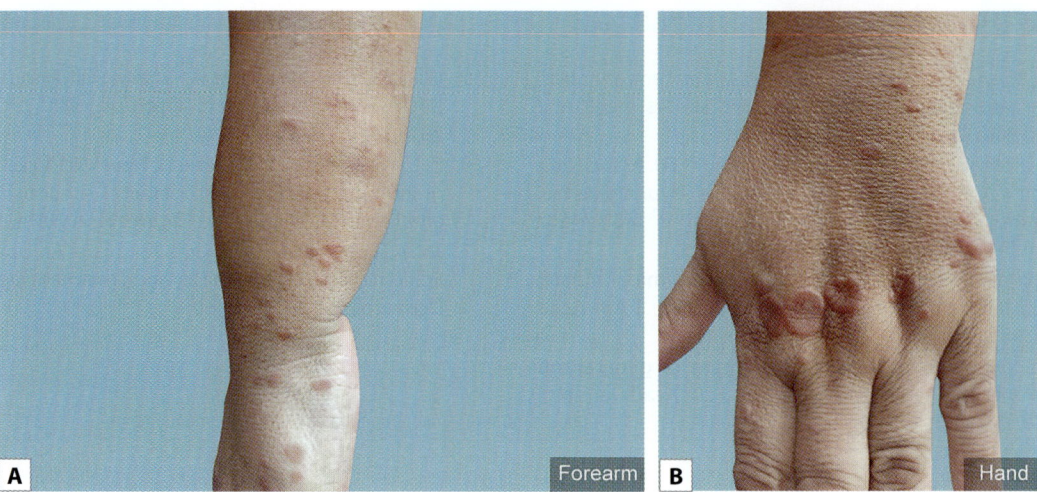

FIGS. 7A AND B: Similar annular and arcuate papules and plaques involving the extremities.

DIAGNOSIS

The diagnosis is primarily clinical, based on the characteristic morphology and distribution of the lesions. In atypical or ambiguous cases, a skin biopsy can confirm the clinical suspicion and exclude other dermatoses.[1,5]

DIFFERENTIAL DIAGNOSIS

Disseminated GA must be distinguished from other annular skin conditions, including:
- Tinea corporis
- Erythema annulare centrifugum
- Annular lichen planus
- Porokeratosis
- Secondary syphilis
- Erythema multiforme
- Annular elastolytic giant cell granuloma
- Cutaneous sarcoidosis[1,5]

MANAGEMENT

Treating disseminated GA can be difficult, particularly in cases that are widespread or resistant to therapy.[2,5,6]
- *Topical treatments:*
  - Potent corticosteroids
  - Calcineurin inhibitors such as tacrolimus[5,6]
- *Systemic therapies:*
  - Short courses of oral corticosteroids for severe exacerbations
  - Methotrexate or hydroxychloroquine for persistent or extensive disease
  - Biologic agents [e.g., tumor necrosis factor alpha (TNF-α) inhibitors] in cases unresponsive to conventional therapy.[2,5,6]
- *Phototherapy:* Narrowband ultraviolet B (UVB) or psoralen ultraviolet A (PUVA) may be considered for widespread disease.[2,5,6]
- *Metabolic management:* Optimizing blood glucose control in diabetic patients can facilitate improvement or even resolution of lesions.[3,7]

PROGNOSIS

Disseminated GA usually runs a chronic, relapsing course and is less likely to resolve spontaneously than its localized counterpart. With appropriate systemic treatment and management of underlying metabolic issues, gradual improvement is expected. Residual postinflammatory hyperpigmentation may persist after the lesions resolve.[1,5]

Clinical Pearls

- The presence of multiple annular lesions with raised edges and central clearing, distributed symmetrically, is typical of disseminated GA.[1]
- A strong association with type 2 diabetes mellitus points to a role for immune dysregulation and microvascular changes.[3,4,7]
- Histopathological examination is essential for diagnosis and to exclude similar-appearing conditions.[1,5]
- Effective glycemic control is an important aspect of management and may speed up lesion clearance.[3,7]

REFERENCES

1. Dabski K, Winkelmann RK. Generalized granuloma annulare: clinical and laboratory findings in 100 patients. J Am Acad Dermatol. 1989;20(1):39-47.
2. Lukács J, Schliemann S, Elsner P. Treatment of generalized granuloma annulare - a systematic review. J Eur Acad Dermatol Venereol. 2015;29(8):1467-80.
3. Pathave H, Barve V, Gadade H, Nayak C. A case of generalized granuloma annulare with diabetes mellitus: regressed with antidiabetic therapy. Turk J Dermatol. 2020;14(3):79-81.
4. Barbieri JS, Rosenbach M, Rodriguez O, Margolis DJ. Association of Granuloma Annulare With Type 2 Diabetes, Hyperlipidemia, Autoimmune Disorders, and Hematologic Malignant Neoplasms. JAMA Dermatol. 2021;157(7):817-23.
5. Joshi TP, Duvic M. Granuloma Annulare: An Updated Review of Epidemiology, Pathogenesis, and Treatment Options. Am J Clin Dermatol. 2022;23(1):37-50.
6. Wang J, Khachemoune A. Granuloma Annulare: A Focused Review of Therapeutic Options. Am J Clin Dermatol. 2018;19(3):333-344.
7. Agrawal P, Pursnani N, Jose R, Farooqui M. Granuloma annulare: A rare dermatological manifestation of diabetes mellitus. J Family Med Prim Care. 2019;8(10):3419-21.

Case 4: Generalized Granuloma Annulare in a Diabetic Patient

■ PRESENTATION

A 57-year-old female with a 9-year history of type 2 diabetes mellitus presented with multiple asymptomatic annular skin lesions of several months' duration. Glycemic control was optimal [glycated hemoglobin (HbA1c): 6.28%], and she denied any systemic symptoms.

■ EXAMINATION

- Multiple skin-colored to erythematous annular plaques with central clearing and slightly raised borders were observed on the abdomen, chest, back, and proximal limbs (Figs. 8A to C).
- No scaling or mucosal involvement was noted.

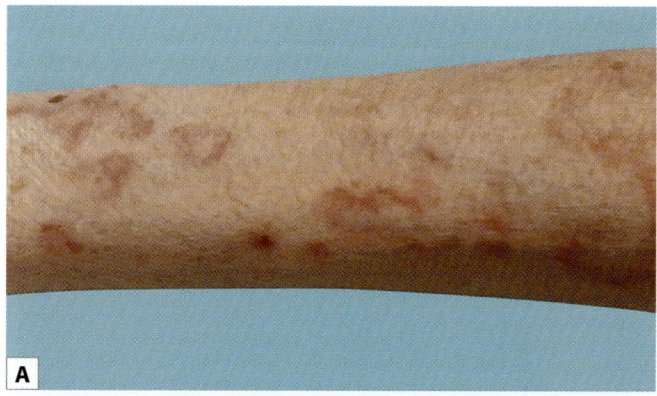
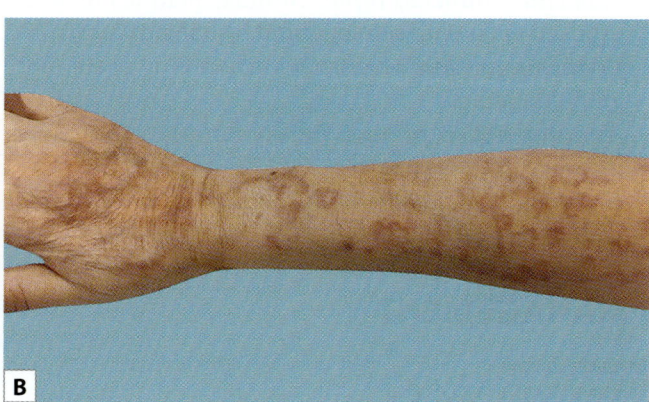
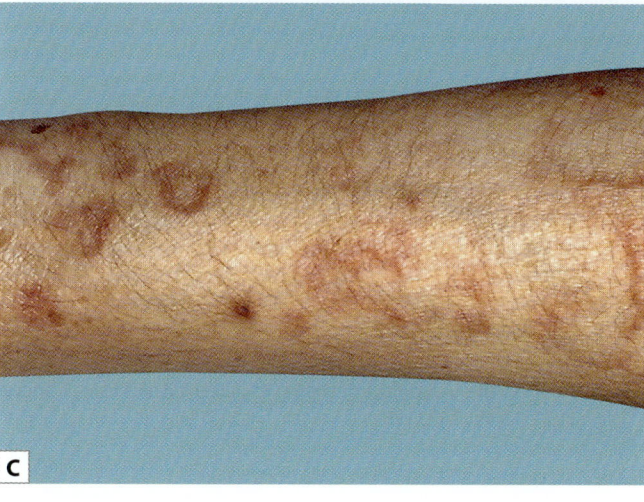

FIGS. 8A TO C: Annular and skin-colored to erythematous plaques with central clearing and slightly raised borders observed over the proximal limbs.

- Nailfold capillaroscopy revealed altered tortuosity, dilated loops, and giant capillaries, suggesting diabetic microangiopathy.
- There was no clinical evidence of diabetic retinopathy or nephropathy.

INVESTIGATIONS

Skin biopsy confirmed the diagnosis of interstitial-type GA, demonstrating dermal palisaded granulomas with mucin deposition and collagen necrobiosis.

DIAGNOSIS

Generalized GA (interstitial type) in a patient with type 2 diabetes mellitus.[1-5]

DIFFERENTIAL DIAGNOSIS

- *Necrobiosis lipoidica diabeticorum:* Shiny, atrophic, yellow-brown plaques, more common on the shins.
- *Sarcoidosis:* May mimic GA; histology shows non-caseating granulomas without mucin.
- *Tinea corporis:* Annular lesions with peripheral scale; KOH positive.
- *Subacute cutaneous lupus:* Annular plaques in sun-exposed areas with serologic and histologic clues.
- *Erythema annulare centrifugum:* Trailing scale, not granulomatous.
- *Annular lichen planus:* Rarely annular, intensely pruritic, and violaceous.
- *Granulomatous infections:* Ruled out by lack of systemic features and negative cultures.[5]

MANAGEMENT

Topical therapy:
- High-potency topical corticosteroids (e.g., clobetasol) applied to active lesions.
- Calcineurin inhibitors (e.g., tacrolimus) considered for sensitive areas or as steroid-sparing agents.[5,6]

Systemic therapy (for widespread or refractory cases):
- Hydroxychloroquine as a first-line systemic agent
- Phototherapy [PUVA or narrow-band ultraviolet-B (NB-UVB)], where available
- Retinoids (acitretin or isotretinoin), dapsone, or methotrexate in select cases
- Biologic agents (e.g., TNF-α inhibitors) used with caution due to variable responses.[4,6]

Metabolic care:
- Continued glycemic control and lipid management
- Monitoring for associated autoimmune conditions, especially thyroid dysfunction
- Regular screening for microvascular complications (retina, kidneys, and neuropathy)[7]

PROGNOSIS

Generalized GA is benign but chronic, with frequent relapses. Some cases may resolve spontaneously over 1–2 years. Lesions may stabilize or regress with improved metabolic control. Long-term dermatologic follow-up is advised for resistant or recurrent cases.[2-4]

> **Clinical Pearls**
> - Symmetrical, annular, nonscaly plaques with central clearing on the trunk and limbs
> - More common in middle-aged women with metabolic comorbidities
> - Histopathology shows palisading granulomas and mucin-rich collagen degeneration.
> - Diabetic microangiopathy is often present.[2,4,7]

REFERENCES

1. Agrawal P, Pursnani N, Jose R, Farooqui M. Granuloma annulare: A rare dermatological manifestation of diabetes mellitus. J Family Med Prim Care. 2019;8(10):3419-21.
2. Granuloma Annulare [Internet]. www.hopkinsmedicine.org. 2019. Available from: https://www.hopkinsmedicine.org/health/conditions-and-diseases/granuloma-annulare.
3. Thornsberry LA, English JC 3rd. Etiology, diagnosis, and therapeutic management of granuloma annulare: an update. Am J Clin Dermatol. 2013;14(4):279-90.
4. Alghamdi MA. Therapeutic Options for Granuloma Annulare: An Updated Review. J Pharm Res Int. 2023;35(15):1-10.
5. Lobo C, Kaimal S. Generalized granuloma annulare. CMAJ. 2024;196(29):E1013.
6. Barbieri JS, Rosenbach M, Rodriguez O, Margolis DJ. Association of Granuloma Annulare With Type 2 Diabetes, Hyperlipidemia, Autoimmune Disorders, and Hematologic Malignant Neoplasms. JAMA Dermatol. 2021;157(7):817-23.
7. Fornons-Servent R, Bauer-Alonso A, Llobera-Ris C, Penín RM, Marcoval J. Granuloma Annulare: a Case-control Study of Possible Associated Diseases. Dermatol Pract Concept. 2022;12(4):e2022173.

CHAPTER 24

Eruptive Xanthomas in Uncontrolled Diabetes Mellitus

NK Singh, Akashkumar N Singh, Anuradha Kapoor

■ PRESENTATION

A 25-year-old woman with a known history of hypothyroidism and irregular medical follow-up presented with a 1-month history of asymptomatic, discrete, yellowish papules on the palms, soles, and trunk. The lesions were monomorphic, measuring approximately 2–4 mm in diameter, and some were surrounded by an erythematous halo.

She denied any systemic symptoms or mucosal involvement.

■ EXAMINATION

- Multiple discrete, yellow-red papules (~2-4 mm), some with an erythematous halo, were observed on the palms **(Figs. 1A and B)**, soles, and trunk.
- No systemic signs or mucosal lesions were noted.

■ INVESTIGATIONS

- *Thyroid-stimulating hormone (TSH):* >100 mIU/L—Markedly elevated, indicating poorly controlled hypothyroidism, which is associated with disturbances in lipid metabolism.
- *Random blood sugar (RBS):* Elevated—suggesting hyperglycemia, potentially related to an underlying insulin resistance state.
- *Serum triglycerides (TG):* Very high (>1,000 mg/dL)—significantly elevated, supporting the clinical suspicion of hypertriglyceridemia, a common trigger for eruptive xanthomas.
- *Skin biopsy:* Confirmed the clinical suspicion of "eruptive xanthoma", demonstrating characteristic foamy macrophages within the dermis.

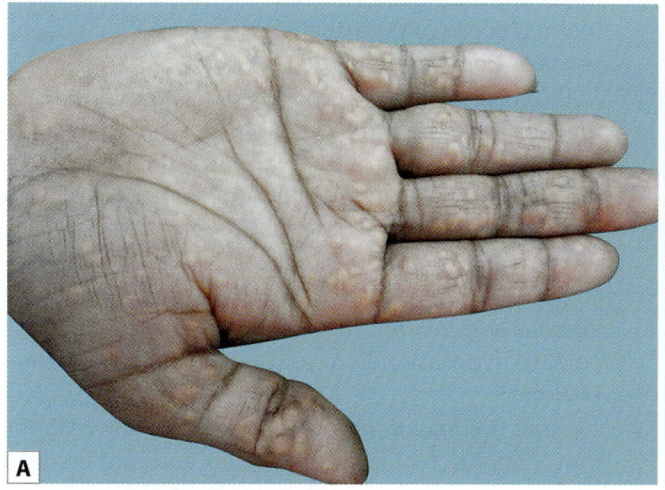
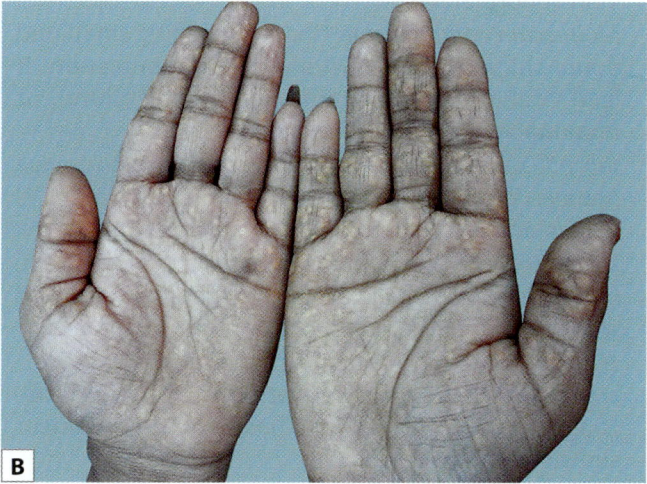

FIGS. 1 A AND B: Multiple discrete yellow-red papules (approximately 2–4 mm in size), some surrounded by an erythematous halo, noted on the palms.

DIAGNOSIS

Eruptive xanthoma associated with severe hypertriglyceridemia due to uncontrolled hypothyroidism and undiagnosed diabetes. The clinical diagnosis is based on the sudden appearance of discrete, yellow-red, dome-shaped papules, typically distributed over extensor surfaces. Histopathology confirms the presence of foamy macrophages within the dermis. A comprehensive metabolic evaluation is essential for identifying and managing the underlying hypothyroidism, hypertriglyceridemia, and glucose dysregulation.[1-5]

PATHOGENESIS

Eruptive xanthomas result from profound hypertriglyceridemia and systemic lipid dysregulation. They are a distinctive dermatologic indicator of this state, most frequently observed in the context of poorly controlled diabetes mellitus.[1] These lesions are characterized by the abrupt emergence of yellow-red papules due to lipid accumulation within the dermis. Their presence signals underlying systemic lipid derangement and serves as a crucial marker for heightened cardiovascular risk.[1,4] The pathologic process involves the excessive infiltration of lipoproteins into the subendothelial space, leading to the accumulation of lipid-laden macrophages (foam cells) within the dermis—a process reminiscent of early atherogenesis.[6,7]

DIFFERENTIAL DIAGNOSIS

- *Granuloma annulare:* Presents as annular (ring-shaped) and non-yellow papules. It is not associated with any lipid abnormalities.[1]
- *Molluscum contagiosum:* Characterized by small and dome-shaped papules with central umbilication. It is of viral origin and commonly affects children or immunocompromised individuals.[1]
- *Juvenile xanthogranuloma:* Appears as yellow to orange nodules, primarily in infants and young children. It is benign and usually resolves spontaneously.[1]
- *Necrobiotic xanthogranuloma:* Presents as yellowish, indurated plaques that may ulcerate. It is often associated with monoclonal gammopathy or paraproteinemia.[2]
- *Histoid leprosy:* Identified by smooth and skin-colored nodules appearing over clinically normal skin. Diagnosis is confirmed by a positive slit-skin smear showing acid-fast bacilli.[3]
- *Lichen amyloidosis:* Characterized by intensely itchy, hyperpigmented papules, usually on the shins. Histopathological examination reveals amyloid deposits in the dermis.[4]

PATHOPHYSIOLOGY

Eruptive xanthomas are cutaneous manifestations of severe hypertriglyceridemia, typically when serum triglyceride levels exceed 1,000 mg/dL.[8] The condition is triggered by an excess of circulating chylomicrons or very-low-density lipoproteins (VLDL), leading to lipoprotein deposition in the skin.[5] This process activates dermal macrophages, which transform into foam cells upon engulfing lipids.[6,7] Diabetes mellitus contributes via insulin resistance, which promotes increased lipolysis and elevated free-fatty acids, while also impairing the clearance of triglyceride-rich lipoproteins.[5] Concurrent hypothyroidism further aggravates the disturbance in lipid metabolism, compounding the risk.[2]

MANAGEMENT

Dermatology Management

- Confirmation of diagnosis via skin biopsy is definitive but often unnecessary when clinical features and laboratory findings are classical.[7,8]
- Topical therapies are ineffective, as there is no direct topical intervention for these lesions.
- Serial photographic documentation is recommended to monitor lesion evolution, which typically resolves in parallel with normalization of lipid levels.[8]

Diabetology/Physician Management

- *Glycemic control:* Initiate or optimize antidiabetic therapy, such as metformin, dipeptidyl-peptidase 4 (DPP-4) inhibitors, or insulin as indicated.[8] Frequent blood glucose monitoring is essential, with a target of glycated hemoglobin (HbA1c) of <7%.[8]
- *Lipid-lowering therapy:* Fibrates (e.g., fenofibrate 145 mg/day) are the cornerstone for rapid triglyceride reduction.[5,8] Omega-3 fatty acids [2–4 g/day eicosapentaenoic acid (EPA)/docosahexaenoic acid (DHA)] may be added.[8] Statins are considered for long-term cardiovascular protection.[5] Niacin and bile acid sequestrants may be used selectively.[5]
- *Thyroid dysfunction:* Initiate levothyroxine therapy to correct hypothyroidism and facilitate lipid normalization.[2]
- *Lifestyle modifications:* Advise a low-fat, low-carbohydrate diet, strict avoidance of alcohol and simple sugars, and regular physical activity (at least 150 minutes of moderate-intensity exercise per week).[5,8] Avoid drugs that may exacerbate hypertriglyceridemia, such as estrogens and corticosteroids.[5]

- *Pancreatitis risk mitigation:* For triglyceride levels exceeding 1,000 mg/dL, assess for symptoms of acute pancreatitis (abdominal pain and elevated lipase). Hospitalization may be warranted for high-risk individuals.[5,8]

■ PROGNOSIS

With prompt metabolic correction, eruptive xanthoma lesions typically resolve within 2–4 weeks, once triglyceride levels fall below 500 mg/dL.[8] Cosmetic improvement closely follows metabolic stabilization. The overall prognosis is excellent with early diagnosis and intervention, though recurrences may occur if metabolic control lapses.[5]

> **Clinical Pearls**
>
> ▶ Eruptive xanthomas may be the initial visible sign of severe metabolic dysfunction, including previously undiagnosed diabetes mellitus.[1,2]
> ▶ Always evaluate lipid profile, thyroid function, and fasting glucose in patients presenting with such lesions.[1,4]
> ▶ Early, aggressive intervention prevents complications such as pancreatitis and cardiovascular disease.[5,8]
> ▶ Lesions are commonly symmetrical, pruritic, and localized to extensor surfaces.[1]
> ▶ Patient education is vital regarding the risk of recurrence with dietary indiscretions or medication of nonadherence.[8]

REFERENCES

1. Kanitakis J. Eruptive xanthoma. Clin Dermatol. 1994;12(2):131-6.
2. Sharma A, Bansal A, Gupta A. Eruptive xanthomas as a cutaneous sign of severe hypertriglyceridemia in undiagnosed diabetes. Indian J Dermatol. 2020;65(1):67-8.
3. Rader DJ, Hovingh GK. Remnant lipoproteins and atherothrombosis. Circulation. 2014;131(16):1673-6.
4. Sharma V, Handa S. Disorders of lipid metabolism and the skin. Indian J Dermatol Venereol Leprol. 2007;73(2):72-7.
5. Goldberg RB. Hypertriglyceridemia: risk and management. Am J Cardiol. 1998;81(4A):7B-12B.
6. Fredrickson DS, Levy RI, Lees RS. Fat transport in lipoproteins—An integrated approach to mechanisms and disorders. N Engl J Med. 1967;276:34-44.
7. Kurban AK, Mehregan AH. Histopathology of eruptive xanthomas. Arch Dermatol. 1963;88:725-30.
8. Das SK, Das S. Metabolic syndrome in skin tags: a hospital-based observational study. Int J Res Dermatol. 2021;7(5):708-12.

CHAPTER 25

Abdominal Pseudohernia due to Diabetic Truncal Neuropathy

Santosh B

■ PRESENTATION

A 49-year-old male with a 10-year history of type 2 diabetes and hypertension presented with a 2-month history of localized right upper abdominal pain and a noticeable bulge in the same area. He also reported unintentional weight loss and paresthesia affecting both lower limbs and the right upper abdominal region.

The patient weighed 68 kg and was on metformin, glimepiride, and amlodipine. The pain was dull to burning in nature, intensifying at night, and there was no significant trauma or cough impulse associated with the swelling.

■ EXAMINATION

- On inspection, a soft, reducible bulge was noted over the right upper abdominal wall, with no cough impulse **(Fig. 1)**.

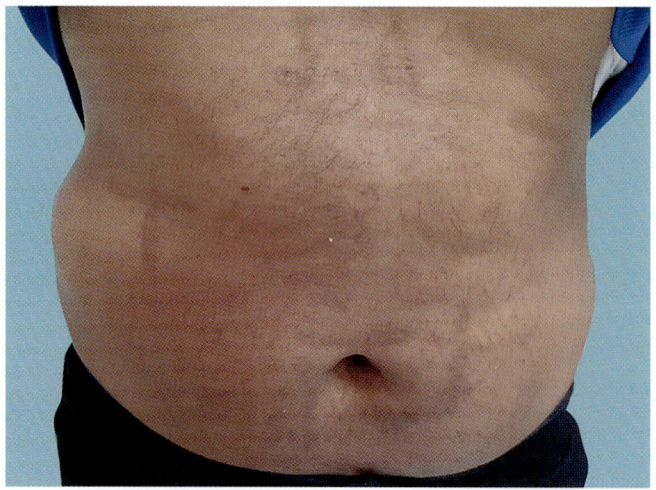

FIG. 1: Soft, reducible bulge over the right upper abdominal wall with no cough impulse.

- Sensory examination revealed decreased touch and temperature sensation across the T7–T10 dermatomes.
- In the lower limbs, clinical examination confirmed bilateral distal symmetric peripheral neuropathy.

■ INVESTIGATIONS

To assess the clinical presentation and rule out other causes, a comprehensive evaluation was performed.
- *Abdominal imaging [ultrasound/computed tomography (CT)]:* This excludes structural causes such as hernias or intra-abdominal pathology. Muscle thinning may be observed, but no mass or true hernia is detected.
    - *Ultrasound result:* Grade I fatty liver; no hernia or mass
- *Electrophysiological studies:* Nerve conduction studies (NCS) and electromyography confirm truncal neuropathy and peripheral sensorimotor involvement.
    - *Nerve conduction studies result:* Truncal polyradiculopathy and sensorimotor neuropathy in all limbs
- *Laboratory tests:* Glycemic control [glycated hemoglobin (HbA1c)], lipid profile, and vitamin B12 levels are essential for metabolic assessment.
    - *Results:* HbA1c—10.3%, low-density lipoprotein cholesterol (LDL-C)—176 mg/dL, and triglycerides—243 mg/dL

■ ETIOPATHOGENESIS

Abdominal pseudohernia results from segmental denervation and subsequent weakness of the abdominal musculature due to truncal motor neuropathy. In diabetes, this leads to flaccid weakness and focal protrusion of the abdominal wall, mimicking a hernia. Chronic, poorly controlled diabetes is a major risk factor.

DIAGNOSIS

Abdominal pseudohernia due to diabetic truncal neuropathy: Diagnosis is clinical, supported by imaging and electrophysiological studies. The absence of a true hernia on imaging and the presence of segmental sensory/motor deficits are diagnostic clues.[1,2,3]

DIFFERENTIAL DIAGNOSES

Differentiating abdominal pseudohernia from other causes of abdominal pain and swelling is crucial:
- True abdominal wall hernias (umbilical, incisional, and Spigelian)
- Abdominal wall hematomas
- Intra-abdominal masses (tumors, lipomas, and abscesses)
- Herpes zoster-related pseudohernia
- Discogenic radiculopathy (T7–T12)
- Other causes of abdominal muscle denervation (thoracic/lumbar disc prolapse, spinal cord injury, and surgical trauma)[3]

Pain of neuropathic origin should be distinguished from pain due to cardiac, pulmonary, or gastrointestinal causes.

MANAGEMENT

Neurology/Dermatology

- *Neuropathic pain:* Pregabalin, gabapentin, duloxetine, carbamazepine; amitriptyline as an alternative[3]
- Vitamin B12 supplementation if deficient
- Avoid unnecessary surgical interventions unless imaging confirms a true hernia.

Diabetology/Physician

- Intensify glycemic control; consider insulin glargine, continue metformin and glimepiride, and add sitagliptin if needed.[4]
- Address dyslipidemia with statins (e.g., rosuvastatin 20 mg).
- Advise regular self-monitoring of blood glucose, lifestyle modification, and follow-up every 3 months.

PROGNOSIS

With improved glycemic control and appropriate symptomatic treatment, diabetic truncal neuropathy and the associated pseudohernia typically resolve gradually over 3–6 months. Most cases do not require surgical intervention, as the abdominal bulge subsides with reinnervation and metabolic correction.[2,3]

> ### Clinical Pearls
>
> ▶ Suspect diabetic truncal neuropathy in patients with poorly controlled, long-standing diabetes presenting with segmental abdominal pain and bulging.[3]
> ▶ Features such as a reducible swelling without a cough impulse and normal imaging suggest pseudohernia rather than a true hernia.[2,3]
> ▶ Early recognition avoids unnecessary investigations and surgical procedures.[3]
> ▶ Electrophysiological studies are crucial for confirmation.[2,3]
> ▶ Most patients improve with correction of metabolic derangements and neuropathy-directed therapy.[3]

REFERENCES

1. Ellenberg M. Diabetic neuropathic cachexia. Diabetes. 1974;23(5):418-23.
2. Tashiro S, Akaboshi K, Kobayashi Y, Mori T, Nagata M, Liu M. Herpes zoster–induced trunk muscle paresis presenting with abdominal wall pseudohernia, scoliosis, and gait disturbance and its rehabilitation: A case report. Arch Phys Med Rehabil. 2010;91(2):321-5.
3. Franklin GM. Truncal neuropathies and their evaluation. Neurol Clin. 2007;25(1):45-57.
4. Vinik AI, Nevoret ML, Casellini C, et al. Diabetic neuropathies: A statement by the American Diabetes Association. Diabetes Care. 2005;28(4):956-62.

CHAPTER 26

Porphyria Cutanea Tarda in Patients with Type 2 Diabetes Mellitus

Suhas Gopal Erande, Anil Patki

▪ PRESENTATION

A 53-year-old male farmer presented with fragile skin, blisters, and darkening over the dorsum of the hands and face for the past 6 months. The blisters appeared gradually on sun-exposed areas, ruptured easily, and healed slowly, leaving erosions, crusts, and hyperpigmented patches. He reported no systemic symptoms such as jaundice or fatigue. The patient has had type 2 diabetes mellitus for the past 10 years, treated with metformin and glimepiride. There is no history of liver disease, hepatitis, or human immunodeficiency virus (HIV) infection. He has occasional alcohol use but no tobacco exposure.

▪ EXAMINATION

- On inspection, there were multiple hyperpigmented macules, shallow erosions, and crusted areas on the dorsum of the hands and nasal bridge **(Fig. 1)**.

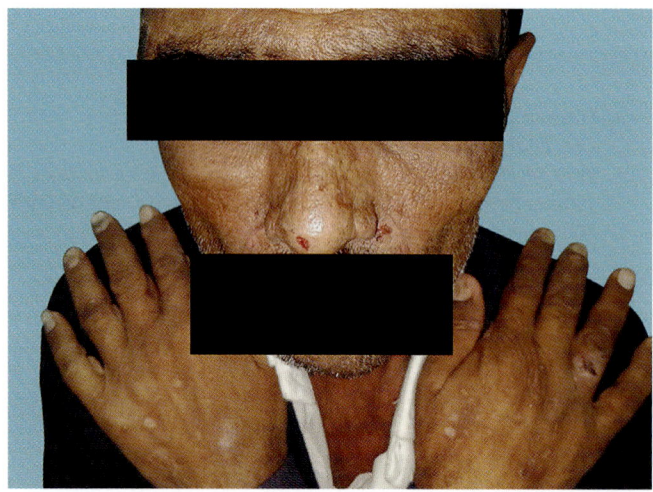

FIG. 1: Multiple hyperpigmented macules, shallow erosions, and crusted areas on the dorsum of the hands and nasal bridge.

- The facial skin showed atrophic scarring and mild hypertrichosis over the malar region. Several vesicles and bullae were noted on the dorsal hands, some intact and others ruptured. The surrounding skin appeared fragile.
- There were no systemic signs suggestive of acute hepatic dysfunction, such as hepatomegaly, jaundice, or ascites.

▪ INVESTIGATION

A clinical diagnosis of porphyria cutanea tarda (PCT) was suspected based on photosensitive blistering, skin fragility, and hyperpigmentation.

- *Wood's lamp examination:* It revealed pink–red fluorescence of urine.
- *Urinary porphyrin profile:* Elevated levels of uroporphyrin and heptacarboxyl porphyrins confirmed the diagnosis.
- *Serum ferritin:* Elevated, suggesting hepatic iron overload
- *Liver function tests:* Mildly elevated transaminases
- *Hepatitis B and C serology:* Negative, helping to exclude common secondary triggers of PCT.
- *Skin biopsy (if performed):* Showed subepidermal bullae with festooning of dermal papillae and minimal dermal inflammation.

▪ PATHOPHYSIOLOGY

Porphyria cutanea tarda results from decreased activity of the hepatic enzyme uroporphyrinogen decarboxylase, a key step in the heme biosynthesis pathway.[1,2,3] This enzymatic deficiency leads to the accumulation of photosensitizing porphyrins—particularly uroporphyrins—in the plasma and skin.[1,2] Upon exposure to ultraviolet (UV) light, these porphyrins generate reactive oxygen species, causing oxidative damage to the epidermis and dermal–epidermal junction, which manifests as skin fragility, blistering, and hyperpigmentation.[1,2,4]

In patients with diabetes, factors such as hepatic iron overload, insulin resistance, and disrupted heme metabolism further predispose to enzyme inhibition and contribute to the onset and progression of PCT.[4,5]

■ DIAGNOSIS

Porphyria cutanea tarda in a patient with type 2 diabetes mellitus, presenting as photosensitive blistering, skin fragility, and characteristic porphyrin abnormalities[1,2]

■ DIFFERENTIAL DIAGNOSES

Several conditions can mimic the presentation of PCT. Careful clinical, laboratory, and histopathological evaluation helps in distinguishing these:
- *Epidermolysis bullosa acquisita:* It is characterized by deeper subepidermal bullae, more prominent scarring, and positive anti-collagen VII antibodies.[2]
- *Bullous pemphigoid:* It presents with tense bullae and widespread distribution, often with an eosinophil-rich inflammatory infiltrate on histology.[2]
- *Pseudoporphyria:* It resembles PCT clinically but lacks porphyrin elevation on laboratory testing.[2]
- *Systemic lupus erythematosus (SLE):* It may show photosensitivity and blistering but is accompanied by other systemic features and positive antinuclear antibody (ANA) testing.[2]

■ MANAGEMENT

Effective management of PCT in the context of type 2 diabetes requires collaboration between dermatologists and diabetologists/physicians to address both the cutaneous manifestations and underlying metabolic contributors.[1,2,6]

Dermatologist Management

- *Strict photoprotection:* Advise use of broad-spectrum sunscreen (SPF >50) and protective clothing to minimize UV exposure.[1,2]
- *Hydroxychloroquine*: Low-dose mobilization therapy (100 mg twice weekly) helps promote porphyrin excretion while minimizing hepatotoxicity.[6]
- *Phlebotomy (if iron overload present):* Remove 500 mL of blood every 2–3 weeks until serum ferritin is reduced to <50 ng/mL.[1,2,6]

Diabetologist's/Physician's Management

- *Optimize glycemic control:* Intensify diabetes management; consider switching to insulin or adding a GLP-1 receptor agonist to improve metabolic parameters and reduce hepatic iron load.[5]
- *Avoid iron supplements and hepatotoxic drugs:* These may exacerbate hepatic injury and worsen PCT.[1,2,4]
- *Monitor liver function tests (LFTs) and serum ferritin:* Regular monitoring is essential to assess response to treatment and detect complications early.[1,2]
- *Lifestyle advice:* Counsel on limiting alcohol intake and avoiding estrogens, both of which can trigger or worsen PCT.[1,2]

■ PROGNOSIS

- Excellent with regular phlebotomy or hydroxychloroquine[1,2,6]
- Recurrences are common without continued management of underlying diabetes, hepatic iron, or UV exposure.[1,2,5]
- Long-term hepatic monitoring is essential due to the increased risk of fibrosis or hepatocellular carcinoma.[1,2,4]

Clinical Pearls

▶ Suspect PCT in diabetic patients who present with fragile skin, vesicles, and erosions on sun-exposed areas such as the hands and face.[5]
▶ Always screen for hepatic dysfunction, iron overload, and potential secondary triggers, including hepatitis C virus (HCV) infection.[1,2,4]
▶ Both hydroxychloroquine (low-dose mobilization) and phlebotomy are effective treatments; the choice should be guided by ferritin levels and hepatic status.[6]
▶ Porphyria cutanea tarda may be the first clinical clue to underlying occult liver disease, including HCV infection or subclinical hepatic siderosis.[1,2,4]

REFERENCES

1. Elder GH, Hift RJ, Meissner PN. The porphyrias: Recent advances. Clin Med (Lond). 2013;13(6):629-32.
2. Puy H, Gouya L, Deybach JC. Porphyrias. Lancet. 2010;375(9718):924-37.
3. Anderson KE, Sassa S, Bishop DF, Desnick RJ. Disorders of heme biosynthesis: X-linked sideroblastic anemia and the porphyrias. In: Scriver CR, Beaudet A, Sly WS, Valle D (Eds). The Metabolic and Molecular Bases of Inherited Disease, Volume 2, 8th edition. New York: McGraw-Hill; 2001. pp. 2991-3062.
4. Jalil S, Grady JJ, Lee C, Anderson KE. Associations among behavior-related susceptibility factors in porphyria cutanea tarda. Clin Gastroenterol Hepatol. 2010;8(3):297-302.
5. Ventura P, Cappellini MD, Rocchi E. The porphyrias: Clinical presentation, diagnosis and management. Blood Rev. 2009;23(1):1-15.
6. Singal AK, Kormos-Hallberg C, Lee C, Sadagoparamanujam VM, Grady JJ, Freeman DH, et al. Low-dose hydroxychloroquine is as effective as phlebotomy in treatment of patients with porphyria cutanea tarda. Clin Gastroenterol Hepatol. 2012;10(12):1402-9.

SECTION 6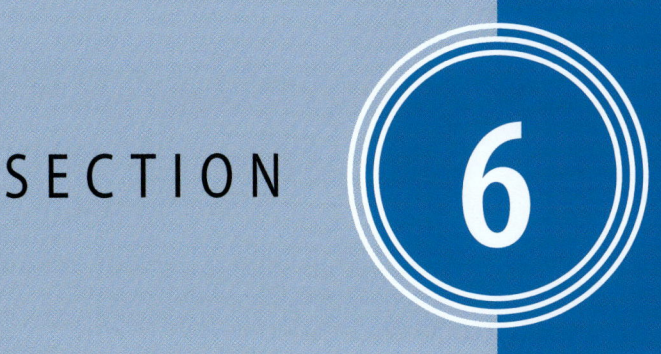

Psychosocial and Cosmetic Skin Conditions in Diabetes

▶ Section Outline

Chapter 27: Vitiligo in Diabetes (Autoimmune Pigmentary Changes)
Nipul Vara, Vishwa Marvania

Chapter 28: Hidradenitis Suppurativa in Diabetes
Bharat Bhushan Kukreja

Chapter 29: Alopecia in Diabetes Mellitus (Hair Loss Associations)
Nipul Vara, Vishwa Marvania

Chapter 30: Postinflammatory Hyperpigmentation in Diabetes: Truncal Distribution
Suhas Gopal Erande, Anil Patki

CHAPTER 27

Vitiligo in Diabetes (Autoimmune Pigmentary Changes)

Nipul Vara, Vishwa Marvania

■ PRESENTATION

A 45-year-old woman with a 10-year history of type 2 diabetes mellitus presented with progressively enlarging depigmented macules and patches over the past 4 years, primarily affecting the dorsal aspects of her hands and feet. The lesions were asymptomatic but cosmetically distressing. She reported glycemic variability, with glycated hemoglobin (HbA1c) levels ranging between 7.8 and 9.5%. Additionally, she experienced chronic stress and anxiety, for which she was prescribed escitalopram 10 mg and clonazepam 0.5 mg at bedtime. She had been on optimal dermatological treatment since the onset of vitiligo lesions.

■ EXAMINATION

- Well-demarcated depigmented macules and patches on the hands **(Fig. 1)** and feet **(Fig. 2)**.
- Symmetrical distribution with some areas showing perifollicular repigmentation.
- Positive Koebner phenomenon observed at sites of minor trauma.

■ INVESTIGATIONS

- *Wood's lamp examination:* Lesions exhibited bright blue-white fluorescence, confirming complete depigmentation.
- Skin biopsy was not performed due to the classical clinical presentation.
- *Laboratory investigations:*
  - HbA1c: 8.4%
  - *Thyroid-stimulating hormone (TSH):* Within normal limits
  - *Antinuclear antibody (ANA):* Negative
  - *Vitamin B12:* Normal

■ DIAGNOSIS

- Vitiligo in diabetes mellitus
- Vitiligo, an autoimmune depigmenting disorder, is commonly seen in patients with diabetes mellitus due to shared autoimmune mechanisms.

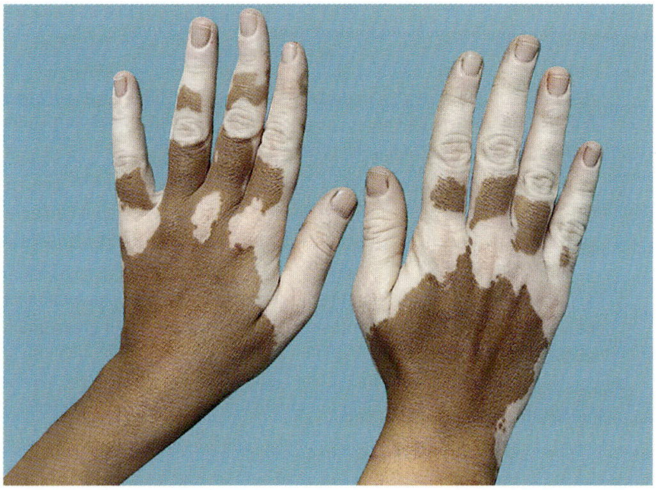

FIG. 1: Well-demarcated depigmented macules and patches on the hands.

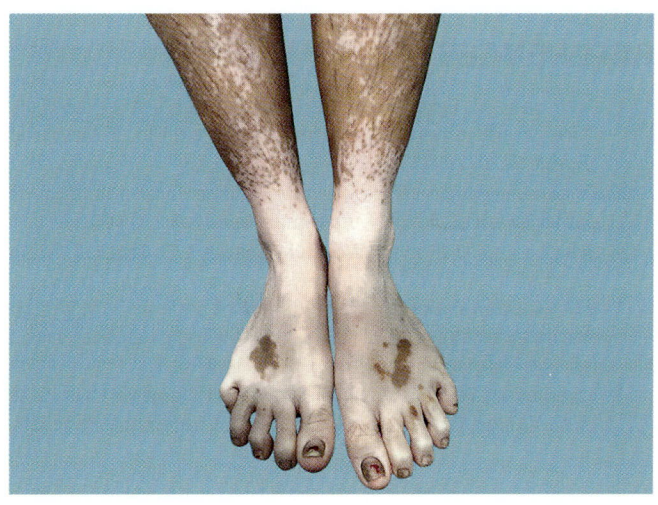

FIG. 2: Well-demarcated depigmented macules and patches on the feet.

DIFFERENTIAL DIAGNOSIS

- *Tinea versicolor:* A superficial fungal infection presenting with fine scaling, hypopigmented or hyperpigmented patches; diagnosis is confirmed by a positive KOH test showing yeast cells.
- *Pityriasis alba:* Common in children; manifests as ill-defined, slightly scaly hypopigmented patches, often on the face.
- *Postinflammatory hypopigmentation:* Occurs after a skin injury or inflammation, with irregular borders and a history of preceding dermatitis or trauma.
- *Idiopathic guttate hypomelanosis:* Appears as small, round, white macules mainly on sun-exposed areas of older adults; lesions are stable and asymptomatic.
- *Lichen sclerosus:* Presents as atrophic, white plaques with a wrinkled surface, commonly affecting the genital and perianal regions, often with itching or discomfort.

MANAGEMENT

Dermatological Approach

- Topical tacrolimus 0.1% ointment applied to facial and flexural lesions.[1]
- Topical corticosteroids (e.g., mometasone furoate 0.1%) for acral areas, used intermittently.[1]
- Narrowband ultraviolet B (NB-UVB) phototherapy administered biweekly for 3 months, resulting in partial perifollicular repigmentation.[1-3] Phototherapy was monitored cautiously due to potential risks associated with diabetic neuropathy and altered skin barrier function.[1]
- Camouflage cosmetics are recommended for cosmetically sensitive areas.[1]
- Psychosocial support is provided to address emotional distress associated with visible lesions.[4-7]

Diabetological Considerations

- Optimization of glycemic control through insulin titration and continuous glucose monitoring.
- Introduction of glucagon-like peptide-1 (GLP-1) receptor agonist (e.g., liraglutide) to aid in weight management and reduce glycemic variability.
- Coordination with psychiatric care to manage stress and anxiety, potentially benefiting vitiligo management.[5,7]

PROGNOSIS

- Partial response observed, with perifollicular repigmentation in some areas.[1]
- Stabilization of lesion progression noted.[1]
- *Prognostic factors:*
  - *Positive:* Early initiation of treatment, adherence to phototherapy, absence of other autoimmune conditions.[1,2]
  - *Negative:* Acral location of lesions, glycemic variability, and chronic stress.[1,5]

> ### Clinical Pearls
> - Vitiligo onset in diabetic patients may indicate underlying autoimmune processes, even in the absence of type 1 diabetes mellitus.[2,4]
> - Psychiatric comorbidities, such as stress and anxiety, can influence the course of vitiligo and should be addressed concurrently.[5,7]
> - Koebner phenomenon underscores the importance of minimizing skin trauma, especially in diabetic patients with peripheral neuropathy.[6]

REFERENCES

1. Rodrigues M, Ezzedine K, Hamzavi I, Pandya AG, Harris JE. Current and emerging treatments for vitiligo. J Am Acad Dermatol. 2017;77(1):17-29.
2. Ongenae K, Van Geel N, Naeyaert JM. Evidence for an autoimmune pathogenesis of vitiligo. Autoimmun Rev. 2003;2(3):163-72.
3. Schallreuter KU, Moore J, Wood JM, Beazley WD, Gaze DC, Tobin DJ, et al. In vivo and in vitro evidence for hydrogen peroxide (H_2O_2) accumulation in the epidermis of patients with vitiligo and its successful removal by a UVB-activated pseudocatalase. J Investig Dermatol Symp Proc. 1999; 4(1): 91-6.
4. Ezzedine K, Lim HW, Suzuki T, Katayama I, Hamzavi I, Lan CCE, et al. Vitiligo Global Issues Consensus Conference Panelists. Revised classification/nomenclature of vitiligo and related issues: the Vitiligo Global Issues Consensus Conference. Pigment Cell & Melanoma Research. 2012;25(3):E1-13.
5. Papadopoulos L, Bor R, Legg C, Hawk JL. Impact of life events on the onset of vitiligo in adults: preliminary evidence for a psychological dimension in aetiology. Clinical and Experimental Dermatology. 1998; 23(6):243-8.
6. Krüger C, Schallreuter KU. A review of the worldwide prevalence of vitiligo in children/adolescents and adults. Int J Dermatol. 2012;51(10):1206-12.
7. Gawkrodger DJ. Psychosocial aspects of vitiligo. Clin Exp Dermatol. 1997;22(6):406-8.

CHAPTER 28

Hidradenitis Suppurativa in Diabetes

Bharat Bhushan Kukreja

CLINICAL PRESENTATION

Hidradenitis suppurativa (HS) is a *chronic, relapsing inflammatory skin disorder* affecting apocrine gland-bearing regions. It typically presents with:
- *Deep-seated, painful nodules*
- Recurrent abscesses and *malodorous discharge*
- Formation of *draining sinus tracts* and extensive scarring
- *Common sites:* Axillae, groin, perineum, perianal, and inframammary areas.
- Significant impact on quality of life, particularly in women of reproductive age.[1-5]

CLASSIFICATION

Hurley staging system (1989) stratifies patients with HS into three stages based on the presence and extent of lesions, scarring and sinus tracts.

Hurley Stage I—Mild
- Solitary or multiple *isolated abscesses*
- No sinus tracts or scarring (*Refer* **Figs. 1A and B**)

Hurley Stage II—Moderate
- Recurrent abscesses
- *Sinus tract formation,* scarring, and widely separated lesions (*Refer* **Figs. 2A and B**)

Hurley Stage III—Severe
- *Diffuse involvement* of the area
- Multiple *interconnected sinus tracts* and abscesses
- Extensive *fibrosis and drainage* (*Refer to* **Fig. 3**)[1,3]

EXAMINATION

On clinical examination, the following findings may be seen:
- *Tender, erythematous nodules or abscesses* in apocrine-rich areas
- *Papules, pustules,* and *fluctuant nodules*
- *Interconnecting sinus tracts* and rope-like scarring in chronic disease
- *Foul-smelling discharge* from ruptured abscesses
- Postinflammatory pigmentation and fibrosis

These findings correspond to the severity outlined in the *Hurley staging system* (**Figs. 1 to 3**).

INVESTIGATIONS

- *CBC, ESR, CRP:* Detect systemic inflammation

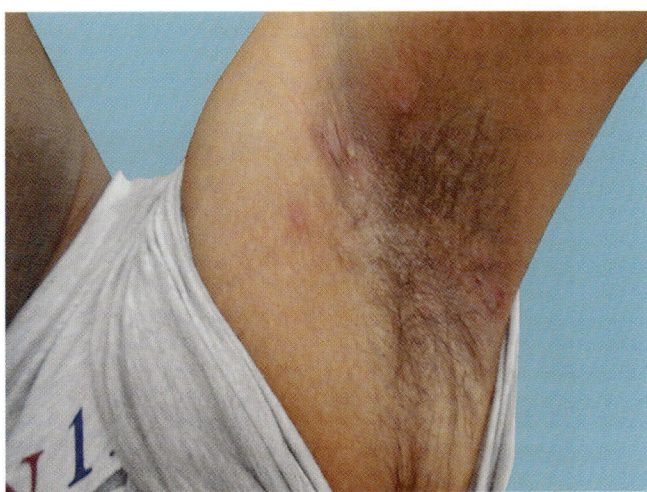

FIG. 1A: Multiple inflamed nodules and papules with mild hyperpigmentation and scarring in the axillary region.

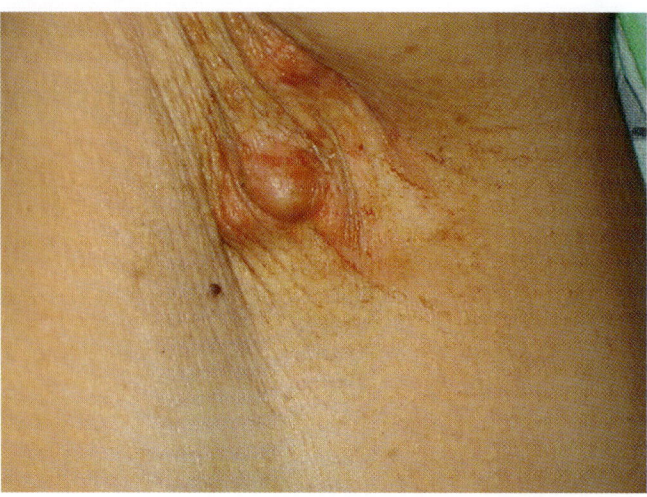

FIG. 1B: Multiple inflamed nodules and abscesses, coalescing.

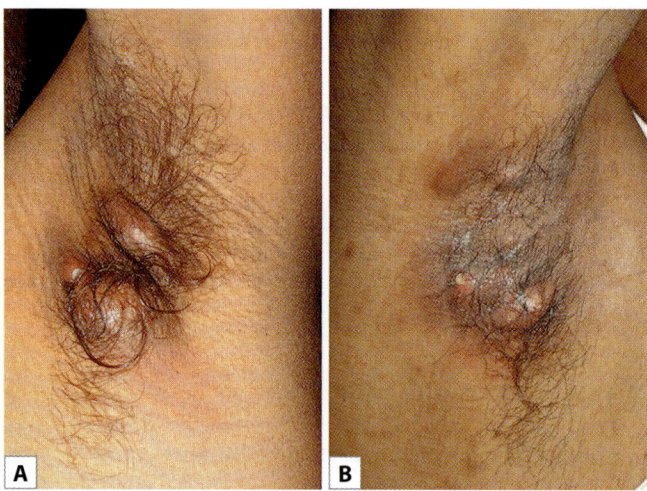

FIGS. 2A AND B: Multiple inflammatory nodular lesions, abscesses with fibrotic scarring.

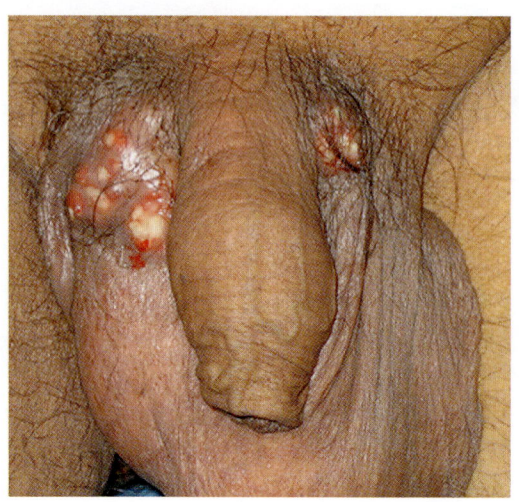

FIG. 3: Nodular, fluctuant, inflamed lesions in the groin area bilaterally. Draining sinuses and pustules are prominent.

- *Culture/sensitivity:* If infection suspected
- *Glycated hemoglobin (HbA1c), fasting glucose*: Evaluate for diabetes/insulin resistance.
- *Hormonal profile, pelvic USG:* For polycystic ovary syndrome (PCOS) screening
- *Ultrasound or MRI:* Sinus tract mapping in moderate/severe cases.[2,5]

DIAGNOSIS

Diagnosis is *clinical,* based on the triad:
- *Typical lesions:* Nodules, abscesses, and sinus tracts
- *Typical sites:* Axillae, groin, perineal/inframammary
- *Chronic course:* Recurrent episodes over ≥6 months[3,6]

DIFFERENTIAL DIAGNOSIS

In considering the differential diagnosis of chronic nodular or ulcerative skin lesions, several conditions should be evaluated:
- *Cutaneous Crohn's disease* often presents with gastrointestinal symptoms, perianal ulcers, and histologic evidence of granulomas.
- *Carbuncles* are typically acute, localized infections that are nonrecurrent and lack chronicity.
- *Epidermoid cysts* generally display a central punctum, are not clustered, and do not present as chronic lesions.
- *Scrofuloderma,* a manifestation of cutaneous tuberculosis, is characterized by a tubercular etiology with caseating granulomas.
- *Acne conglobata* usually affects the trunk, features comedones, and has an earlier onset, commonly in younger individuals.

Each diagnosis can be distinguished by these hallmark features, aiding in clinical differentiation.

MANAGEMENT

Dermatology Management

General Measures (All Stages)
- Educate patient on skin hygiene and encourage the use of loose clothing.
- Recommend antiseptic washes (e.g., chlorhexidine).
- Promote weight loss and smoking cessation as part of skin care.
- Counsel on avoiding skin friction and trauma.

Stage I (Mild)
- Prescribe topical clindamycin 1%.
- Use antiseptic washes regularly.

- Start short-course oral antibiotics like doxycycline during flare-ups.
- Screen for metabolic comorbidities.

Stage II (Moderate)

- Oral combination antibiotics: Clindamycin + rifampicin for 8–12 weeks
- Hormonal therapy such as oral contraceptives or spironolactone in women (especially with PCOS)
- Intralesional corticosteroids for inflamed nodules
- Use ultrasound for evaluating deep-seated lesions before referring to surgery.

Stage III (Severe)

- Start biologic therapy with *adalimumab* [the only Food and Drug Administration (FDA)-approved biologic for HS]
- Coordinate with surgeons for patients requiring surgical intervention.

Diabetology/Physician Management

- Ensure *tight glycemic control* in diabetic and insulin-resistant patients.
- Assess and manage *metabolic comorbidities* such as obesity, PCOS, and dyslipidemia.
- Guide patients through a structured *weight loss program*.
- Offer *nutritional counseling* and address insulin resistance.
- Support *smoking cessation* and lifestyle changes.

- Help to prepare patient medically before surgery (preoperative optimization).
- Monitor for adverse effects of long-term antibiotics, hormonal therapy, or biologics.

Surgical Management

Primarily in Stage III (Severe or Refractory Disease)

- *Wide excision* of affected areas to prevent recurrence
- CO_2 *laser deroofing* for sinus tracts and chronic lesions
- *Skin grafting* to cover large defects postsurgery

Preoperative Optimization (in Coordination with Physician)

- Achieve good glycemic control.
- Ensure the patient is infection-free.
- Provide *nutritional support* and assess healing capacity.

Clinical Pearls

▶ Hidradenitis suppurativa often masquerades as "recurrent boils"—suspect it when persistent in apocrine areas.
▶ Use *Hurley stage* to guide treatment planning.
▶ Address comorbidities: *Obesity, diabetes, PCOS, and smoking.*
▶ *Adalimumab* improves remission in moderate-to-severe HS.
▶ *Surgical intervention* is key for sinus tracts in Hurley Stage III.
▶ Avoid long-term empirical antibiotics without clear infection.[1,4]

REFERENCES

1. Zouboulis CC, Desai N, Emtestam L, Hunger RE, Ioannides D, Juhász I, et al. European S1 guideline for the treatment of hidradenitis suppurativa/acne inversa. J Eur Acad Dermatol Venereol. 2015;29(4):619-44.
2. Krajewski AC, Mikulska M, Matusiak L, Szepietowski JC. Ultrasonographic examination of hidradenitis suppurativa: Clinical utility and correlation with histopathological findings. Dermatol Surg. 2018;44(4):557-63.
3. Garg A, Kirby JS, Lavian J, Lin G, Strunk A. Sex- and age-adjusted population analysis of comorbidities in hidradenitis suppurativa. JAMA Dermatol. 2017;153(9):853-9.
4. Grant A, Gonzalez T, Montgomery MO, Cardenas V, Kerdel FA. Infliximab therapy for patients with moderate to severe hidradenitis suppurativa: A retrospective report of 20 patients. J Am Acad Dermatol. 2010;62(3):397-402.
5. Jemec GBE. Clinical practice. Hidradenitis suppurativa. N Engl J Med. 2012;366(2):158-64.
6. Alavi A, Anooshirvani N, Kim WB, Coutts P, Ghazarian D. Quality-of-life impairment in patients with hidradenitis suppurativa: A Canadian study. Am J Clin Dermatol. 2015;16(1):61-5.

CHAPTER 29

Alopecia in Diabetes Mellitus (Hair Loss Associations)

Nipul Vara, Vishwa Marvania

■ PRESENTATION

A 42-year-old male, a business executive with a 7-year history of type 2 diabetes mellitus (T2DM) and well-controlled hypertension, presented with a gradually progressive, painless patch of hair loss over the right temporoparietal scalp.

- The lesion was asymptomatic, with no redness, scaling, itching, or pustules.
- There was no recent history of stress, illness, drug changes, or family history of alopecia or autoimmune diseases.
- The patient reported no involvement of other body hair and had no systemic complaints.

■ EXAMINATION

- Clinical examination revealed a single, smooth, well-circumscribed alopecic patch measuring approximately 4.5 × 3 cm over the right temporoparietal scalp **(Fig. 1)**.

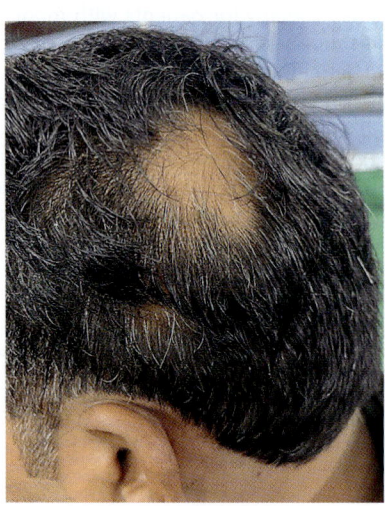

FIG. 1: Alopecia areata in diabetes mellitus.

- The surrounding skin was normal, with no signs of erythema or pustules.
- A positive pull test at the lesion margins indicated active hair shedding.
- Nails showed no pitting or ridging.
- Other body hair was unaffected.

■ INVESTIGATIONS

- *Glycated hemoglobin (HbA1c) level* was 8.2% (reference <7%), indicating poor long-term glycemic control.[1]
- *Fasting blood sugar* was 152 mg/dL (reference 70–99 mg/dL), which is elevated and suggests inadequate short-term glucose control.
- *Antithyroid peroxidase (TPO) antibodies* were elevated at 146 IU/mL (reference <35 IU/mL), suggestive of autoimmune thyroiditis.
- *Antinuclear antibody (ANA) test* was negative, indicating no evidence of systemic autoimmunity.
- *Vitamin D3 level* was 18 ng/mL (reference 30–100 ng/mL), confirming vitamin D deficiency.
- *Serum ferritin* was 78 ng/mL (reference 30–400 ng/mL), which falls within the normal range.
- *Trichoscopy* revealed yellow dots and exclamation mark hairs, which are diagnostic features of alopecia areata (AA).

■ DIAGNOSIS

- The patient was diagnosed with AA in the setting of uncontrolled T2DM.[1-3]
- Alopecia areata AA is an autoimmune, nonscarring hair loss disorder that typically presents as discrete, smooth patches of hair loss on the scalp.[2,3] It is well-documented in individuals with autoimmune conditions, particularly type 1 diabetes mellitus (T1DM), and less commonly in patients with long-standing T2DM, where immune

dysregulation and chronic inflammation play a contributing role.[2-4]
- This case was also associated with autoimmune thyroiditis, as indicated by elevated anti-TPO antibodies, and vitamin D deficiency, both of which are known to coexist with autoimmune dermatological conditions such as AA.[2-4]

■ DIFFERENTIAL DIAGNOSIS

- *Tinea capitis:* A fungal infection of the scalp that can cause scaly patches of hair loss, often with broken hairs and inflammation[2,3]
- *Trichotillomania:* A psychological condition characterized by compulsive hair pulling, leading to irregular patches of hair loss with varying hair lengths[2,3]
- *Telogen effluvium:* A form of diffuse hair shedding triggered by stress, illness, or nutritional deficiencies, without clearly demarcated patches[2,3]
- *Secondary syphilis:* Can present with "moth-eaten" patchy alopecia, often accompanied by other systemic signs of syphilitic infection[2,3]
- *Androgenetic alopecia:* A patterned, progressive form of hair loss influenced by genetic and hormonal factors, typically with gradual thinning[2,3]

■ PATHOPHYSIOLOGY

Alopecia areata is a T-cell mediated autoimmune disorder in which autoreactive CD8+ cytotoxic T lymphocytes target the hair follicles in the anagen (growth) phase, leading to nonscarring hair loss.[2,3] The immune system mistakenly recognizes components of the hair follicle as foreign, triggering an inflammatory response that disrupts normal hair growth.[2,3] In patients with diabetes mellitus, particularly T1DM and some cases of long-standing T2DM, there is a breakdown of immune tolerance due to dysregulated immune checkpoints and elevated levels of proinflammatory cytokines such as interleukin-2 (IL-2) and interferon-gamma (IFN-γ).[1-3] These changes impair the immune privilege of hair follicles, making them more susceptible to autoimmune attack.[2,3] As a result, diabetes-induced immune dysregulation increases the patient's vulnerability to autoimmune conditions, including alopecia areata.[1-3]

■ MANAGEMENT

Dermatologist Management

The primary dermatological treatment involves reducing inflammation and promoting hair regrowth.[2,3]
- Topical corticosteroids such as clobetasol propionate 0.05% lotion are applied twice daily to suppress local autoimmune activity.[2,3]
- Intralesional triamcinolone acetonide (5 mg/mL) is injected at a dose of 0.1 mL/cm^2 once a month for up to 3 months to target resistant patches.[2,3]
- Topical minoxidil 5% is used once daily to stimulate hair follicle activity and promote regrowth.[2,3]
- Diphenylcyclopropenone (DPCP) immunotherapy may be considered if there is no satisfactory response after 3–4 months of standard therapy.[2,3]

■ DIABETOLOGIST/PHYSICIAN MANAGEMENT

Optimal diabetes control is crucial for improving autoimmune regulation and treatment outcomes:[1]
- Glycemic control should be optimized by switching to a basal–bolus insulin regimen temporarily and adding metformin SR 1g twice daily, if not already prescribed.[1]
- Patients should be screened annually for associated autoimmune conditions, including thyroid dysfunction [Thyroid-stimulating hormone (TSH) and anti-TPO], vitamin B12 deficiency, and celiac disease if clinically indicated.[1]
- Blood glucose levels should be closely monitored during steroid therapy to detect and manage steroid-induced hyperglycemia.[1]

Nutritional and Supportive Care

Nutritional support and stress management are important adjuncts to medical therapy:[1-3]
- Vitamin D supplementation should be initiated at 60,000 IU once weekly for 8 weeks to correct deficiency.[2,3]
- Biotin and zinc supplements may be given daily for 3–6 months to support hair health.[2,3]
- Psychological support should be offered to address cosmetic concerns and any related anxiety or stress.[2-4]

- Patients should be advised to avoid unnecessary topical irritants that may exacerbate inflammation or damage the scalp.[2,3]

PROGNOSIS AND FOLLOW-UP

- Hair regrowth typically begins within 4–6 weeks after starting treatment.[2,3]
- Relapse rates are high (approximately 30–50%), especially in patients with poorly controlled diabetes.[2-4]
- Regular follow-up with both dermatology and diabetology is essential, ideally every 3 months during the initial phase of treatment, to monitor progress and adjust therapy accordingly.[1-3]

Clinical Pearls

- Always suspect autoimmune overlap in diabetic patients presenting with new-onset alopecia.[1-3]
- Poor glycemic control aggravates autoimmune processes and delays recovery.[1-3]
- Early dermatology referral improves cosmetic outcomes and psychological well-being.[2-4]
- Avoid high-potency topical steroids on broken or atrophic skin, and monitor blood glucose during systemic or potent local steroid therapy.[1-3]
- Rule out autoimmune thyroiditis and vitamin D deficiency in all cases of alopecia areata.[2-4]

REFERENCES

1. American Diabetes Association. Standards of Medical Care in Diabetes—2024. Diabetes Care. 2024;47:S1-4.
2. Alkhalifah A, Alsantali A, Wang E, McElwee KJ, Shapiro J, et al. Alopecia areata update: Part I. Clinical picture, histopathology, and pathogenesis. J Am Acad Dermatol. 2010;62(2):177-88.
3. Ito T. The role of immune privilege in the pathogenesis of alopecia areata. J Investig Dermatol Symp Proc. 2013.
4. Villasante Fricke AC, Miteva M. Epidemiology and burden of alopecia areata: A systematic review. Clin Cosmet Investig Dermatol. 2015;8:397-403.

CHAPTER 30

Postinflammatory Hyperpigmentation in Diabetes: Truncal Distribution

Suhas Gopal Erande, Anil Patki

■ PRESENTATION

A 62-year-old woman with an 18-year history of type 2 diabetes mellitus presented with persistent dark pigmented spots over the trunk, mainly on the flanks and back. These lesions developed over the past 3 months following a febrile illness associated with a generalized pruritic rash. The rash gradually resolved but left behind dark discoloration of the skin. The patient denied any history of drug allergy or contact with potential allergens.

■ EXAMINATION

On detailed skin examination, the following findings were noted:
- Multiple dark brown macules and postinflammatory marks are distributed over the lateral trunk, particularly the flanks and back **(Fig. 1)**.

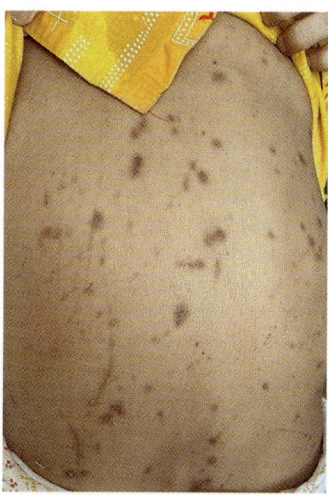

FIG. 1: Multiple dark brown macules and postinflammatory marks over the abdomen, particularly the flanks and back.

- Lesions varied in size from 0.3 to 1.2 cm, with irregular borders; some appeared slightly linear, consistent with healed excoriations.
- No active papules, ulcers, signs of infection, or mucosal involvement were present.
- There were no systemic symptoms.

■ INVESTIGATION

Relevant laboratory and dermatological investigations were performed to support the diagnosis and rule out other causes:
- *Laboratory tests:*
  - *Glycated hemoglobin (HbA1c):* 10.2% (indicating poor glycemic control)
  - *C-reactive protein (CRP):* 22 mg/L (suggesting mild residual inflammation)
  - *Complete blood count (CBC):* Normalizing white blood cell count
  - *Liver and renal function panels:* Within normal limits
- *Skin biopsy (if performed):* Basal layer hyperpigmentation with increased melanophages in the superficial dermis.
- *Dermoscopy (if done):* Patchy pigment network without any features suggestive of malignancy.

■ PATHOPHYSIOLOGY

Postinflammatory hyperpigmentation (PIH) develops as a consequence of cutaneous injury or inflammation. In this condition, inflammatory mediators stimulate melanocytes, leading to excessive melanin production and deposition in the epidermis or dermis.[1,2] In individuals with diabetes, the persistence and severity of pigmentation are often worsened by delayed wound healing, a sustained proinflammatory cytokine environment, and underlying microvascular insufficiency.[1,2] The pathogenesis of PIH also involves complex hormonal and molecular pathways, including the roles of estrogen, progesterone, endothelins, nitric oxide, and various signaling cascades that regulate melanogenesis.[2-4]

DIAGNOSIS

Based on the clinical features, history, and supporting investigations, the patient was diagnosed with PIH secondary to resolving necrotizing fasciitis and diabetic gangrene. The pattern and distribution of pigmentation, along with the absence of active inflammation or systemic symptoms, support this diagnosis in the context of long-standing diabetes.[1,2,4]

DIFFERENTIAL DIAGNOSIS

Other conditions that can mimic the presentation of truncal hyperpigmentation and should be considered include:
- *Fixed drug eruption:* Typically localized, recurrent, and associated with drug exposure[1,2,4]
- *Acanthosis nigricans:* Presents as velvety, hyperpigmented plaques in symmetrical, intertriginous areas[1,2,4]
- *Lichen planus pigmentosus:* Characterized by slate-gray macules that are more diffusely distributed[2,4]
- *Pigmented purpuric dermatoses:* Shows petechiae and purpura with hemosiderin deposition[1,2]

MANAGEMENT

Management of PIH in diabetic patients involves a combination of dermatological care, wound surveillance, and systemic metabolic control[1,2,4]

Dermatological Approach

Treatment includes topical depigmenting agents such as azelaic acid, kojic acid, or short-term use of hydroquinone to reduce pigmentation.[1,2,5]
- Retinoids or creams containing alpha- or beta-hydroxy acids (AHA/BHA) may be prescribed for mild exfoliation to improve skin texture.[1,2,5]
- Combination therapies, including triple combination creams (hydroquinone, tretinoin, and corticosteroids), and newer agents such as tranexamic acid and niacinamide, have also shown efficacy.[5,6]
- A broad-spectrum sunscreen is essential to prevent further darkening of the lesions due to ultraviolet exposure.[1,2,5]

Surgical Management (If Ulcer was Previously Present)

If the wound has fully healed, no further surgical intervention is typically necessary. However, in patients with associated venous insufficiency, compression therapy may be advised to improve circulation and prevent recurrence.[1,2]

Diabetology/Physician Approach

Glycemic control should be intensified using agents such as insulin or glucagon-like peptide-1 (GLP-1) receptor agonists to support skin healing and reduce inflammation.[1,2] Physicians should monitor previous wound sites regularly and address any early signs of recurrence. Concurrent microvascular complications such as diabetic retinopathy and nephropathy should also be evaluated and managed accordingly.[1,2]

PROGNOSIS

The prognosis of PIH in diabetes is generally benign, with pigmentation gradually lightening over several months.[1,2,4] However, complete resolution is unlikely when dermal melanin deposits are present.[1,2,4] The most important factor influencing long-term outcome is the achievement of sustained glycemic and vascular control, which helps prevent recurrence and supports overall skin health.[1,2,4]

> **Clinical Pearls**
>
> When evaluating and managing PIH in diabetic patients, keep the following key points in mind:
> - Postinflammatory hyperpigmentation in diabetics can be more intense and prolonged due to impaired healing and persistent inflammation.[1,2,4]
> - Ulcer-related pigmentation must not be mistaken for melanoma or fixed drug eruption, as misdiagnosis can lead to unnecessary anxiety or procedures.[1,2,4]
> - Always consider a history of prior infection, trauma, or gangrene when assessing new areas of hyperpigmentation.[1,2,4]
> - Consistent use of sunscreen and optimal glycemic control are fundamental in preventing progression or recurrence of PIH.[1,2-6]

REFERENCES

1. Davis EC, Callender VD. Postinflammatory hyperpigmentation: A review of the epidemiology, clinical features, and treatment options in skin of color. J Clin Aesthet Dermatol. 2010;3(7):20-31.
2. Khunger N, Kandhari R. Postinflammatory hyperpigmentation: Etiopathogenesis, prevention, and treatment. Pigment Int. 2016;3(2):41-6.
3. Taylor SC, Cook-Bolden F, Rahman Z, Strachan D. Acne vulgaris in skin of color. J Am Acad Dermatol. 2002;46(2 Suppl Understanding):S98-106.
4. Callender VD, Alexis AF, Daniels SR, Woolery-Lloyd H, Williams K, Andriessen A, et al. Racial differences in acne: Implications for treatment and skin care recommendations. Am J Clin Dermatol. 2012;13(6):407-14.
5. Gupta AK, Gover MD, Nouri K, Taylor S. The treatment of melasma: A review of clinical trials. J Am Acad Dermatol. 2006;55(6):1048-65.
6. Sheth VM, Pandya AG. Melasma: A comprehensive update: Part II. J Am Acad Dermatol. 2011;65(4):699-714.

SECTION 7

Dermatology of Diabetic Foot

▶ Section Outline

Chapter 31: Nonhealing Foot Ulcer in Diabetes Mellitus
Nipul Vara, Vishwa Marvania

Chapter 32: Nonhealing Trophic Ulcer in a Diabetic Male
Bela J Shah

Chapter 33: Difficult-to-Treat Diabetic Foot Ulcer Complicated by Osteomyelitis
Amalkumar Bhattacharya, Pradnya Gatkal, Dipali Rahirkar, Arjun Khadse, Chaitanya Bhandekar

Chapter 34: Maggot Infestation in a Diabetic Foot Ulcer: Clinical Case and Review
Bharat Bhushan Kukreja

Chapter 35: Diabetic Toe Gangrene (Dry Gangrene) in Uncontrolled Diabetes
Suhas Gopal Erande, Anil Patki

Chapter 36: Diabetic Foot Gangrene with Heel Ulceration and Digital Necrosis
Suhas Gopal Erande, Anil Patki

Chapter 37: Extensive Dry Gangrene of the Foot in a Diabetic Smoker
Nipul Vara

CHAPTER 31

Nonhealing Foot Ulcer in Diabetes Mellitus

Nipul Vara, Vishwa Marvania

■ PRESENTATION

A 63-year-old male presented with a large chronic nonhealing ulcer over the lateral aspect of the right lower leg extending to the dorsum of the foot. The ulcer had been present for the past 3 weeks. It initially began as a blister that ruptured and rapidly progressed into an open wound with yellow discharge, pain, and surrounding skin discoloration.
- The patient denied any history of trauma or systemic symptoms such as fever or chills.
- He has a 15-year history of type 2 diabetes mellitus with poor glycemic control [glycated hemoglobin (HbA1c) > 9%], irregular use of medication, and nonadherence to dietary and exercise advice.
- He was also suspected to have hypertension and showed signs of malnutrition.
- There were no previous episodes of diabetic foot ulcers, amputations, or diabetic retinopathy.

■ EXAMINATION

- On examination, the patient was afebrile with a blood pressure of 134/84 mm Hg and pulse of 88 beats/minute.
- The ulcer measured approximately 10 × 6 cm, involving the lateral aspect of the lower leg and extending to the dorsum of the foot **(Figs. 1A and B)**.
- The wound bed showed a mix of yellow slough, necrotic tissue, and exposed subcutaneous structures.
- The margins were irregular and thickened. The surrounding skin displayed hyperpigmentation, thickening, and signs of chronic inflammation.
- Peripheral pulses were palpable but weak.
- Sensory testing confirmed diabetic neuropathy with decreased vibration and reduced response to the monofilament test.
- There was no crepitus and no systemic signs of sepsis.

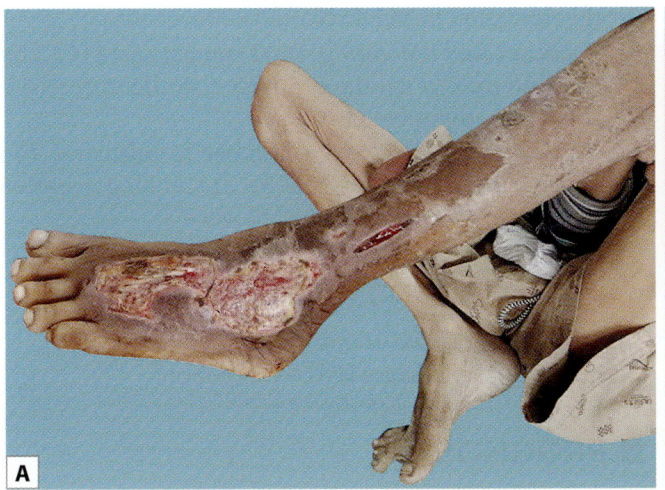
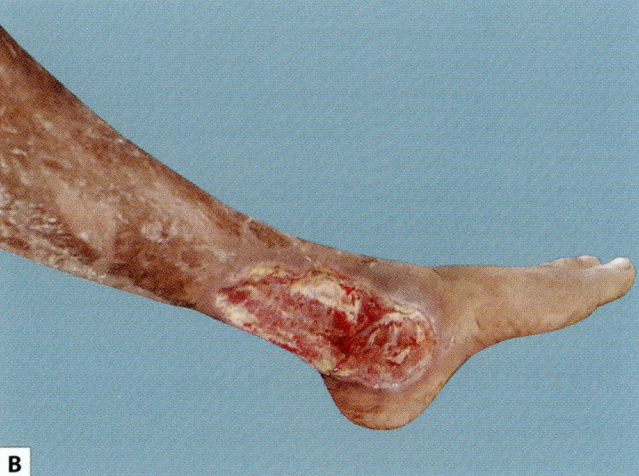

FIGS. 1A AND B: Extensive ulceration over the lateral right leg and foot. Wound bed is covered with yellow slough, granulation tissue, and necrotic zones. Surrounding skin shows postinflammatory hyperpigmentation, thickening, and scarring consistent with chronicity.

INVESTIGATIONS

- Investigations revealed poor glycemic control with an HbA1c of 9.4%, fasting blood glucose of 162 mg/dL, and postprandial blood glucose of 245 mg/dL.
- Hemoglobin was low at 9.8 g/dL, and total white blood cell count was elevated at 14,200/mm³, suggesting anemia and active infection.
- *Inflammatory markers were raised:* C-reactive protein (CRP) at 38 mg/L and erythrocyte sedimentation rate (ESR) at 65 mm/h
- Serum albumin was 2.8 g/dL, indicating protein malnutrition
- A wound swab culture isolated *Pseudomonas aeruginosa* sensitive to piperacillin–tazobactam.
- A Doppler ultrasound showed moderate peripheral arterial disease.
- X-ray of the leg ruled out osteomyelitis.
- Monofilament and vibration tests confirmed the presence of diabetic peripheral neuropathy.

PATHOPHYSIOLOGY

Diabetic ulcers result from a triad of factors: Neuropathy (leading to sensory loss and unrecognized trauma), peripheral arterial disease (compromised healing due to ischemia), and infection (impaired immunity with rapid microbial overgrowth).[1-3] Chronic hyperglycemia induces oxidative stress, endothelial dysfunction, and inhibits fibroblast activity and angiogenesis, all of which are crucial for wound healing.[2,3]

DIAGNOSIS

Diabetic foot ulcer: It is a chronic, nonhealing wound that develops in patients with diabetes, typically as a result of peripheral neuropathy, peripheral arterial disease, and impaired immunity.[1,3,4] These ulcers most commonly occur on the plantar aspect of the foot or over pressure points and are characterized by a loss of protective sensation, poor wound healing, and a high risk of infection and subsequent complications, including osteomyelitis and amputation.[1,3,4]

DIFFERENTIAL DIAGNOSIS

When evaluating a chronic nonhealing ulcer in a diabetic patient, the following differential diagnoses should be considered:[1,3,4]

- *Chronic venous ulcer with secondary infection:* Ulcers are usually located over the medial malleolus, often associated with varicosities and venous insufficiency.[1,3]
- *Tropical ulcer:* These are typically seen in tropical climates, presenting as rapidly progressing ulcers with undermined edges.[1,3]
- *Pyoderma gangrenosum:* A rare, inflammatory ulcerative condition often associated with systemic diseases such as inflammatory bowel disease and characterized by rapidly enlarging, painful ulcers with violaceous borders.[1,3]
- *Ischemic ulcer:* Resulting from severe peripheral arterial disease, these ulcers are usually painful, located on the toes or pressure points and exhibit poor granulation tissue formation.[1,3]

Each of these conditions must be differentiated from a diabetic foot ulcer based on clinical features, patient history, and relevant investigations.[1,3,4]

MANAGEMENT STRATEGY

Diabetology/Physician Management

- Glycemic optimization with a basal–bolus insulin regimen and frequent glucose monitoring[1,3,5]
- *Nutrition:* High-protein diabetic diet with oral supplements such as zinc, vitamin C, and L-arginine[2,3,5]

Management by General Surgeons

- Surgical debridement of necrotic tissue[4,5]
- *Dressings:* Alternate saline and hydrocolloid/honey dressings; consider collagen matrix dressing; and avoid occlusive dressings due to infection risk[4,5]
- Negative pressure wound therapy (NPWT) after infection control[4,5]
- Empirical intravenous piperacillin–tazobactam, with de-escalation based on wound culture[3-5]
- *Footwear and offloading:* Total contact cast (TCC) not feasible due to exudate; advised semicompression dressing with limb elevation[5]
- *Patient education:* Strict glucose monitoring, foot hygiene, use of protective footwear, smoking cessation, hydration, and exercise postrecovery[1,5]

Vascular Surgery Management

Initiation of cilostazol 100 mg twice daily and referral for peripheral artery disease (PAD) evaluation[5]

PROGNOSIS

With the current management approach, slow but steady healing is expected, but there remains a risk of recurrence or progression to deep-tissue infection.[3-5] Long-term limb salvage depends on strict glycemic and vascular care.[3,5]

Clinical Pearls

- Comprehensive foot examination and risk assessment are essential for early identification and prevention of diabetic foot complications.[1,5]
- Optimal glycemic control is crucial for wound healing and reducing the risk of ulcer recurrence.[2,3,5]
- Multidisciplinary care involving diabetologists, surgeons, vascular specialists, and wound care nurses improve outcomes in diabetic foot ulcer management.[3,5]
- Early surgical intervention and appropriate antibiotic therapy are key to preventing limb loss.[3-5]
- Patient education on foot care, footwear, and lifestyle modification significantly reduces the risk of new ulcer formation and amputation.[1,5]
- Regular follow-up and monitoring for signs of infection or ischemia are vital for long-term limb salvage.[3,5]

REFERENCES

1. Boulton AJM, Armstrong DG, Albert SF, Frykberg RG, Hellman R, Kirkman MS, et al.; American Diabetes Association; American Association of Clinical Endocrinologists. Comprehensive Foot Examination and Risk Assessment: A report of the Task Force of the Foot Care Interest Group of the American Diabetes Association. Diabetes Care. 2008;31(8):1679-85.
2. Brem H, Tomic-Canic M. Cellular and molecular basis of wound healing in diabetes. J Clin Invest. 2007;117(5):1219-22.
3. Armstrong DG, Boulton AJM, Bus SA. Diabetic foot ulcers and their recurrence. N Engl J Med. 2017;376(24):2367-75.
4. Lipsky BA, Berendt AR, Deery HG, Embil JM, Joseph WS, Karchmer AW, et al. Diagnosis and treatment of diabetic foot infections. Clin Infect Dis. 2004;39(7):885-910.
5. International Working Group on the Diabetic Foot (IWGDF). (2023). Guidelines on the prevention and management of diabetes-related foot disease. [online] Available from https://iwgdfguidelines.org/wp-content/uploads/2023/07/IWGDF-2023-01-Practical-Guidelines.pdf [Last accessed August, 2025].

CHAPTER 32

Nonhealing Trophic Ulcer in a Diabetic Male

Bela J Shah

■ PRESENTATION

A 42-year-old male, employed as a salesman and diagnosed with type 2 diabetes mellitus for the past 8 years, presented with persistent, nonhealing ulcers on both feet, with occasional purulent discharge, over a 9-month duration. He denied systemic complaints such as fever, weight loss, or limb pain. Despite consistent wound care and regular dressing by a surgeon, there was no evidence of healing. His diabetes management consisted of metformin 500 mg twice daily, though adherence to dietary recommendations and foot care was suboptimal. There was no history of trauma, surgical intervention, or neurovascular incidents.

■ EXAMINATION

On examination, both great toes exhibited single, deep, well-circumscribed, punched-out ulcers with clean bases **(Figs. 1 and 2)**. The surrounding skin was indurated but nontender, and there were no signs of cellulitis or gangrene. The patient's body mass index (BMI) was 29.6 kg/m^2, indicating an overweight status.

Peripheral pulses were palpable, and there was no pedal edema.

■ LABORATORY INVESTIGATIONS

Laboratory investigations revealed fasting blood glucose of 188 mg/dL, postprandial glucose of 256 mg/dL, and a glycated hemoglobin (HbA1c) of 7.5%. Complete blood count, liver and renal function tests, thyroid profile, and lipid profile were within normal limits. Viral markers for hepatitis B virus (HBV), hepatitis C virus (HCV), and human immunodeficiency virus (HIV) were negative.

■ DIAGNOSIS

Nonhealing trophic ulcer associated with poorly controlled type 2 diabetes mellitus.[1]

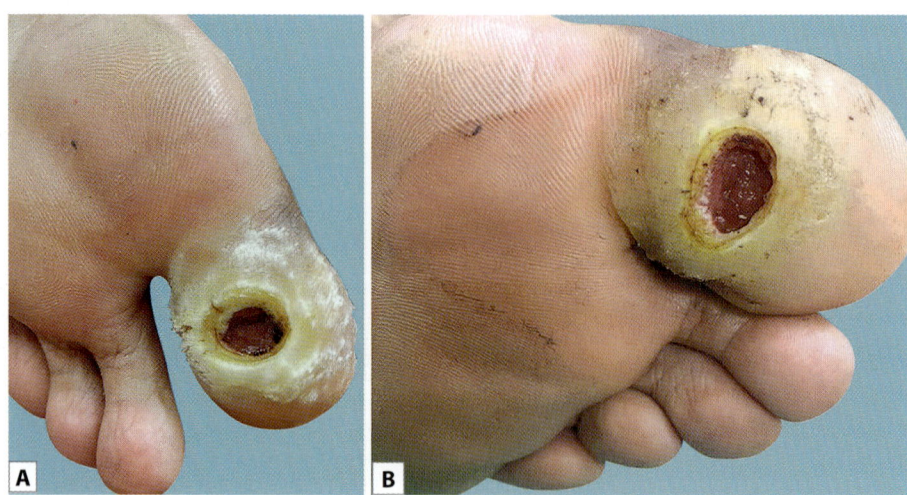

FIGS. 1A AND B: Single, deep, well-circumscribed, punched-out ulcers with clean bases on both great toes.

DIFFERENTIAL DIAGNOSES

- *Syphilitic gumma:* Characterized by deep ulcers with indurated margins; excluded by negative serology
- *Pyoderma gangrenosum:* Rapidly progressing, painful ulcers with undermined borders
- *Venous ulcers:* Typically found near the medial malleolus, often with hemosiderin pigmentation
- *Ulcers related to hemoglobinopathies:* Chronic ulcers in conditions such as sickle cell anemia.
- *Vasculitic ulcers:* Painful lesions with purpuric bases, often accompanied by systemic symptoms
- *Neoplastic ulcers (e.g., Marjolin ulcer):* Nonhealing, exophytic, and may bleed

PATHOPHYSIOLOGY

Trophic ulcers in diabetes result from a combination of factors:
- Peripheral neuropathy leads to loss of protective sensation, predisposing to unnoticed trauma.
- Microvascular disease (diabetic microangiopathy) impairs local blood supply and healing.
- Immunosuppression in diabetes delays wound repair and increases infection risk.
- Repetitive mechanical stress and pressure, particularly over bony prominences or weight-bearing areas, contribute to ulcer formation.

These ulcers commonly develop under areas of callus, which subsequently fissure and ulcerate, often progressing to deeper tissue layers with minimal symptoms due to neuropathy.[1]

MANAGEMENT

Wound Care and Dermatological Management

- Surgical debridement to remove necrotic tissue and promote a healthy wound bed[2-4]
- Topical antibiotics such as mupirocin or fusidic acid for localized infection control[2-5]
- Moist wound dressings, including hydrocolloid or foam-based materials, to maintain optimal healing environment[2-4]
- Offloading using specialized footwear or orthotic devices to redistribute pressure away from ulcerated sites[2-4]
- Advanced modalities for refractory ulcers include:
  - Negative pressure wound therapy (NPWT)[2-4]
  - Hyperbaric oxygen therapy (HBOT)[2-4]
  - Application of topical growth factors [e.g., platelet-derived growth factor (PDGF)][2-4]

Diabetology and Systemic Management

- *Adjustment of antidiabetic therapy:* Metformin was increased to 500 mg 3 times daily, with the addition of glimepiride 1 mg once daily, to optimize glycemic control.[1]
- Emphasis was made on strict glycemic regulation to facilitate wound healing[1]
- Daily foot inspection and avoidance of barefoot walking were advised.[1]
- Screening for other diabetic complications (e.g., retinal and renal involvement) was performed and found to be normal.[1]
- Patient education regarding foot hygiene, skin moisturization, and early recognition of infection was reinforced.[1]

Additional Considerations

- In chronic, nonhealing ulcers, underlying osteomyelitis should be excluded using clinical assessment and imaging as needed.[6,7]
- Smoking cessation, regular foot care, daily self-examination, use of custom footwear, and ongoing patient education are critical for both healing and prevention of future complications.[7]

PROGNOSIS

The likelihood of healing is influenced by ulcer depth, infection control, and the degree of glycemic management. With comprehensive care, chronic diabetic ulcers may heal within 8–12 weeks, though there is a risk of scarring and recurrence. Delayed or inadequate intervention can result in severe complications, including osteomyelitis and limb amputation.[1]

Clinical Pearls

▶ Trophic ulcers typically occur at pressure points (e.g., great toe, heel, and metatarsal heads).[1] These ulcers are often painless due to underlying neuropathy, leading to delayed presentation.[1]
▶ Always consider and rule out osteomyelitis in chronic, nonhealing ulcers.[6,7]
▶ Core management strategies include offloading, debridement, infection control, and metabolic optimization.[1-4]
▶ Preventive measures such as custom footwear, regular podiatric care, and patient education are essential to minimize recurrence.[8]

REFERENCES

1. Boulton AJM, Armstrong DG, Albert SF, Frykberg RG, Hellman R, Kirkman MS, et al.; American Diabetes Association; American Association of Clinical Endocrinologists. Comprehensive foot examination and risk assessment: A report of the task force of the foot care interest group of the American Diabetes Association, with endorsement by the American Association of Clinical Endocrinologists. Diabetes Care. 2008;31(8):1679-85.
2. Game FL, Attinger C, Hartemann A, Hinchliffe RJ, Löndahl M, Price PE, et al; International Working Group on the Diabetic Foot. IWGDF guidance on use of interventions to enhance the healing of chronic ulcers of the foot in diabetes. Diabetes Metab Res Rev. 2016;32(S1):75-83.
3. Armstrong DG, Lavery LA; Diabetic Foot Study Consortium. Negative pressure wound therapy after partial diabetic foot amputation: A multicentre, randomised controlled trial. Lancet. 2005;366(9498):1704-10.
4. Frykberg RG, Banks J. Challenges in the Treatment of Chronic Wounds. Adv Wound Care. 2015;4(9):560-82.
5. Lipsky BA, Berendt AR, Cornia PB, Pile JC, Peters EJ, Armstrong DG, et al.; Infectious Diseases Society of America. 2012 Infectious Diseases Society of America clinical practice guideline for the diagnosis and treatment of diabetic foot infections. Clin Infect Dis. 2012;54(12):e132-73.
6. Jeffcoate WJ. Wound healing: A practical algorithm. Diabetes Metab Res Rev. 2012;28(S1):58-61.
7. Singh N, Armstrong DG, Lipsky BA. Preventing foot ulcers in patients with diabetes. JAMA. 2005;293(2):217-28.
8. Lavery LA, Higgins KR, Lanctot DR, Constantinides GP, Zamorano RG, Athanasiou KA, et al. Preventing diabetic foot ulcer recurrence in high-risk patients: use of temperature monitoring as a self-assessment tool. Diabetes Care. 2007;30(6):14-20.

CHAPTER 33

Difficult-to-Treat Diabetic Foot Ulcer Complicated by Osteomyelitis

Amalkumar Bhattacharya, Pradnya Gatkal, Dipali Rahirkar, Arjun Khadse, Chaitanya Bhandekar

■ PRESENTATION

A 35-year-old rural male with a 4-year history of poorly controlled type 2 diabetes mellitus presented to the outpatient department with a 2-month-old nonhealing ulcer on the anteromedial aspect of the right distal leg, extending toward the great toe. The ulcer originated following minor trauma sustained while working in the field. Despite over-the-counter antibiotics, traditional herbal remedies, and oral antibiotics, the wound progressively enlarged, continuing to discharge minimal amounts of fluid and pus. The patient reported foul-smelling discharge, surrounding redness, and minimal pain, with no systemic symptoms such as fever, chills, malaise, or rest pain. His medical history includes dyslipidemia, obesity [body mass index (BMI) 26 kg/m²], chronic smoking, and alcoholism.[1,2]

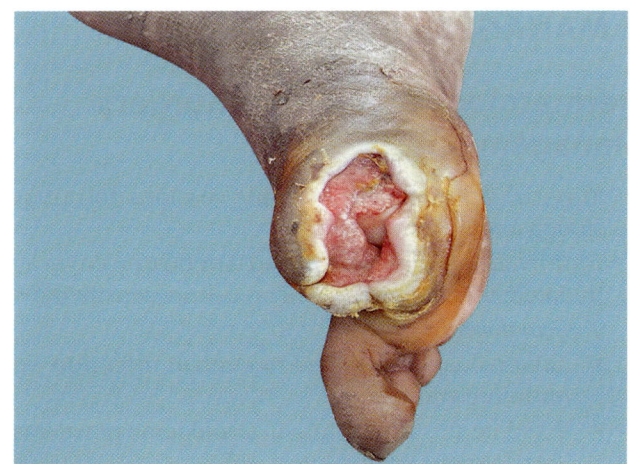

FIG. 1: Single 5 × 5 cm ulcer with punched-out edges, necrotic base, surrounding erythema, and signs of active local infection.

■ EXAMINATION

On examination, the following clinical findings were noted:
- The patient was alert, oriented, and afebrile. Both lower limbs were dry, and there were no visible signs of trophic changes such as brittle nails or loss of hair. No systemic signs of sepsis or evidence of rest pain were observed.
- There was a single ulcer measuring 5 × 5 cm with punched-out edges and a necrotic base, surrounded by erythematous skin. Visible signs of active local infection were present **(Fig. 1)**.
- Peripheral pulses were palpable in all limbs and capillary refill time was <2 seconds, indicating preserved peripheral perfusion.
- Peripheral sensory neuropathy was confirmed using a 10 g monofilament test and vibration sense loss over the feet (bilateral neuropathic feet with loss of protective sensation).

■ INVESTIGATIONS

On investigation, the following findings were observed:
- *Glycemic status:*
  - *Glycated hemoglobin (HbA1c):* 10.8%
  - *Random blood sugar:* 240 mg/dL
- *Infective/inflammatory markers:*
  - *Total WBC count:* 17,000/mm³
  - *C-reactive protein (CRP):* 18 mg/L.
- *Wound evaluation:* Wound swab cultures were collected before initiating antibiotic therapy to guide appropriate antimicrobial management.
- *Radiology:* X-ray of the right foot showed osteopenia with a periosteal reaction at the first metatarsophalangeal (MTP) joint, suggestive of underlying osteomyelitis.
- *Other laboratory parameters:*
  - *Hemoglobin:* 11 g/dL
  - *Blood urea nitrogen (BUN):* 20 mg/dL

DIAGNOSIS

Diabetic foot ulcer with underlying osteomyelitis involving the first MTP joint, confirmed by imaging and consistent clinical progression.[3,4]

DIFFERENTIAL DIAGNOSES

- Chronic neuropathic ulcer without bone involvement[4,5]
- Trophic ulcer from peripheral vascular disease[4,5]
- Tubercular osteomyelitis (ruled out by imaging and negative systemic features)[3]
- Deep fungal or atypical mycobacterial infection[3]

MANAGEMENT

Dermatology and Wound Surgery Management

- *Surgical debridement:* Multiple sessions to remove slough and necrotic tissue[3,4]
- *Empirical antibiotics:* Broad-spectrum coverage initiated, then tailored based on culture sensitivity[3]
- *Topical therapy:*
  - Silver-based dressings to control infection and promote granulation[6]
  - Exudate-absorbing dressings and ionic powders to form a moist wound interface[6]
  - Advanced wound-care techniques, including negative pressure wound therapy (NPWT) and ideal wound healing dressings, were employed as needed to enhance healing and granulation tissue formation.[6]
- *Wound follow-up:* Regular wound clinic visits; dressing changes every 48 hours
- *Surgical consultation:* Plastic surgery considered split-thickness skin grafting, deferred based on progressive granulation.[6]
- *Outcome:* Healthy granulation tissue formed within 1 month, ulcer size reduced. The patient was admitted twice, each time for <2 weeks, with a total hospital stay of approximately 28 days.[2]

Diabetology/Physician Management

- *Glycemic optimization:* Insulin started for immediate control (not detailed but implied from setting).[1,2]
- *Lifestyle advice:* Counseling on alcohol cessation, smoking cessation, diet, and weight reduction.[1,2]
- *Neuropathy management:* Initiation of foot care education, protective footwear, and daily foot checks[4,5]
- *Multidisciplinary care:* Involvement of endocrinologist, plastic surgeon, orthopedic specialist, and wound-care nurse.[6]
- *Long-term monitoring:* Scheduled HbA1c every 3 months and vascular/neuro assessment[6]

PROGNOSIS

With a structured, team-based, multimodal approach, the patient's foot ulcer improved significantly. Osteomyelitis was controlled, granulation tissue formed adequately, and the need for amputation was avoided.[2,3,6] This case underscores the importance of optimizing the general medical condition, including nutritional status and glycemic control, before and during wound management for best outcomes.[4,6] However, given the neuropathic background and poor initial glycemic control, the risk of recurrence remains unless strict glycemic and lifestyle modifications are sustained.[3,4]

Clinical Pearls

- Diabetic foot ulcers often result from the triad of neuropathy, trauma, and ischemia.[4,5]
- Osteomyelitis should be suspected in any chronic diabetic ulcer with exposed bone, sinus tracts, or unresponsive infection.[3]
- Early signs like loss of protective sensation, even without pain, must be actively screened.[4,5]
- Multidisciplinary wound care, including aggressive debridement and optimized systemic status, is key to limb salvage.[6]
- Use of advanced dressing technologies (silver-based, moisture-control powders, and NPWT) aids healing in deep, complex wounds.[6]

REFERENCES

1. Mandewo W, Edodge E, Chideme-Munodawafa A, Mandewo G. Non-adherence to treatment among diabetic patients attending outpatient clinic at Mutare provincial hospital, Zimbabwe. Int J Sci Technol Res. 2014;3:66-86.
2. Subhash C. Diabetic foot ulcer–a case study. J Exerc Sci Physiol. 2005;1:98-9.
3. Lipsky BA, Berendt AR, Cornia PB, Pile JC, Peters JG, Armstrong DG, et al. 2012 IDSA clinical practice guideline for the diagnosis and treatment of diabetic foot infections. Clin Infect Dis. 2012;54(12):132-73.
4. Jeffcoate WJ, Harding KG. Diabetic foot ulcers. Lancet. 2003;361(9368):1545-51.
5. Boulton AJM, Vileikyte L, Ragnarson-Tennvall G, Apelqvist J. The global burden of diabetic foot disease. Lancet. 2005;366(9498):1719-24.
6. Bakker K, Apelqvist J, Lipsky BA, Van Netten JJ. The 2015 IWGDF guidance on the prevention and management of foot problems in diabetes. Diabetes Metab Res Rev. 2016;32(S1):7-15.

CHAPTER 34

Maggot Infestation in a Diabetic Foot Ulcer: Clinical Case and Review

Bharat Bhushan Kukreja

■ PRESENTATION

A 62-year-old woman with type 2 diabetes mellitus for over 20 years presented to the emergency department with complaints of extreme weakness, inability to walk, loss of appetite, and fever for the past 3 days. She had discontinued her diabetes medication for the last 3 months due to personal and financial difficulties.[1,2] She worked as an agricultural laborer and was the primary earner for her family.[2] Over time, her general health had progressively declined.

This case reflects the challenges of managing an advanced diabetic foot ulcer with secondary maggot infestation (myiasis) in an elderly, socioeconomically disadvantaged patient.

■ EXAMINATION

On arrival, she appeared dehydrated, febrile, and disoriented. Her pulse rate was 110 beats/min, and her supine blood pressure was 100/60 mm Hg. She was pale and severely undernourished, showing signs of sarcopenia. Systemic examination was unremarkable except for findings in the right lower limb.

Foot Examination

Her right foot was swollen from the ankle to the toes. A large ulcer with gangrene was observed over the dorsum of the right great toe, extending up to the nail margin **(Fig. 1)**. The ulcer base was covered with thick, greyish-yellow discharge, exposing fascia and tendons. Multiple live maggots were visible within the wound. Peripheral pulses in the affected limb were palpable and equal on both sides **(Fig. 2)**.

■ INVESTIGATIONS

Initial investigations were conducted to assess the extent of infection, metabolic control, renal function, and to identify any systemic complications. The following findings were noted:
- *Random blood glucose:* 410 mg/dL—indicating severe hyperglycemia

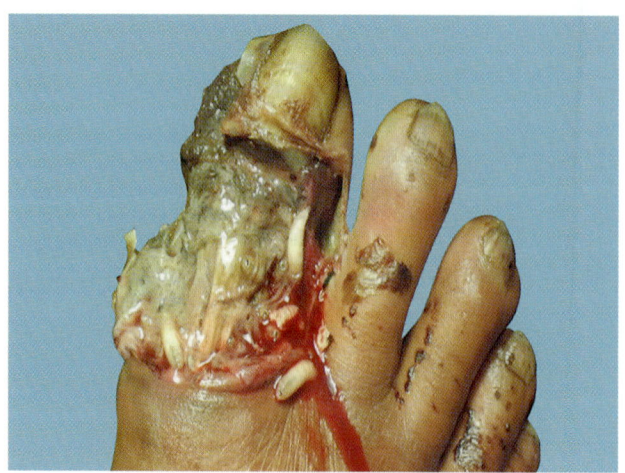

FIG. 1: Wound with maggots.
Courtesy: Dr Sudhir Jain, diabetic foot surgeon, Guwahati, Assam.

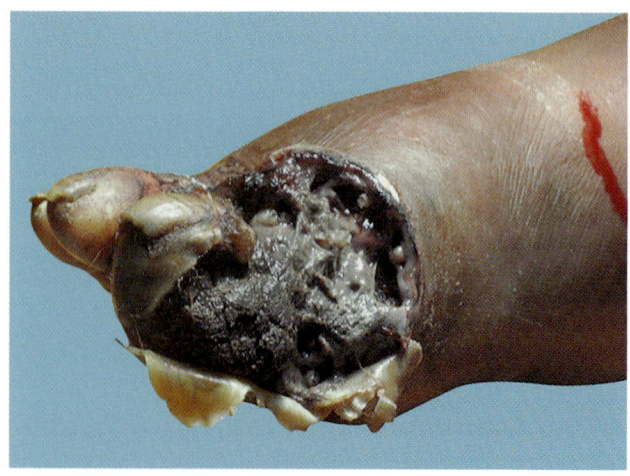

FIG. 2: Gangrenous base of the wound.
Courtesy: Dr Sudhir Jain, diabetic foot surgeon, Guwahati, Assam.

- *Urine output:* Anuria for the past 8 hours, suggesting possible acute kidney injury
- *Urinalysis:*
  - *Protein:* Trace
  - *Sugar:* ++++
  - *Ketones:* Negative—consistent with poor glycemic control
- *Complete blood count (CBC):*
  - *Total leukocyte count (TLC):* 21,000/mm³ with 90% neutrophils—pointing to severe infection
  - *Erythrocyte sedimentation rate (ESR):* 55 mm/h
  - *Hemoglobin:* 10 g%, indicating anemia of chronic disease
- *Renal function:*
  - *Creatinine:* 1.4 mg/dL
  - *Estimated glomerular filtration rate (eGFR):* 40.17 mL/min/1.73 m²—suggestive of mild renal impairment
- *Electrolytes:*
  - *Sodium:* 136 mmol/L
  - *Potassium:* 3.6 mmol/L—within normal range but needs monitoring
- *Liver function tests:* Serum glutamic oxaloacetic transaminase (SGOT) 37 U/L, serum glutamate pyruvate transaminase (SGPT) 42 U/L—mildly elevated, possibly due to systemic stress or medication
- *Electrocardiogram (ECG):* Sinus tachycardia—reflecting dehydration, infection, or metabolic stress
- *Wound swab:* Sent for culture and sensitivity—essential for guiding targeted antibiotic therapy

These investigations confirmed the presence of sepsis, uncontrolled diabetes, and early kidney dysfunction, requiring urgent multidisciplinary intervention.

DIAGNOSIS

Diabetic foot ulcer with gangrene and secondary maggot infestation (myiasis): The final diagnosis was based on clinical presentation, local examination, and was supporting laboratory investigations. The presence of a chronic nonhealing ulcer, signs of gangrene, visible live maggots, and systemic sepsis in a poorly controlled diabetic patient confirmed the diagnosis. Myiasis, though rare, was indicative of poor wound hygiene and advanced neglect, requiring urgent surgical and medical intervention.[3-5,1]

DIFFERENTIAL DIAGNOSES

A few other conditions were considered based on the clinical picture:
- *Diabetic foot ulcer with secondary infection:* It is common in uncontrolled diabetes; however, the presence of maggots pointed to a more advanced, neglected wound.[3-5]
- *Dry or wet gangrene of the toe:* It can be differentiated by the extent of tissue involvement; in this case, wet gangrene was present with superadded infestation.[2,3,6]
- *Necrotizing fasciitis:* It is ruled out due to the absence of crepitus, skin discoloration beyond the ulcer margins, and rapid systemic deterioration.[2,3,6]
- *Tropical ulcer or infected traumatic wound:* These were less likely due to the chronicity of the ulcer, absence of recent trauma, and a long history of diabetes.[3-5]
- *Onychomycosis:* Chronic fungal nail infection can be a precursor or contributor to diabetic foot ulcers, especially in the great toe. Though not prominent in this case, it should be considered in the differential due to its known association with poor nail health in diabetics.[6]

Accurate differentiation was essential to avoid delay in surgical management and to ensure appropriate use of antimicrobial therapy.

MANAGEMENT

- Immediate fluid resuscitation and intravenous insulin for hyperglycemia
- Empiric broad-spectrum intravenous antibiotics
- *Emergency surgical intervention:* Amputation of the right great toe under regional block, with meticulous removal of maggots and debridement **(Figs. 3 to 6)**
- Postoperative intensive care, ongoing glycemic control, and wound management
- Gradual clinical improvement; transferred to the general ward after 4 days

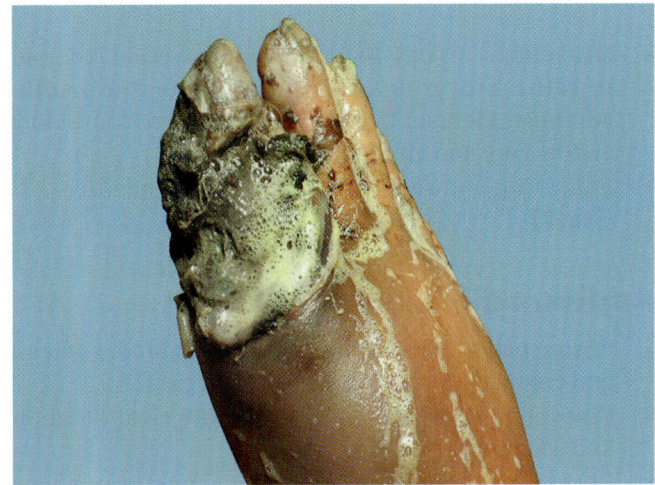

FIG. 3: Intensive cleaning.
Courtesy: Dr Sudhir Jain, diabetic foot surgeon, Guwahati, Assam.

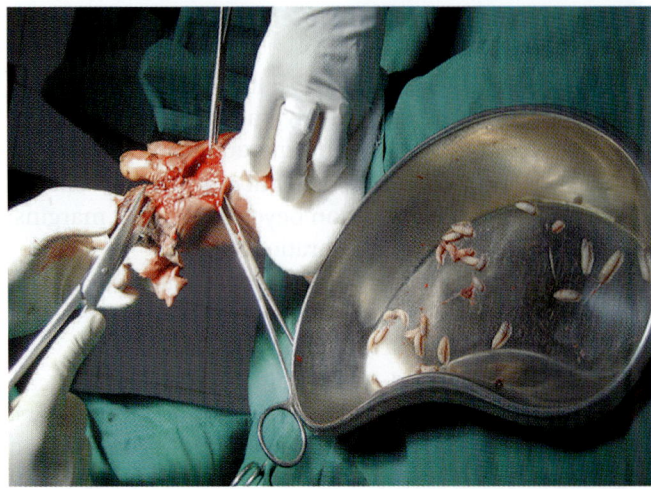

FIG. 4: Maggots being removed.
Courtesy: Dr Sudhir Jain, diabetic foot surgeon, Guwahati, Assam.

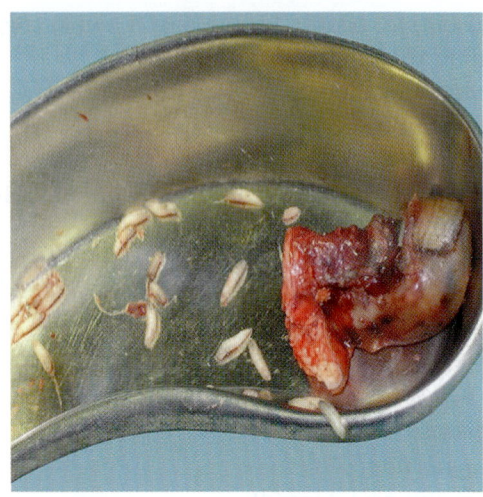

FIG. 5: Amputated great toe with maggots.
Courtesy: Dr Sudhir Jain, diabetic foot surgeon, Guwahati, Assam.

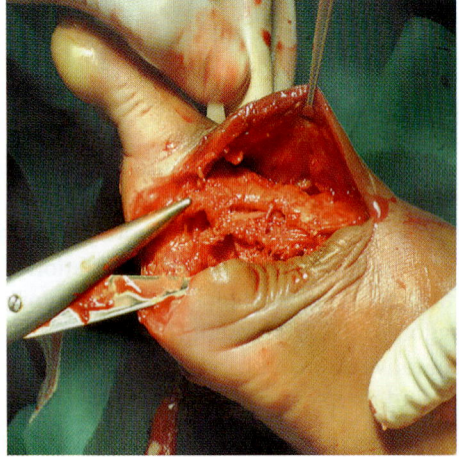

FIG. 6: Post extensive debriment and amputation, healthy tissue.
Courtesy: Dr Sudhir Jain, Diabetic foot surgeon, Guwahati, Assam.

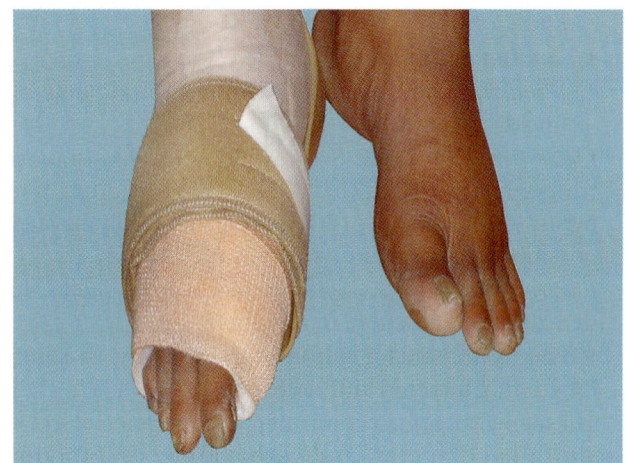

FIG. 7: Recovered foot.
Courtesy: Dr Sudhir Jain, diabetic foot surgeon, Guwahati, Assam.

- Discharged on day 10 with a stable wound, trained in self-monitoring of blood glucose and insulin administration, and given comprehensive counseling on foot care and glycemic control
- Follow-up showed satisfactory wound healing[3-5,7,1] **(Fig. 7)**

Additional Recommendations

- Ensure patient's history includes occupation, address, and contact information for completeness.
- Chief complaints should be listed with clear duration and sequence.
- Consider adding details on social support, previous foot-care education, and access to healthcare facilities to contextualize barriers and guide prevention strategies.[2]

Clinical Pearls

- *Diabetic foot ulcers* are a serious and common complication of long-standing, poorly controlled diabetes, especially when associated with peripheral neuropathy and peripheral vascular disease.[1-3,8]
- *Neglect, poor glycemic control, and socioeconomic hardship* often contribute to late presentation and advanced disease, as demonstrated in this case.[1,2]
- *Myiasis (maggot infestation)* is a rare but striking indicator of extreme neglect and inadequate wound hygiene. Although maggots may contribute to the natural debridement of necrotic tissue, their presence should prompt immediate surgical and medical attention.[4,5]
- The case highlights the *urgent need for early recognition* and *aggressive intervention* in diabetic foot infections to prevent limb- or life-threatening complications.[1-3]

- *Multidisciplinary management* involving physicians, surgeons, nurses, and diabetic educators is essential for optimal outcomes.[1-3]
- *Patient education* is critical, particularly in rural and underserved areas, to improve self-care, adherence to treatment, and timely medical consultation.[8]
- *Comprehensive care* should include glycemic control, appropriate wound care, antibiotic therapy, and surgical intervention when indicated.[1,3,7]
- *Preventive strategies* such as routine foot examinations, proper footwear, and structured diabetes education programs can significantly reduce the incidence of such advanced presentations.[3,2,8]

REFERENCES

1. Zubair M, Malik A, Ahmad J. Clinico-microbiological study and antimicrobial drug resistance profile of diabetic foot infections in North India. Foot (Edinb). 2011;21(1):6-14.
2. World Health Organization. Global report on diabetes. Geneva: WHO; 2016.
3. Lipsky BA, Berendt AR, Cornia PB, Pile JC, Peters EJ, Armstrong DG, et al.; Infectious Diseases Society of America. 2012 IDSA clinical practice guideline for the diagnosis and treatment of diabetic foot infections. Clin Infect Dis. 2012;54(12):e132-73.
4. Tileklioğlu E, Yıldız İ, Bozkurt-Kozan F, Malatyali E, Ertuğrul MB, Ertabaklar H. Wound Myiasis in Diabetic Foot Ulcer: Calliphoridae and Sarcophagidae Family. Iran J Parasitol. 2021;16(4):678-685.
5. Sherman RA. Maggot therapy for treating diabetic foot ulcers unresponsive to conventional therapy. Diabetes Care. 2003;26(2):446-451.
6. Hay RJ, Baran R. Onychomycosis: A proposed revision of the clinical classification. J Am Acad Dermatol. 2011;65(6):1219-27.
7. Robson MC, Steed DL, Franz MG. Wound healing: Biologic features and approaches to maximize healing trajectories. Curr Probl Surg. 2001;38(2):72-140.
8. Boulton AJ, Armstrong DG, Albert SF, Frykberg RG, Hellman R, Kirkman MS, et al. Comprehensive foot examination and risk assessment: A report of the task force of the Foot Care Interest Group of the American Diabetes Association, with endorsement by the American Association of Clinical Endocrinologists. Diabetes Care. 2008;31(8):1679-85.

CHAPTER 35

Diabetic Toe Gangrene (Dry Gangrene) in Uncontrolled Diabetes

Suhas Gopal Erande, Anil Patki

■ PRESENTATION

A 47-year-old male presented with black discoloration of the second toe for 2 weeks, associated with dull pain and numbness. The symptoms started gradually, and there was no history of trauma or preceding infection. The patient has a 10-year history of type 2 diabetes mellitus, poorly controlled with a glycated hemoglobin (HbA1c) of 10.3%, and he admits to nonadherence to treatment. He is a 20-pack-year smoker and also has hypertension and dyslipidemia.

■ EXAMINATION

- On local examination, the second toe was found to be dry, black, and shrivelled, with a clear line of demarcation, which is typical of dry gangrene **(Fig. 1)**. There was no purulence, erythema, or evidence of soft-tissue infection. On clinical examination, the appearance was consistent with dry, mummified necrosis without features of infection.

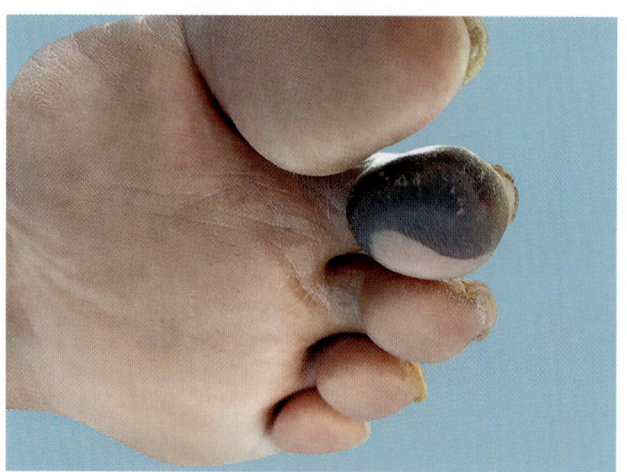

FIG. 1: Dry, black, shrivelled second toe with a clear line of demarcation, characteristic of dry gangrene.

- Vascular examination revealed weak dorsalis pedis and posterior tibial pulses, capillary refill time greater than 3 seconds, and dry, scaly skin over the foot.
- Neurologically, the patient had numbness of the foot, consistent with diabetic peripheral neuropathy.

■ INVESTIGATIONS

- The lipid profile showed a low-density lipoprotein (LDL) of 142 mg/dL and high-density lipoprotein (HDL) of 34 mg/dL, indicating an atherogenic lipid profile.
- Serum creatinine was mildly elevated at 1.3 mg/dL, raising concern for early nephropathy.
- The complete blood count showed mild leukocytosis, while C-reactive protein (CRP) and erythrocyte sedimentation rate (ESR) were mildly raised, suggesting chronic inflammation rather than acute infection.
- The ankle-brachial index (ABI) was 0.4, indicating moderate-to-severe peripheral arterial disease (PAD).
- An X-ray of the foot showed no gas in soft tissues but revealed bone erosion.
- Doppler ultrasound of the lower limb showed severely diminished blood flow in the arteries of the foot.
- A skin biopsy, if performed, would show coagulative necrosis without neutrophilic infiltration. Laboratory investigations revealed an HbA1c of 10.3%, fasting glucose of 180 mg/dL, and postprandial glucose of 286 mg/dL.

■ PATHOPHYSIOLOGY

The development of dry gangrene in this patient is the result of multiple pathophysiological mechanisms associated with diabetes. These mechanisms act together to impair blood flow, delay healing, and increase susceptibility to tissue necrosis.

Peripheral Arterial Disease

Diabetes accelerates atherosclerosis in the lower limb arteries, with a 2–7 times increased risk of PAD compared to nondiabetics.[1-3] Atherosclerotic plaque formation narrows or blocks arteries, severely reducing blood supply to the distal tissues. This results in critical limb ischemia and sets the stage for tissue necrosis.

Microangiopathy

Persistent hyperglycemia causes endothelial dysfunction and thickening of the capillary basement membrane, impairing perfusion and tissue oxygenation and delaying wound healing. Microvascular damage also limits the formation of collateral vessels, making it harder for the body to compensate for arterial blockages.[2,4]

Neuropathy

Diabetic neuropathy results in sensory loss, so patients are often unaware of minor trauma, pressure points, or repetitive stress injuries.[5] In addition, motor neuropathy can cause foot deformities, increasing areas of high pressure and the risk of skin breakdown. Autonomic neuropathy contributes by reducing sweating, leading to dry, cracked skin that is more vulnerable to injury.[2]

Ischemic Necrosis

Critical ischemia leads to tissue death by coagulative necrosis, resulting in dry gangrene in the absence of infection.[4] The affected tissue becomes dry, black, and shriveled, with a clear line of demarcation from healthy tissue. Without intervention, secondary infection may occur, converting dry gangrene into wet gangrene, which carries a higher risk of sepsis.[2,4]

■ DIAGNOSIS

Dry gangrene of the toe is caused by critical limb ischemia from PAD in a patient with uncontrolled diabetes and smoking history. The condition has developed as a result of severe PAD in the setting of uncontrolled diabetes and significant smoking history.[1,2] The presence of a clear line of demarcation, absence of pus or swelling, and dry, mummified tissue support this diagnosis.[2,4]

■ DIFFERENTIAL DIAGNOSES

Several conditions may mimic or overlap with the presentation of dry gangrene. It is important to consider these possibilities to ensure accurate diagnosis and appropriate management.

- *Wet gangrene:* It is characterized by infected, moist, foul-smelling tissue with purulent discharge and surrounding edema.[4] It progresses rapidly and is often accompanied by systemic signs such as fever and tachycardia.
- *Diabetic foot ulcer:* It typically presents as a superficial, nonhealing sore over pressure points or trauma sites. The surrounding skin may show signs of callus formation, and there is usually no distinct line of demarcation as seen in dry gangrene.[2]
- *Acute limb ischemia:* It presents suddenly with severe pain, pallor, pulselessness, paresthesia, paralysis, and poikilothermia (the six Ps). It is often caused by embolism or in situ thrombosis and represents a surgical emergency.[3]
- *Acral melanoma:* It may appear as a dark, irregularly pigmented lesion on the toe, resembling gangrene. However, it tends to have asymmetrical borders, color variation, and slow progressive enlargement rather than tissue necrosis.[4]
- *Peripheral embolic infarction:* It occurs due to embolic occlusion of distal arteries, leading to localized tissue death. Unlike dry gangrene from chronic PAD, embolic infarction presents abruptly and may not show gradual demarcation or chronic skin changes.[3]

■ MANAGEMENT

The management of dry gangrene in this patient focuses on local control of necrotic tissue, restoring limb perfusion, preventing complications, and addressing underlying risk factors. A multidisciplinary approach involving surgery, vascular intervention, and medical therapy is essential for optimal outcomes.

Surgical/Local

- *Amputation:* It indicated for confirmed or impending dry gangrene. A decision between conservative management or surgical removal (toe amputation) depends on the extent of necrosis and risk of progression.[1,6,7]
- *Revascularization:* Angioplasty or bypass surgery may be considered to restore perfusion to the affected limb and prevent further tissue loss.[2,3]
- *Wound care:* The affected area should be kept dry and clean. Debridement is avoided unless there is conversion to wet gangrene or secondary infection.[4]

Diabetologist/Physician Management

- *Glycemic control:* Basal-bolus insulin should be initiated to achieve rapid and sustained reduction in HbA1c.[2,3]
- *Antiplatelet therapy:* Aspirin 75–150 mg daily or clopidogrel is recommended to reduce vascular risk.[2]
- *Statin:* High-intensity statin therapy (e.g., atorvastatin 40–80 mg) should be prescribed to manage dyslipidemia and lower cardiovascular risk.[2,3]
- *Antibiotics:* Reserved for cases where secondary infection is present or suspected.[4]
- *Smoking cessation and foot protection:* The patient must be counseled to stop smoking, and proper foot care measures should be implemented to prevent new ulcers or trauma.[2,3]

■ PROGNOSIS

The prognosis of dry gangrene depends on the severity of ischemia, the presence of infection, and the timeliness of intervention. Early recognition and management can prevent serious complications.

- Dry gangrene may auto-amputate if perfusion is adequately restored.[5]
- Without timely intervention, the condition can progress to wet gangrene, leading to spread of necrosis, sepsis, and the need for major amputation.[1,4,6]

Clinical Pearls

▸ Always assess pedal pulses and ABI during diabetic foot evaluations.[2]
▸ Dry gangrene with a clear demarcation indicates sterile ischemic necrosis—antibiotics are not required unless there are features of wet gangrene.[4]
▸ The combination of neuropathy and peripheral arterial disease significantly increases the risk of limb loss.[2]
▸ Use standardized classifications such as Fontaine, Rutherford, or WIfI to guide treatment decisions.[1,3]
▸ Early collaboration with vascular specialists improves patient outcomes and helps preserve limb function.[2,3]

REFERENCES

1. Jude EB, Lu J, Fisher R. Diabetes and peripheral artery disease: A review. Diabetes. 2022.
2. Buttolph A, Marietta M, Sapra A. Gangrene. In: StatPearls [Internet]. Treasure Island (FL): StatPearls Publishing; 2025 PMID: 32809387.
3. American Diabetes Association. Peripheral arterial disease in people with diabetes. Diabetes Care. 2003;26(12):3333-41.
4. Khan T, Lopez Rowe V. Medscape. (2025). Diabetic foot ulcers: Practice essentials. [online] Available from https://emedicine.medscape.com/article/460282-overview [Last accessed August, 2025].
5. Kim Jiyoun. The pathophysiology of diabetic foot: A narrative review. Journal of Yeungnam Medical Science. 2023;40(4): 328-334.
6. Cross S. Gangrene. Elsevier Health Sci. 2018.
7. Murphy-Lavoie HM, Ramsey A, Nguyen M, Vadakekut ES. Diabetic Foot Infections. In: StatPearls [Internet]. Treasure Island (FL): StatPearls Publishing; 2025.

CHAPTER 36

Diabetic Foot Gangrene with Heel Ulceration and Digital Necrosis

Suhas Gopal Erande, Anil Patki

■ PRESENTATION

A 64-year-old male presents with blackening of the great and second toes, a foul-smelling discharge, and swelling of the right foot for 10 days. The condition started as a blister on the plantar surface, progressed to an ulcer, and then to digital gangrene. The patient has long-standing type 2 diabetes (14 years), peripheral neuropathy (3 years), and hypertension. Medical compliance has been irregular. Social history includes habitual barefoot walking and long-standing tobacco use.

■ EXAMINATION

- On examination, the right foot shows dry gangrene of the great and second toes and a necrotic heel ulcer with slough and undermined margins **(Figs. 1A and B)**.

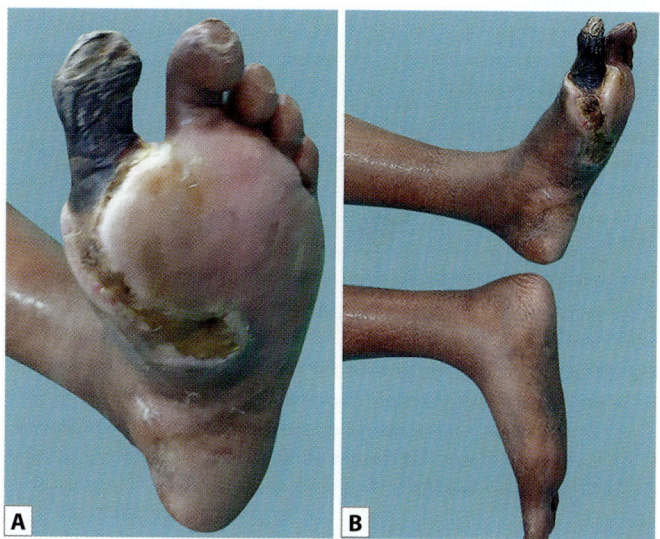

FIGS. 1A AND B: Dry gangrene of the great and second toes, and a necrotic heel ulcer with slough and undermined margins on the right foot.

- The foot appears shiny and discolored with minimal hair growth, indicating chronic ischemia.
- Palpation confirms feeble or absent dorsalis pedis and posterior tibial pulses.
- The foot is cold to the touch, and sensory loss is present below the ankle, suggesting neuropathy, although motor function is preserved.

■ INVESTIGATIONS

To assess the extent of infection, ischemia, and systemic status, the following investigations were performed:

- *Laboratory tests*:
  - *Glycated hemoglobin (HbA1c)*: 11.3% (indicating poorly controlled diabetes)
  - *White blood cell (WBC) count*: 14,200/mm^3, suggesting infection
  - *C-reactive protein (CRP)*: 140 mg/L, elevated, indicative of significant infection/inflammation
  - *Erythrocyte sedimentation rate (ESR)*: 92 mm/h, highly elevated, suggesting chronic inflammatory state
  - *Random blood sugar (RBS)*: 340 mg/dL, confirming hyperglycemia
  - *Serum creatinine*: 1.5 mg/dL, indicating mild renal impairment
  - *Lipid profile*: Elevated low-density lipoprotein (LDL) and triglyceride levels
- *Microbiology*: *Wound swab culture*: Growth of *Klebsiella pneumoniae* and *Pseudomonas aeruginosa*, suggesting gram-negative infection
- *Imaging studies*: *Doppler ultrasound*: Ankle–brachial index (ABI) of 0.55, suggesting significant arterial disease; posterior tibial artery shows a nontriphasic waveform
  - *X-ray foot*: No evidence of bony erosion (osteomyelitis)
  - *Additional imaging*: Magnetic resonance imaging (MRI) if needed, to rule out underlying osteomyelitis

PATHOPHYSIOLOGY

Prolonged hyperglycemia in diabetes leads to both microvascular and macrovascular damage. Chronic hyperglycemia damages peripheral nerves, resulting in neuropathy and loss of protective sensation, making the foot susceptible to repeated trauma and unnoticed injuries. At the same time, peripheral arterial disease compromises perfusion, leading to tissue ischemia.[1-3] Impaired immunity in diabetic patients facilitates polymicrobial invasion, infection, and tissue necrosis, progressing to gangrene.[1,4]

DIAGNOSIS

The clinical examination, laboratory results, and Doppler findings confirm the diagnosis of a diabetic foot (Wagner Grade 4) presenting with dry gangrene of the great and second toes and a necrotic heel ulcer.[1,2,5]

DIFFERENTIAL DIAGNOSIS

- *Critical limb ischemia without diabetes*: Similar clinical picture due to arterial insufficiency, presenting with rest pain, gangrene, and nonhealing wounds[3]
- *Leprous trophic ulcer*: Chronic plantar ulcer due to sensory loss in leprosy, typically painless and located over pressure points
- *Pyoderma gangrenosum*: A rare neutrophilic dermatosis presenting with painful, rapidly enlarging ulceration and a violaceous border
- *Cutaneous mucormycosis*: Fungal infection presenting with necrotic, black eschar, and rapid progression, usually in immunocompromised patients
- *Arterial embolism*: Acute loss of perfusion due to arterial blockage, presenting with severe pain, pallor, pulselessness, and gangrene[3]

MANAGEMENT

Surgical management

- Debridement of necrotic tissue to control infection and prevent its spread[1,5,6]
- Forefoot or ray amputation if required, based on clinical and vascular assessment[6]
- Negative pressure wound therapy (NPWT) and skin grafting after achieving infection control and a clean granulating bed[5]

- *Antibiotics*: Empirical intravenous (IV) therapy with meropenem and clindamycin until culture results guide targeted therapy.[4] Adjust regimen based on sensitivity and clinical response.[4]

Diabetologist/Physician Management

- Intensive insulin therapy with a basal-bolus regimen; discontinue oral antidiabetic medications[1,5]
- Close monitoring and management of blood glucose, kidney function, acid–base status, and signs of diabetic ketoacidosis[1]
- Optimization of cardiovascular status and comorbidities[6]

Multidisciplinary Management

- Vascular surgery consultation for possible revascularization or bypass if indicated[3,6]
- Plastic surgery for reconstructive procedures and advanced wound care[6]
- Physiotherapy and diabetic education for rehabilitation, prevention of complications, and long-term foot care[1,5]

PROGNOSIS

The outcome depends largely on adequate revascularization, effective infection control, and tight glycemic management.[3,6] Without timely intervention, progression to a major amputation is highly likely.[1,5] Even after healing, the risk of recurrence remains high unless meticulous foot care, patient education, and optimal metabolic control are maintained.[1,7]

> **Clinical Pearls**
>
> ▶ An ABI < 0.7 indicates significant arterial disease and warrants early vascular consultation for possible revascularization.[2,3]
> ▶ Dry gangrene may be painless due to neuropathy, delaying patient presentation and increasing risk of complications.[1]
> ▶ Timely surgical debridement is critical for managing ischemic or infected diabetic foot wounds and preserving viable tissue.[1,6]
> ▶ Education and regular foot care can reduce the risk of reulceration and amputation by 40–50%.[1,7]
> ▶ Annual Doppler screening is recommended for high-risk diabetic patients to detect early arterial disease and guide timely intervention.[3,7]

REFERENCES

1. Lipsky BA, Berendt AR, H Gunner Deery, John M Embil, Warren S Joseph, et al.; Infectious Diseases Society of America. Diagnosis and treatment of diabetic foot infections. Plastic and Reconstructive Surgery. 2006;117(7 Suppl):212S-238S.
2. Prompers L, Huijberts M, Apelqvist J, Jude E, Piaggesi A, Bakker K, et al. High prevalence of ischemia, infection and serious comorbidity in patients with diabetic foot disease in Europe. Baseline results from the Eurodiale study. Diabetologia. 2007;50(1):18-25.
3. Hinchliffe RJ, Forsythe RO, Apelqvist J, Boyko EJ, Fitridge R, Hong JP; International Working Group on the Diabetic Foot (IWGDF), et al. Guidelines on diagnosis, prognosis, and management of peripheral artery disease in patients with foot ulcers and diabetes (IWGDF 2019 update). Diabetes Metab Res Rev. 2020;36 Suppl 1:e3276.
4. International Working Group on the Diabetic Foot (IWGDF). Diagnosis and treatment of foot infection in persons with diabetes (IWGDF 2019 update). Diabetes/Metabolism Research and Reviews. 2020;36(Suppl 1):e3280.
5. Wang X, Yuan CX, Xu B, Yu Z. Diabetic foot ulcers: Classification, risk factors and management. World Journal of Diabetes. 2022;13(12):1049-1065.
6. Hingorani A, LaMuraglia GM, Henke P, Meissner MH, Loretz L, Zinszer KM, et al. The management of diabetic foot: A Clinical practice guideline by the Society for Vascular Surgery in collaboration with the American Podiatric Medical Association and the Society for Vascular Medicine. J Vasc Surg. 2016;63(2 Suppl):3S-21S.
7. van Netten JJ, Bus SA, Apelqvist J, Lipsky BA, Hinchliffe RJ, Game F; International Working Group on the Diabetic Foot, et al. Definitions and criteria for diabetic foot disease. Diabetes Metab Res Rev. 2020;36 Suppl 1:e3268.

CHAPTER 37

Extensive Dry Gangrene of the Foot in a Diabetic Smoker

Nipul Vara

■ PRESENTATION

This patient, who is a 54-year-old female with long-standing, poorly controlled type 2 diabetes mellitus and a significant smoking history, presented with a 4-week history of blackening and hardening of the left foot. The patient noticed decreased pain and sensation despite the discoloration, along with weight loss and intermittent low-grade fever. No overt purulent discharge was observed. The condition originated from a minor injury sustained while walking barefoot.

■ EXAMINATION

- On clinical examination, the patient exhibited signs consistent with advanced dry gangrene. The affected area involved approximately two-thirds of the left foot, with black, leathery, mummified skin and a well-demarcated line above the ankle **(Fig. 1)**.
- Palpation revealed absent dorsalis pedis and posterior tibial pulses, indicating critical ischemia [ankle–brachial index (ABI): 0.3].
- There was no crepitus or fluctuance, suggesting absence of gas or deep abscess. Surrounding areas demonstrated mild erythema and slough, indicating early signs of a secondary infection.
- Neurological examination confirmed loss of protective sensation (10 g monofilament test).

■ INVESTIGATIONS

A range of laboratory and diagnostic investigations were performed to assess the patient's status and to plan further treatment.
- *Glycemic parameters*: Glycated hemoglobin (HbA1c): 10.2%; fasting blood sugar: 184 mg/dL; postprandial blood sugar: 320 mg/dL, indicating long-standing hyperglycemia
- *Inflammatory markers*: White blood cell (WBC) count: 13,200/mm^3; C-reactive protein (CRP): 92 mg/L, suggesting active infection/inflammation
- *Lipid profile*: Low-density lipoprotein (LDL) cholesterol: 162 mg/dL, indicating dyslipidemia and increased cardiovascular risk
- *Renal parameters*: Serum creatinine: 1.5 mg/dL; urine protein: 1+ and microalbuminuria present, suggesting early diabetic nephropathy
- *Vascular studies*: ABI: 0.3 (critical ischemia), Doppler study confirming absence of tibial flow
- *Cardiac evaluation*: Electrocardiogram (ECG) revealed sinus rhythm with evidence of left ventricular hypertrophy (LVH).

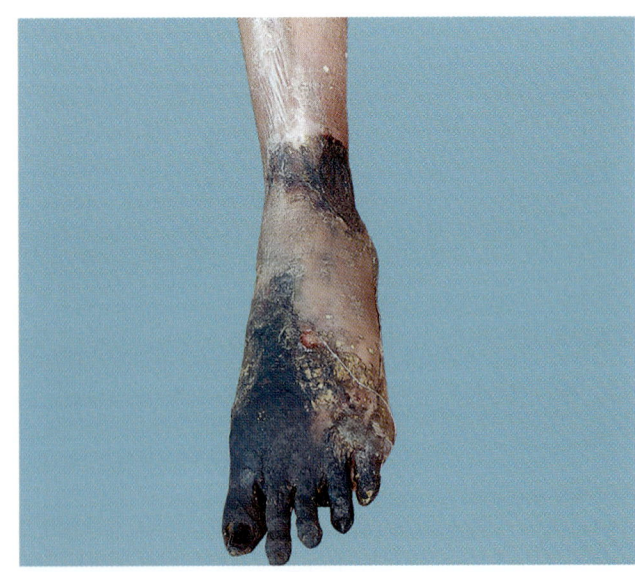

FIG. 1: Advanced dry gangrene involving two-thirds of the left foot, with black, leathery, mummified skin and a well-demarcated line above the ankle.

PATHOPHYSIOLOGY

Dry gangrene occurs due to chronic, severe ischemia caused by advanced peripheral arterial disease (PAD).[1,2] In this patient, long-standing diabetes and heavy smoking have accelerated the atherosclerosis of lower limb arteries, leading to critical arterial narrowing and blockage.[1,2] Chronic hyperglycemia damages the microvasculature and contributes to neuropathy, which prevents early detection of trauma and allows wounds to progress unnoticed.[2,3] As arterial blood flow becomes critically reduced, the affected tissue becomes dehydrated, mummified, and ultimately necrotic.[1,2] The well-demarcated area of dead tissue may later autoamputate if left untreated, making early vascular assessment and intervention crucial.[1-3]

DIAGNOSIS

Based on clinical examination and investigations, the patient is diagnosed with extensive dry gangrene of the foot in a long-standing diabetic smoker, associated with critical limb ischemia (ABI: 0.3).[1,2] This presentation is characteristic of advanced PAD compounded by diabetic neuropathy.[1-3]

DIFFERENTIAL DIAGNOSIS

Several conditions can mimic or present similarly to dry gangrene, and it is vital to distinguish them for appropriate management. The use of standardized outcome definitions, as recommended in diabetic foot care guidelines, improves diagnostic consistency and treatment planning.[4]

- *Wet gangrene*: It is associated with purulence, spreading cellulitis, and systemic signs of sepsis.[2,5]
- *Necrotizing fasciitis*: It is a rapidly progressing infection with severe toxicity, significant pain, and gas within tissue planes.[2,5]
- *Mucormycosis*: It is a fungal infection presenting with black eschar, typically seen in immunocompromised or diabetic patients, and is most common in craniofacial areas.[2,5]
- *Vasculitis*: It presents with livedo reticularis, purpura, and systemic features such as arthritis or nephritis.[2]
- *Cholesterol embolism (blue toe syndrome)*: This presents with discolored toes due to microembolization, often following vascular intervention, and associated with kidney injury.[2]

MANAGEMENT

The patient requires an urgent and multidisciplinary approach to halt disease progression, control infection, and optimize long-term outcomes.[1,2,6] Management includes both surgical and medical interventions.

SURGICAL MANAGEMENT

- *Urgent referral for amputation*: Above-ankle amputation to remove necrotic tissue and prevent the spread of infection[1,2,6]
- *Tissue biopsy*: To rule out fungal infections such as mucormycosis[2,5]
- *Debridement of surrounding slough*: To reduce the risk of superinfection and help delineate viable tissue[2,5,6]

DIABETOLOGIST/PHYSICIAN MANAGEMENT

- *Glycemic control*: Begin intensive insulin therapy (basal-bolus regimen) for tight glucose control[2,3,6]
- *Vascular protection*: Dual antiplatelet therapy (aspirin + clopidogrel) and initiation of a statin for cardiovascular risk reduction[1,6]
- *Renoprotection*: Angiotensin-converting enzyme (ACE) inhibitors for nephropathy and blood pressure control[1,6]
- *Smoking cessation*: Strong counselling and therapy for smoking cessation[1,6]
- *Microvascular screening*: Regular assessment for retinopathy, nephropathy, and neuropathy[1,3]
- *Foot care education*: Guidance on foot hygiene, use of protective footwear, and regular self-inspection to prevent future complications[2,3,6]

PROGNOSIS

Without surgical intervention, there is a high risk of ascending sepsis and systemic complications.[2,5,6] Amputation can be lifesaving in advanced dry gangrene.[1,6] The long-term prognosis depends heavily on adequate vascular control and cessation of smoking.[1,6] Patients remain at risk for recurrence in the contralateral limb.[3,6]

> **Clinical Pearls**
>
> ▶ Dry gangrene often necessitates urgent amputation.[1,2,6]
> ▶ An ABI < 0.4 is indicative of critical limb ischemia.[1,6]
> ▶ The combination of smoking and diabetes significantly accelerates the progression of PAD.[1,2]
> ▶ Do not delay debridement or surgical intervention in gangrenous wounds.[2,5,6]
> ▶ Screen all long-standing diabetic patients for PAD and neuropathy as a part of routine care.[1,3,6]

REFERENCES

1. Hinchliffe RJ, Forsythe RO, Apelqvist J, Boyko EJ, Fitridge R, Hong JP; International Working Group on the Diabetic Foot (IWGDF), et al. Guidelines on diagnosis, prognosis, and management of peripheral artery disease in patients with foot ulcers and diabetes (IWGDF 2019 update). Diabetes Metab Res Rev. 2020;36 Suppl 1:e3276.
2. International Working Group on the Diabetic Foot (IWGDF). Diagnosis and treatment of foot infection in persons with diabetes (IWGDF 2019 update). Diabetes/Metabolism Research and Reviews. 2020;36(Suppl 1):e3280.
3. Armstrong DG, Boulton AJM, Bus SA. Diabetic foot ulcers and their recurrence. N Engl J Med. 2017;376(24):2367-75.
4. van Netten JJ, Bus SA, Apelqvist J, Lipsky BA, Hinchliffe RJ, Game F; International Working Group on the Diabetic Foot. et al. Definitions and criteria for diabetic foot disease. Diabetes Metab Res Rev. 2020;36 Suppl 1:e3268.
5. Lipsky BA, Senneville É, Abbas ZG, Aragón-Sánchez J, Diggle M, Embil JM; International Working Group on the Diabetic Foot (IWGDF), et al. Guidelines on the diagnosis and treatment of foot infection in persons with diabetes (IWGDF 2019 update). Diabetes Metab Res Rev. 2020;36 Suppl 1:e3280.
6. Hingorani A, LaMuraglia GM, Henke P, Meissner MH, Loretz L, Zinszer KM, et al. The management of diabetic foot: A clinical practice guideline by the Society for Vascular Surgery in collaboration with the American Podiatric Medical Association and the Society for Vascular Medicine. J Vasc Surg. 2016;63(2 Suppl):3S-21S.

SECTION 8

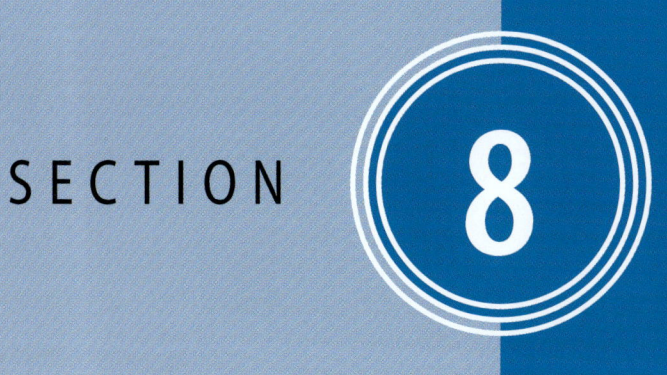

Diagnostic and Special Considerations in Diabetic Dermatology

▶ Section Outline

Chapter 38: Insulin Injection Site Reactions
Arti Muley, Akashkumar N Singh, Sona Mitra, Sudhir Kumar, Gururaj B Sattur, Suhas Gopal Erande, Anil Patki, NK Singh, Leena Singh

Chapter 39: Cutaneous Adverse Effects of Diabetes Therapies
Yashika Doshi, Bela J Shah, Twinkle C Rangnani, Tithi Shah

SECTION 8

Diagnostic and Special Considerations in Pediatric Dermatology

CHAPTER 38

Insulin Injection Site Reactions

Arti Muley, Akashkumar N Singh, Sona Mitra, Sudhir Kumar,
Gururaj B Sattur, Suhas Gopal Erande, Anil Patki, NK Singh, Leena Singh

Part A: Lipohypertrophy and Lipoatrophy

Case 1: Lipoatrophy—Subcutaneous Insulin-induced Localized Lipoatrophy in a Type 1 Diabetic Female

■ PRESENTATION

A 19-year-old woman with a 5-year history of type 1 diabetes mellitus (T1DM) presented with sharply defined, sunken patches at her insulin injection sites over the abdomen, buttocks, thighs, and arm. These areas had started as small depressions and gradually enlarged over time, without associated pain or tenderness.
- She was receiving recombinant human insulin for glycemic control.
- Her medical history was significant for an open cholecystectomy with cystogastrostomy in 2020, performed for cholelithiasis and a pancreatic pseudocyst following an episode of necrotizing pancreatitis.

■ EXAMINATION

On examination, smooth, sharply defined, atrophic lesions measuring 2–5 cm in diameter were noted at insulin injection sites. These included the abdomen (**Figs. 1A to D**), buttocks, thighs, and arm (**Fig. 2**). The largest lesion extended through the subcutaneous fat to the muscle fascia. The overlying skin appeared normal in color and texture but felt firm and fibrous compared to the surrounding tissue.

■ DIAGNOSIS

Subcutaneous insulin-induced localized lipoatrophy (LA) is associated with recombinant human insulin therapy in a T1DM patient.[1-3]

■ DIFFERENTIAL DIAGNOSIS

Dermatological Mimics
- *Morphea*: Sclerotic, indurated plaques
- *Lichen sclerosus*: Porcelain-white, atrophic plaques, and typically genital
- *Lupus panniculitis*: Inflammatory nodules progressing to atrophic depressions
- *Atrophoderma of Pasini and Pierini*: Noninflammatory, sharply demarcated depressions with "cliff-drop" borders

Injection/Drug-related Atrophy
- *Steroid-induced atrophy*: Superficial, telangiectatic, and linear atrophy

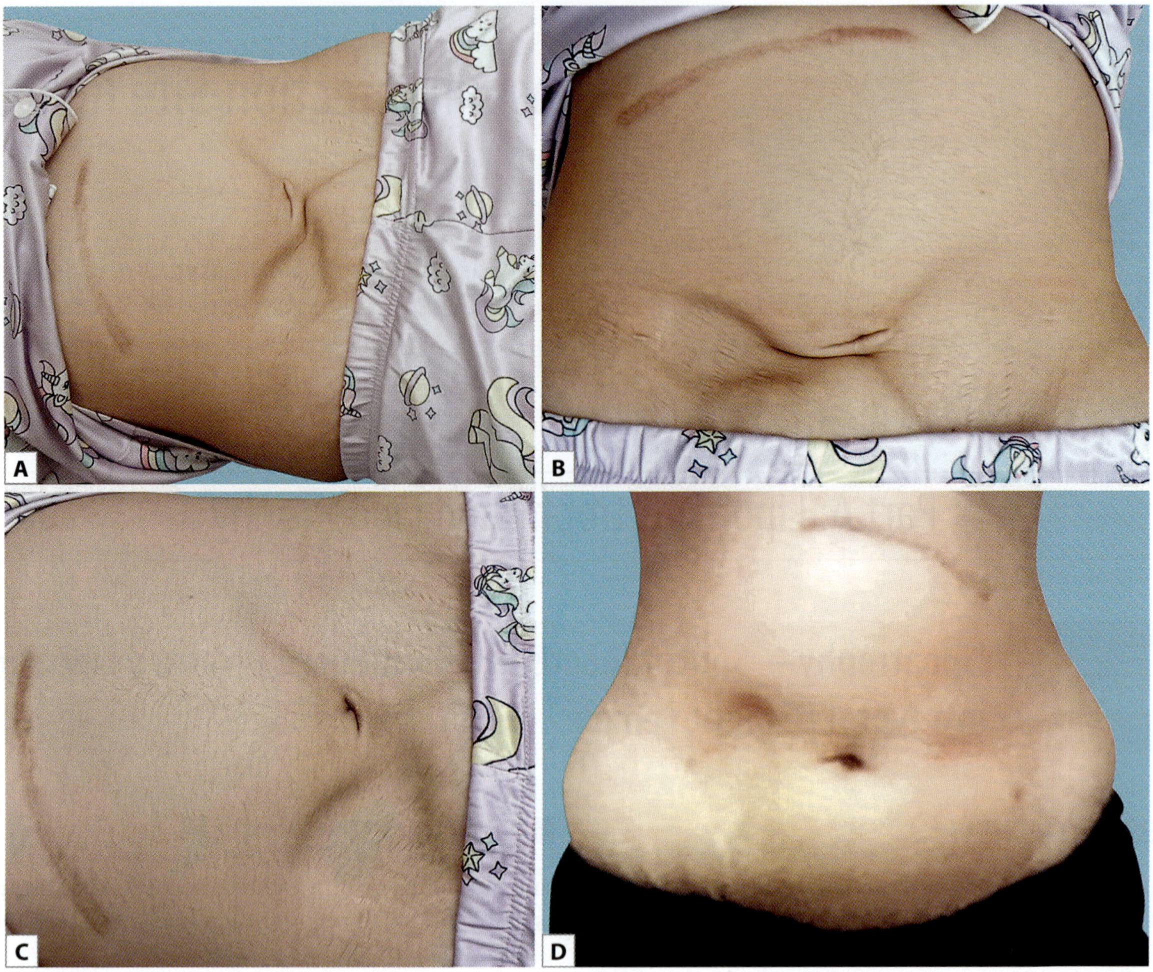

FIGS. 1A TO D: Lipoatrophy at the abdomen: (A) Lateral view, with scar of past cholecystectomy; (B) Coronal view; (C) Superior view; (D) Frontal view.

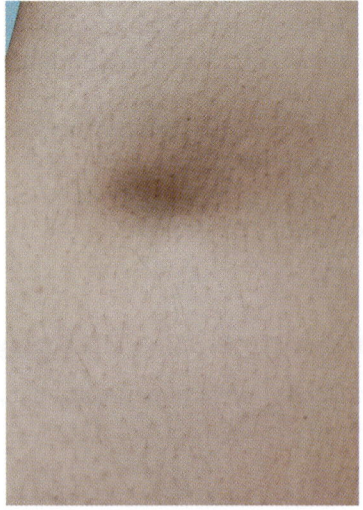

FIG. 2: Lipoatrophy in the posterior arm.

- *Postinjection granulomas*: Central depression following vaccine or drug injection

Lipodystrophic Syndromes

- *Partial lipodystrophy (LD)*: Autoimmune or familial fat loss, not restricted to injection sites
- *Postsurgical atrophy*: Depression resulting from surgical scars
- *Neoplastic mimics*: Includes cutaneous T-cell lymphoma, panniculitis

■ PATHOPHYSIOLOGY

The most widely accepted mechanism for insulin-induced LA is immune-mediated injury. Biopsies often reveal anti-insulin antibodies, immune complex deposits, and inflammatory cell infiltrates, including eosinophils and mast cells.[2,4] Elevated cytokines such as tumor necrosis factor alpha (TNF-α) and interleukin 6 (IL-6) disrupt adipocyte differentiation and function, resulting in apoptosis and loss of subcutaneous fat.[4] Histopathology typically demonstrates a lack of subcutaneous fat, lymphocytic infiltration, and mast cell predominance in the affected regions.[2,4]

IMPACT ON DIABETES MANAGEMENT

Erratic insulin absorption from lipoatrophic areas causes unpredictable glycemic fluctuations, increasing the risk of both hypoglycemia and rebound hyperglycemia.[3-5] Patients may require higher insulin doses when injecting into these areas, while switching to normal tissue can lead to excessive insulin action and hypoglycemia. Glycated hemoglobin (HbA1c) may remain elevated despite adherence to therapy due to these absorption abnormalities.[1,5,6]

MANAGEMENT

Dermatology Management

- Discontinue insulin injections at lipoatrophic sites immediately.[1,4,7]
- Rotate injection sites systematically (abdomen, arms, and thighs).[5,7,8]
- Consider topical or intralesional corticosteroids such as dexamethasone.[1,4]
- Topical sodium cromolyn 4% may help by stabilizing mast cells.[1,7]
- In refractory cases, options include topical tacrolimus, phototherapy, or systemic immunomodulators; autologous fat grafting may be considered for cosmetic improvement.

Diabetology/Physician Management

- Switch from recombinant human insulin to insulin analogs (e.g., glargine and lispro).[1,2]
- Use insulin pens with fine needles to minimize trauma.
- Educate patients on proper injection technique, including angle, site rotation, and needle changes.
- Monitor for glycemic variability, lipohypertrophy (LH), and anti-insulin antibody titers.
- Reassess HbA1c after 8–12 weeks of site rotation.

Prognosis

Cosmetic changes may persist even after discontinuing insulin at the affected sites, though some improvement can occur over 6–12 months with proper management and metabolic correction. Relapse is rare if insulin analogs are used and injection hygiene is maintained.[4,5,7] The prevalence of LA is now below 2% due to the use of purified insulin, but awareness remains important.

> **Clinical Pearls**
>
> Suspect localized LA in patients with unexplained glycemic instability or visible skin depressions at insulin injection sites.[4,5] Distinguishing LA from LH is essential, as each affects insulin absorption differently. LA can occur with any type of insulin, including recombinant human insulin, though it is more common with older formulations.[2,4] Young women with autoimmune backgrounds are most frequently affected. Histological confirmation is supportive but not always necessary for diagnosis.

REFERENCES

1. Azriouil M, Guissi L, Kamel F, Moussaid N, Rifai K, Iraqi H, et al. Lipoatrophy in type 1 diabetes treated by human insulin: a case report. EJEA. 2022;81:EP276.
2. Breznik V, Kokol R, Luzar B, Miljković J. Insulin-induced localized lipoatrophy. Acta Dermatovenerol Alp Pannonica Adriat. 2013;22(4):83-5.
3. Kondo A, Nakamura A, Takeuchi J, Miyoshi H, Atsumi T. Insulin-induced distant site lipoatrophy. Diabetes Care. 2017;40(6):e67-8.
4. Gentile S, Strollo F, Ceriello A; AMD-OSDI Injection Technique Study Group. Lipodystrophy in insulin-treated subjects and injection-site reactions: Are we sure everything is clear? Diabetes Ther. 2016;7(3):401-9.
5. Chantelau EA, Praetor R, Praetor J, Poll LW. Relapsing insulin-induced lipoatrophy, cured by prolonged low-dose oral prednisone: a case report. Diabetology & Metabolic Syndrome. 2011;3:33.
6. Singha A, Bhattarcharjee R, Ghosh S, Chakrabarti SK, Baidya A, Chowdhury S. Concurrence of lipoatrophy and lipohypertrophy in children With Type 1 Diabetes using recombinant insulin. Clin Diabetes. 2016;34(1):51-3.
7. Elsayed S, Soliman AT, De Sanctis V, Fawzy D, Ahmed S, Alaaraj N. Insulin-induced lipodystrophy and predisposing factors in children with type 1 diabetes mellitus (T1DM) in a tertiary care Egyptian center. Acta Biomed. 2023;94(3):e2023078.
8. Richardson T, Kerr D. Skin-related complications of insulin therapy: epidemiology and emerging management strategies. American Journal of Clinical Dermatology. 2003;4(10):661-7.

Case 2: Lipohypertrophy

■ PRESENTATION

A 35-year-old female with T1DM for over 18 years, employed in the IT sector, presented with thickened, rubbery swellings over her insulin injection sites. Her diabetes control had been excellent with HbA1c consistently between 6.4 and 6.8%, and she had two successful pregnancies without maternal or fetal complications. Despite glycemic stability, she began noticing firm swellings at injection sites, which had developed insidiously over time.

■ EXAMINATION

On clinical inspection, the patient had multiple, localized, thickened, and rubbery plaques at commonly used subcutaneous insulin injection sites (**Figs. 1A to C**). These swellings were more palpable than visible and showed increased density of subcutaneous tissue without erythema or pain. The lesions were consistent with grade 1–2 LH.

- *Grade 1*: Increased palpable density, and no visible skin changes
- *Grade 2*: Severe hypertrophy, and firm nodular thickening[1,2]

■ INVESTIGATIONS

- *Routine metabolic panel*: HbA1c 6.4–6.8%, glucose variability noted in continuous glucose monitor (CGM)

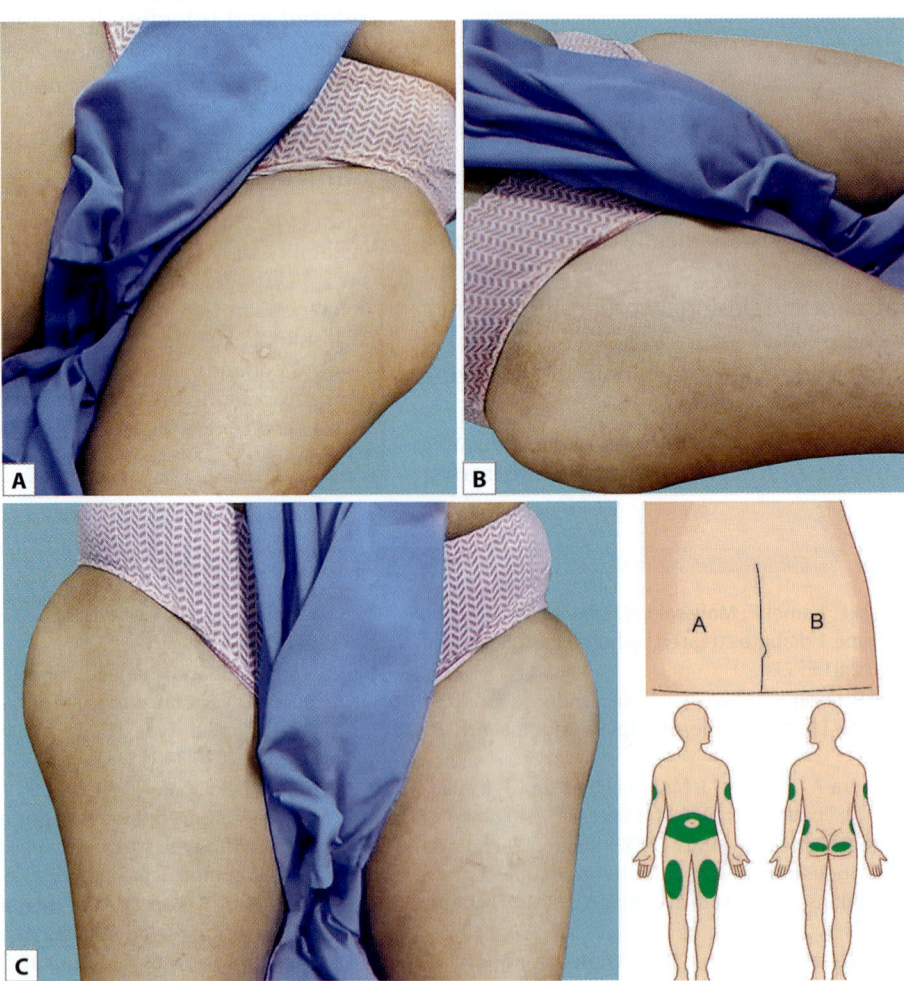

FIGS. 1A TO C: Multiple localized, thickened, and rubbery plaques at commonly used subcutaneous insulin injection sites.

- *Ultrasound of injection sites*: Hyperechoic areas with increased echotexture, confirming subcutaneous fat hypertrophy
- *Optional (if atypical)*:
  - Computed tomography (CT) or magnetic resonance imaging (MRI) if localized amyloidosis suspected
  - Histopathology (rarely indicated) in unresolved or atypical cases

■ DIAGNOSIS

Insulin-induced *LH*—a localized thickening of subcutaneous fat at insulin injection sites due to repeated insulin exposure and poor rotation technique.[1-3]

■ ETIOPATHOGENESIS AND RISK FACTORS

Lipodystrophy is a well-known complication of subcutaneous insulin injections. It can manifest as either *LH* or *LA*.
- *Lipoatrophy* refers to the development of deep, retracted scars on the skin due to damage to subcutaneous fatty tissue.
- *Lipohypertrophy* is characterized by the development of *thickened, rubbery swellings* at insulin injection sites. These are mostly firm but can occasionally appear soft. Due to their subclinical nature, LH lesions are often *missed during routine medical examinations*.

While the exact cause of LH remains unclear, the following mechanisms and associations are implicated:
- *Insulin's growth-promoting properties*: Prolonged exposure of adipose tissue to insulin stimulates local growth of fat cells, leading to hypertrophic swellings.
- *Repeated trauma* from:
  - Poor injection technique
  - Inadequate or infrequent site rotation
  - Reuse of insulin needles, causing localized injury and tissue remodeling

Additional *risk factors* known to be associated with LH include:
- *Female sex*—higher prevalence observed
- *Low socioeconomic status*—may contribute due to limited access to fresh needles and training
- *High body mass index (BMI)*—increased subcutaneous fat layer and potential under-rotation
- *Long-standing diabetes and prolonged insulin use*—cumulative exposure increases the likelihood of LH

■ DIFFERENTIAL DIAGNOSIS

- *Lipoatrophy*: Localized fat loss, retracted scars, and typically seen with older animal insulins[4]
- *Localized insulin-derived amyloidosis ("insulin ball")*: Firm mass, requires imaging or biopsy for differentiation[1]
- *Infectious abscess*: Painful, erythematous, and systemic signs—absent in this case
- *Benign lipoma*: Mobile, soft, slow growing; not typically site-specific or firm/rubbery

■ MANAGEMENT

Dermatologist Management

- *Diagnosis confirmation*: Clinical and imaging support[3]
- *Differentiation*: From amyloidosis or other dermal pathology[1]
- *Rare interventions*:
  - Cosmetic surgery in disfiguring or amyloid cases
  - Trials with *topical steroids* (e.g., dexamethasone)[5] or *cromolyn sodium* in select LA cases[6]

■ PHYSICIAN/DIABETOLOGIST MANAGEMENT

- *Injection technique training*:
  - Rotate injection sites consistently[1,2,7]
  - Avoid injecting into LH areas[3]
  - Discard needles after each use; do not reuse[2]
  - Use shorter, modern needles to reduce trauma[8]
- *Glycemic control optimization*:
  - Adjust insulin dose when shifting away from LH sites to prevent hypoglycemia[3]
  - Educate on erratic absorption risks from LH areas[1]
- *Monitoring*:
  - Periodic inspection and palpation of injection sites at each diabetes visit[1,2]
  - Continuous glucose monitor or self-monitoring blood glucose (SMBG) to assess glucose variability and adjust therapy accordingly[3]

Clinical Pearls

▶ Lipohypertrophy occurs in up to *34% of T1DM* and *49% of insulin-treated* type 2 diabetes mellitus *(T2DM)* patients.[2,9]
▶ Poor site rotation and needle reuse are major contributors.[2,7]

- Lipohypertrophy results in erratic insulin absorption, unpredictable glycemia, and increased insulin requirement.[1,3]
- Early identification and site rotation restore insulin sensitivity and reduce glycemic variability.[3]
- Severe or long-standing LH may require imaging to exclude rare complications such as amyloidosis.[1]
- *Key tip*:
  - Always *palpate—not just inspect—the injection sites* during follow-up.[1]
  - *Missed diagnosis of LD can have significant clinical consequences*: Insulin injected into LD areas can cause wide glucose fluctuations, delayed and erratic absorption, increased insulin requirements, and unexplained hypoglycemic episodes (including rebound hypoglycemia). These glycemic oscillations may not respond to dose changes, increasing both patient and healthcare system burden.
  - *Systematic identification of LH areas is crucial*: Educating patients on good injection habits, proper site rotation, and avoiding affected areas can improve glycemic control, reduce hypoglycemia risk, and decrease economic burden.[1,7]

- *Unusual facts*: In extreme cases, insulin-derived localized amyloidosis ("insulin ball") may occur, requiring cosmetic surgery. Imaging (ultrasound/CT) can differentiate amyloidosis from LH. Early detection of LA with ultrasound is important to prevent further injections at those sites. No specific treatment for LA exists, but anecdotal success has been reported with dexamethasone and cromolyn sodium.
- *Needles and devices*: Faulty or mismatched devices and repeated needle use increase tissue injury risk. Needle lengths should be as short as possible to minimize trauma and avoid inadvertent intramuscular administration, especially in lean individuals.
- The irregular insulin absorption associated with LH can lead to a higher risk of serious hypoglycemic episodes followed by rebound hyperglycemia when patients switch from affected injection sites to unaffected ones. These glucose fluctuations pose significant challenges in achieving stable glycemic control and can have detrimental effects on patients' overall metabolic health.

REFERENCES

1. Gentile S, Strollo F, Ceriello A; AMD-OSDI Injection Technique Study Group. Lipodystrophy in insulin-treated subjects and injection-site reactions: Are we sure everything is clear? Diabetes Ther. 2016;7(3):401-9.
2. Al Hayek AA, Robert AA, Braham RB, Al Dawish MA. Frequency of lipohypertrophy and associated risk factors in young patients with type 1 diabetes: a cross-sectional study. Diabetes Ther. 2016;7(2):259-67.
3. Thewjitcharoen Y, Prasartkaew H, Tongsumrit P, Wongjom S, Boonchoo C, Butadej S, et al. Prevalence, Risk Factors, and Clinical Characteristics of Lipodystrophy in Insulin-Treated Patients with Diabetes: An Old Problem in a New Era of Modern Insulin. Diabetes Metab Syndr Obes. 2020;13:4609-20.
4. Hauner H, Stockamp B, Haastert B. Prevalence of lipohypertrophy in insulin-treated diabetic patients and predisposing factors. Exp Clin Endocrinol Diabetes. 2009;104(2):106-110.
5. Kumar O, Miller L, Mehtalia S. Use of dexamethasone in treatment of insulin lipoatrophy. Diabetes. 1977;26(4):296-9.
6. Phua EJ, Lopez X, Ramus J, Goldfine AB. Cromolyn sodium for insulin-induced lipoatrophy: old drug, new use. Diabetes Care. 2013;36(12):e204-5.
7. Baruah MP, Kalra S, Bose S, Deka J. An audit of insulin usage and insulin injection practices in a large Indian cohort. Indian J Endocrinol Metab. 2017;21(3):443-52.
8. Hirsch L, Byron K, Gibney M. Intramuscular risk at insulin injection sites—measurement of the distance from skin to muscle and rationale for shorter-length needles for subcutaneous insulin therapy. Diabetes Technol Ther. 2014;16(12):867-73.
9. Deng N, Zhang X, Zhao F, Wang Y, He H. Prevalence of lipohypertrophy in insulin-treated diabetes patients: a systematic review and meta-analysis. J Diabetes Investig. 2017;9(3):536-43.

Part B: Allergic Contact Dermatitis from Insulin Pump Adhesive

■ PRESENTATION

A 32-year-old woman with type 1 diabetes mellitus for 10 years, managed with continuous subcutaneous insulin infusion (CSII), presented with recurrent pruritic, erythematous papules and plaques beneath the insulin pump patch on her abdomen. The lesions appeared about 2 days after applying the patch were associated with mild scaling and central crusting, and consistently resolved upon removal of the device. There were no vesicles, pustules, or systemic symptoms such as fever or malaise.

EXAMINATION

- Well-demarcated, erythematous plaques and papules were localized precisely to the area under the adhesive patch **(Fig. 1)**.
- Mild induration and scaling were noted, with central crusting.
- No vesicles, pustules, or signs of secondary infection were present.

INVESTIGATION

- No blood tests were required as clinical evaluation excluded infection. Patch testing (standard allergens and device components) showed a positive reaction to isobornyl acrylate (IBOA), a known allergen in insulin pump adhesives.
- Dermatological assessment confirmed allergic contact dermatitis and differentiated it from irritant contact dermatitis.
- *Histopathology*: Skin biopsy was unnecessary in this typical case. However, if performed (e.g., in atypical or unclear presentations), it would reveal spongiotic dermatitis with a lymphocytic infiltrate, consistent with eczematous contact dermatitis.

PATHOPHYSIOLOGY

The reaction represents a type IV hypersensitivity response to monomers or acrylates, such as isobornyl acrylate (IBOA) and phenoxyethoxy ethyl acrylate, found in insulin pump patch adhesives.[1,2] Sensitization occurs after initial exposure, with elicitation of the immune response upon repeated contact; this results in a localized reaction confined to the adhesive-covered area.[1,3] Adhesive formulations vary between devices, and manufacturers often do not fully disclose component details, making identification and avoidance of specific allergens more challenging.[1]

DIAGNOSIS

- *Allergic contact dermatitis from insulin pump adhesive*: The patient's clinical features, lesion distribution corresponding precisely to the adhesive area, and positive patch test to isobornyl acrylate confirm the diagnosis of allergic contact dermatitis caused by the insulin pump adhesive.[1,2,4]
- *Diabetes correlation*: Adhesive dermatitis is increasingly reported in users of CSII and continuous glucose monitoring (CGM) devices, particularly among individuals with type 1 diabetes, affecting up to 40% of devices.[3,5] This condition can impair glycemic monitoring by reducing wear time, necessitating frequent site rotation, and in some cases, leading to discontinuation of the device.[1,3,5] While poor glycemic control may weaken skin barrier function, the allergic response itself is independent of metabolic status.[1,3]

DIFFERENTIAL DIAGNOSIS

- *Irritant contact dermatitis*: It presents immediately after exposure and does not show a positive patch test.[1,3]
- *Pressure-induced trauma or erythema*: It is typically nonpruritic and lacks spongiosis.[1]
- *Infection (cellulitis)*: It is associated with warmth, tenderness, and systemic signs, which are absent in this case.[1]
- *Lipohypertrophy/lipoatrophy*: Presents as palpable nodules without erythema or features of allergy.[1]

MANAGEMENT

Dermatological Approach

- Immediate removal of the insulin pump patch and initiation of a medium-potency topical corticosteroid for 7–10 days to reduce inflammation[1,3]
- Implementation of barrier strategies such as applying hydrocolloid or silicone-backed dressings under the patch, or using protective barrier sprays/films (e.g., Cavilon® and Brava®) to prevent direct skin contact with the adhesive[1,5,6]
- Recommendation of alternative adhesives, including nonacrylate medical tapes or the use of gateway patches

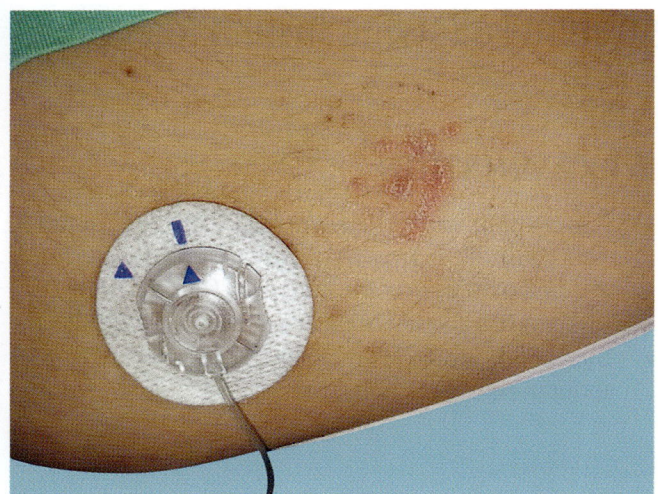

FIG. 1: Well-demarcated, erythematous plaques and papules localized to the area under the adhesive patch.

(e.g., placing a hydrocolloid dressing over the original adhesive)[1,5,6]
- Referral for patch testing in persistent or recurrent cases to identify specific allergens and guide targeted avoidance strategies[1,2,4]

Diabetology/Physician Approach

- Collaborate closely with the dermatologist and device manufacturers to identify and source allergen-free or hypoallergenic devices.[1,3]
- Advise patients on regular rotation of insulin pump sites and routine skin inspections to detect early signs of dermatitis or other local complications.[1,3]
- If allergic reactions persist despite protective measures, consider alternative glucose monitoring or insulin delivery options such as finger-prick blood glucose testing or switching to a different insulin pump system with a more suitable adhesive.[1,3]

PROGNOSIS

Prognosis is favorable with prompt allergen identification and preventive strategies.[1,3] Risks include chronic dermatitis or impaired glycemic control due to nonadherence with CSII/CGM.[1,3] Education reduces recurrence and supports device compliance.[1,3]

Clinical Pearls

▶ Any localized rash under pump patches should raise suspicion of allergic contact dermatitis.[1,3]
▶ Early referral for patch testing is crucial to identify specific adhesive allergens.[1,2,4]
▶ Barrier dressing or nonacrylate tapes are the first-line practical solutions.[1,5,6]
▶ Continue insulin pump use with adapted adhesives unless severe allergy mandates device change.[1,3]

REFERENCES

1. de Groot A, van Oers EM, Ipenburg NA, Rustemeyer T. Allergic contact dermatitis caused by glucose sensors and insulin pumps: A full review: Part 2. Case reports and case series, clinical features, patch test procedures, differentiation from irritant dermatitis, management of allergic patients and (proposed) legislation. Contact Dermatitis. 2025;92(3):164-75.
2. Herman A, de Montjoye L, Baeck M. Adverse cutaneous reaction to diabetic glucose sensors and insulin pumps: Irritant contact dermatitis or allergic contact dermatitis? Contact Dermatitis. 2020;83(1):25-30.
3. Ahrensbøll-Friis U, Simonsen AB, Zachariae C, Thyssen JP, Johansen JD. Contact dermatitis caused by glucose sensors, insulin pumps, and tapes: Results from a 5-year data. Contact Dermatitis. 2021;84(2):75-81.
4. Kamann S, Oppel E, Liu F, Reichl FX, Heinemann L, Högg C. Evaluation of isobornyl acrylate content in medical devices for diabetes treatment. Diabetes Technol Ther. 2019;21(10):533-7.
5. Lombardo F, Passanisi S, Tinti D, Messina MF, Salzano G, Rabbone I. High frequency of dermatological complications in children and adolescents with Type 1 diabetes: a web-based survey. Journal of Diabetes Science and Technology. 2021;15(3):676-83.
6. Dutta N, Crossan D, Munro N, Feher M. Skin Complication of Insulin Pump Therapy-contact dermatitis from patch pump adhesive. Br J Diabetes Vasc Dis. 2014;14:116.

Part C: Postinflammatory Hyperpigmentation Following Insulin Injections

PRESENTATION

A 21-year-old female with a 10-year history of type 1 diabetes presented with multiple, dark brown to black, well-defined macular lesions in a whorled pattern over her abdominal wall. She reported reusing the same insulin syringe (BD) for up to 15 days and had been injecting a premixed insulin combination [isophane/NPH (neutral protamine Hagedorn) 70% and soluble human insulin]. These skin lesions had persisted for >6 months.

EXAMINATION

- Skin examination revealed multiple, discrete, rounded, well-defined brown/black macules arranged in a whorled pattern over the abdomen (Fig. 1).
- No signs of infection or ulceration were noted.
- The patient appeared embarrassed and was concerned about the cosmetic appearance.

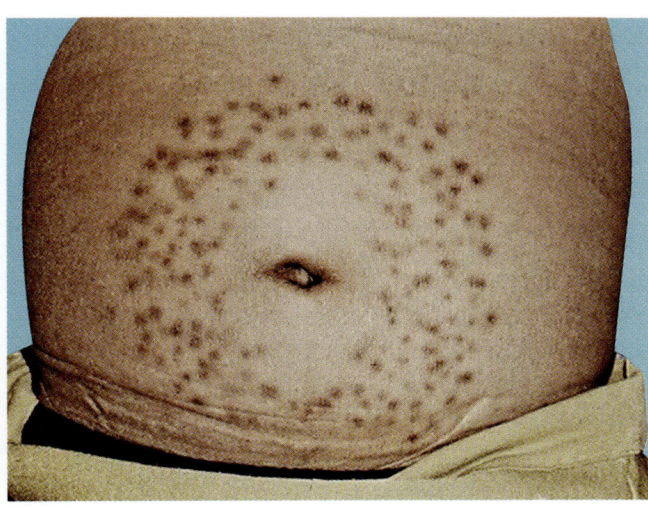

FIG. 1: Multiple discrete, rounded, well-defined brown to black macules arranged in a whorled pattern over the abdomen.

■ INVESTIGATIONS

Skin biopsy showed neutrophilic infiltration, erythrocyte extravasation, and eosinophilic amorphous material surrounded by a neutrophilic infiltrate—supporting a diagnosis of postinflammatory changes.

■ DIAGNOSIS

Postinflammatory hyperpigmentation (PIH) secondary to repeated insulin injections with reused, blunt needles, causing chronic microtrauma.[1,2]

■ DIFFERENTIAL DIAGNOSIS

- *Acanthosis nigricans*: It usually presents as velvety hyperpigmentation in intertriginous areas.
- *Fixed drug eruption*: It typically presents as dusky red to purple plaques that recur at the same site.
- *Lipoatrophy or lipohypertrophy*: It usually involves contour changes, not flat pigmentation.
- *Cutaneous amyloidosis*: It is more likely to be itchy with a rippled appearance.[2,3]

■ MANAGEMENT

Dermatological Approach

- *Counseling* on proper injection techniques to prevent trauma[1,4]
- *Topical treatment*:
  - Emollients twice daily to hydrate and repair the skin
  - Topical betamethasone ointment applied overnight on weekends (Saturday and Sunday) for 4–6 weeks to reduce inflammation and pigmentation[4]
- *Avoidance of further trauma* through patient education
- Monitor for associated conditions such as amyloidosis or acanthosis nigricans[3]

Diabetology/Physician Approach

- *Educate* the patient on safe insulin injection practices:
  - Use of *new syringe/needle* with every injection
  - *Site rotation* to avoid repeated trauma in the same area[1,2]
- *Glycemic control* optimization to prevent further skin complications
- *Assess for metabolic syndrome* or insulin resistance
- *Counsel on hygiene*, including maintaining clean and dry skin before injections
- Address psychological impact and body image concerns sensitively[5]

Clinical Pearls

▶ Postinflammatory hyperpigmentation is a *common but under-recognized* cutaneous complication of insulin injection, especially in patients using poor technique or reusing needles.[2]
▶ *Repeated microtrauma* from blunt needles is a key trigger for hyperpigmentation.[1]
▶ Proper *insulin delivery technique* is as important as the insulin type or dose.[1,4]
▶ *Patient education and counselling* play a central role in preventing such adverse effects.[4]
▶ Although *cosmetically distressing*, PIH is usually reversible over time with appropriate care and behavioral modification.[2,5]
▶ In some cases, *pigmentation may persist* from several months to years, especially if dermal pigment deposition has occurred.[5]

REFERENCES

1. Schuler G, Pelz K, Kerp L. Is the reuse of needles for insulin injection systems associated with a higher risk of cutaneous complications? Diabetes Res Clin Pract. 1992;16(3):209-12.
2. Sawatkar GU, Dogra S, Bhadada SK, Kanwar AJ. Insulin injection: cutaneous adverse effects. Indian J Endocrinol Metab. 2015;19(4):533-4.
3. Sahasrabudhe RA, Limaye TY, Gokhale VS. Insulin Injection Site Adverse Effect in a Type 1 Diabetes Patient: An Unusual Presentation. J Clin Diagn Res. 2017;11(8):OD10-OD11.
4. Schwartz RA, Elston DM. (2023). Postinflammatory Hyperpigmentation. [online] Available from https://emedicine.medscape.com/article/1069191-overview [Last accessed August, 2025].
5. E Lawrence, Syed HA, Al Aboud KM. Postinflammatory hyperpigmentation. In: StatPearls [Internet]. Treasure Island (FL): StatPearls Publishing; 2025.

CHAPTER 39

Cutaneous Adverse Effects of Diabetes Therapies

Yashika Doshi, Bela J Shah, Twinkle C Rangnani, Tithi Shah

Part A: Gliptin-Induced Bullous Pemphigoid

■ PRESENTATION

A 52-year-old male businessman presented with fluid-filled lesions over his trunk and extremities, persisting for 8 months. The lesions were pruritic and developed on erythematous, raised plaques. He also reported painful oral erosions for the past month. There was no history of genital involvement or similar lesions in the past, and no personal or family history of autoimmune disorders.

His medical history included hypothyroidism, managed with levothyroxine 50 µg once daily for 12 years. He was diagnosed with type 2 diabetes mellitus a year prior and started on metformin 500 mg once daily and teneligliptin 20 mg once daily.

■ EXAMINATION

- On examination, multiple tense bullae were observed over urticarial plaques on the upper limbs, hands **(Figs. 1A to D)**, lower limbs **(Fig. 2)**, trunk, and back.
- Oral examination revealed erosions on the soft palate and bilateral buccal mucosa **(Fig. 3)**.
- There were no signs of systemic illness.
- The patient's body mass index (BMI) was 24.6 kg/m².

■ LABORATORY FINDINGS

- Complete blood count, liver and renal function tests, and lipid profile: Within normal limits

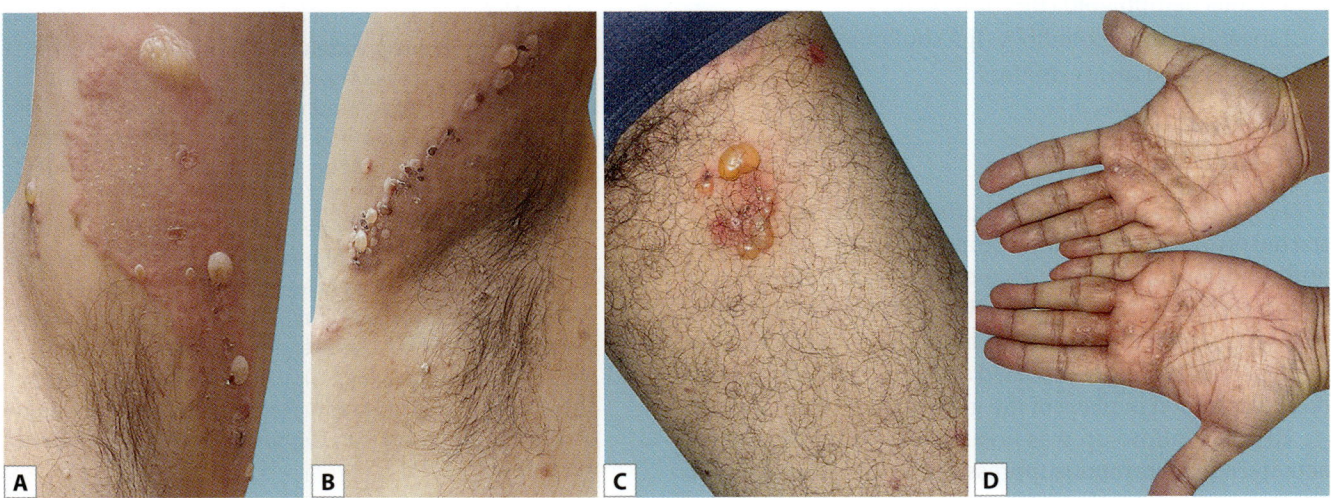

FIGS. 1A TO D: Multiple tense bullae over urticarial plaques on the upper limbs and hands.

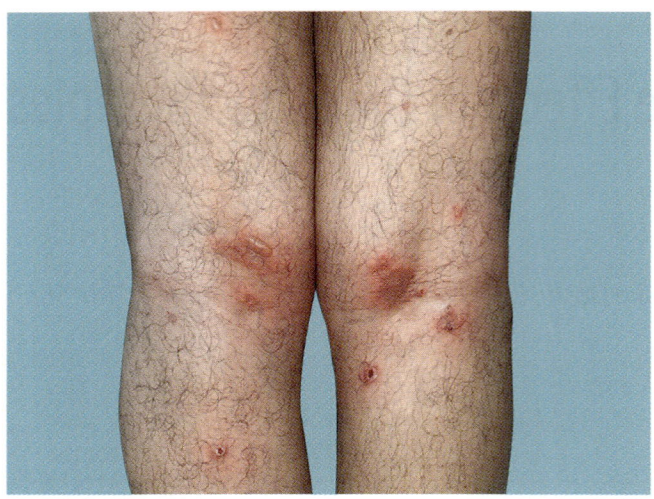

FIG. 2: Tense bullae over urticarial plaques on the lower limbs.

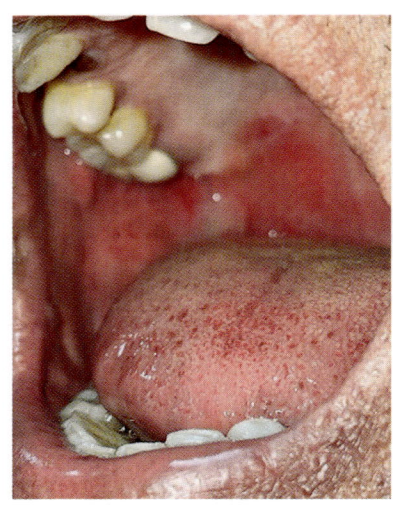

FIG. 3: Erosions on the soft palate and bilateral buccal mucosa.

- Viral markers [hepatitis B virus (HBV), hepatitis C virus (HCV), human immunodeficiency virus (HIV)]: Negative
- *Fasting blood sugar:* 156 mg/dL
- *Postprandial blood sugar:* 256 mg/dL
- *Glycated hemoglobin (HbA1c):* 6.1%
- *Skin biopsy (4 mm punch):* Subepidermal blister with eosinophilic infiltrate, consistent with bullous pemphigoid (BP)

DIAGNOSIS

Gliptin-induced BP is the diagnosis.

DIFFERENTIAL DIAGNOSIS

- Bullous pemphigoid (BP) (idiopathic)
- Linear immunoglobulin A (IgA) bullous dermatosis
- Bullous fixed drug eruption

MANAGEMENT

Teneligliptin was discontinued promptly. The patient was started on oral prednisolone (omnacortil) 20 mg once daily and azathioprine 50 mg twice daily as a steroid-sparing agent. He was referred to his physician for modification of his diabetic regimen, where metformin was continued (increased to 500 mg twice daily) and glimepiride 1 mg once daily was added in place of the gliptin.

Regular follow-up was arranged to monitor disease activity, adjust immunosuppression, and ensure glycemic control.

PROGNOSIS

Within 3 months, the patient's skin and oral lesions resolved with immunosuppressive therapy. Both prednisolone and azathioprine were tapered gradually, and the patient remained in clinical remission. No recurrence of BP was noted after gliptin withdrawal.

Clinical Pearls

- Bullous pemphigoid is a subepidermal autoimmune blistering disorder, typically occurring in the elderly.[1] While most cases are idiopathic, an increasing number have been linked to dipeptidyl peptidase 4 inhibitors (DPP-4i or gliptins) since 2011.[1-3]
- Gliptin-induced BP may present with smaller, less inflammatory bullae, less erythema, and more frequent mucosal involvement compared to classic BP.[2-4]
- Pathogenesis remains unclear, but proposed mechanisms include epitope spreading and DPP-4 receptor inhibition on keratinocytes and immune cells, leading to cytokine-mediated dermoepidermal damage.[3-5] Among gliptins, vildagliptin and linagliptin have shown the strongest association with BP.[6]
- There are no specific guidelines for managing gliptin-induced BP. The mainstay of treatment is discontinuation of the offending drug, often followed by short-term systemic or potent topical corticosteroids.[1,2,3] Most patients achieve remission without relapse after drug withdrawal.[1,2,7]
- Physicians should remain vigilant for BP as a potential adverse effect of gliptins, as early recognition and cessation of the culprit drug can significantly reduce patient morbidity.[1,2,7]

REFERENCES

1. Armanious M, AbuHilal M Gliptin-Induced Bullous Pemphigoid: Canadian Case Series of 10 Patients. Journal of Cutaneous Medicine and Surgery. 2021;25(2):163-8.
2. Kridin K, Bergman R. Association of Bullous Pemphigoid With Dipeptidyl-Peptidase 4 Inhibitors in Patients With Diabetes: Estimating the Risk of the New Agents and Characterizing the Patients. JAMA Dermatology. 2018;154(10):1152–58.
3. Khalaf Kridin, Cohen AD. Dipeptidyl-peptidase IV inhibitor-associated bullous pemphigoid: a systematic review and meta-analysis. Journal of the American Academy of Dermatology. 2021;85(2):501–3.
4. Carnovale C, Mazhar F, Arzenton E, Moretti U, Pozzi M, Mosini G, et al. Bullous pemphigoid induced by dipeptidyl peptidase-4 (DPP-4) inhibitors: a pharmacovigilance-pharmacodynamic/pharmacokinetic assessment through an analysis of the vigibase®. Expert Opin Drug Saf. 2019;18(11):1099–108.
5. Ganeva M, Gancheva T, Manuelyan K, Hristakieva E. Gliptin-induced bullous pemphigoid. Int J Clin Pharmacol Ther. 2024;62(2):89-95.
6. Varpuluoma O, Försti AK, Jokelainen J, Turpeinen M, Timonen M, Huilaja L, et al. Vildagliptin significantly increases the risk of bullous pemphigoid: a Finnish nationwide registry study. J Invest Dermatol. 2018;138(7):1659-61.
7. Béné J, Moulis G, Bennani I, Auffret M, Coupe P, Babai S, et al. French Association of Regional PharmacoVigilance Centres. Bullous pemphigoid and dipeptidyl peptidase-4 inhibitors: a case–noncase study in the French pharmacovigilance database. Br J Dermatol. 2016;175(2):296-301.

Part B: Vildagliptin-Induced Bullous Pemphigoid—Blisters Unveiled

■ PRESENTATION

A 48-year-old woman, weighing 78 kg, presented to the dermatology outpatient department with a 4-month history of severe pruritus and the development of multiple fluid-filled lesions. Her symptoms began after she was diagnosed with type 2 diabetes mellitus during a routine health check and was started on a combination therapy of metformin (1,000 mg) and vildagliptin (100 mg) once daily, taken before meals.

Initially asymptomatic, she soon experienced intense itching across her entire body, followed by the appearance of tense, fluid-filled vesicles on her forehead and oral mucosa. The oral lesions were particularly troublesome, causing significant pain and burning sensations during meals, which led to reduced appetite.

Despite receiving oral corticosteroids (prednisolone 20 mg daily), antibiotic coverage, and topical silver sulfadiazine, her condition did not improve. Over the following weeks, the lesions spread to her shoulders, axillae, flanks, trunk, back, chest, and both upper and lower limbs, eventually involving the palms, soles, face, and neck.

There was no significant personal or family history.

■ EXAMINATION

- The lesions had evolved into well-defined hemorrhagic bullae with erythematous bases, accompanied by intense pruritus and areas of superficial erosions where vesicles and bullae had ruptured.
- Crusted erosions and ill-defined crusts were noted on the face (Figs. 1 and 2), occiput, nape of neck, upper chest (Figs. 3A and B), back and buttocks (Figs. 4A and B), thighs (Fig. 5), and dorsal aspects of both the hands (Figs. 6A and B).
- Nikolsky's sign was notably negative.
- Mucosal examination revealed erythematous superficial crusts on the lower lip mucosa with restricted mouth opening.
- Diffuse erythema and erosions were also noted over the posterior fourchette.

■ INVESTIGATIONS

- Laboratory investigations revealed a markedly elevated serum immunoglobulin E (IgE) level (12,661 IU/mL) and an absolute eosinophil count of 2,160 cells/μL, which decreased with treatment. Her fasting blood glucose was 139 mg/dL, glycated hemoglobin (HbA1c) was 6.8%, and hemoglobin was 10.5 g/dL; other blood and urine parameters were within normal limits.
- A punch biopsy from a hemorrhagic bulla on the dorsum of the hand demonstrated subepidermal blistering with a dense eosinophilic and lymphocytic infiltrate along with perivascular and periadnexal lymphocytic and eosinophilic infiltration (Fig. 7). Direct immunofluorescence (DIF) was performed but returned negative.

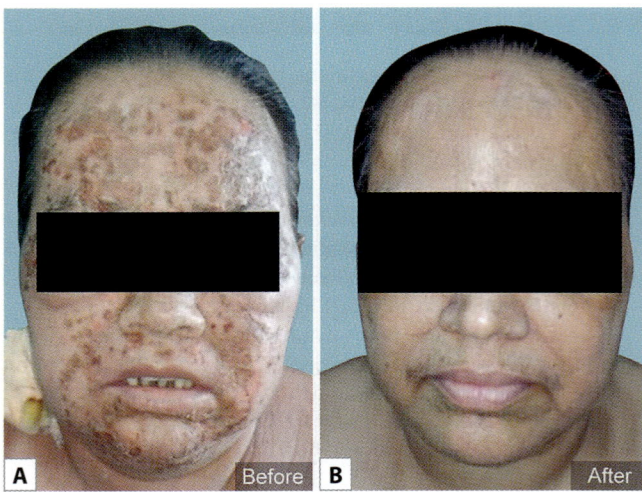

FIGS. 1A AND B: Crusted erosive lesions on face in a patient with drug-associated bullous pemphigoid (DABP).

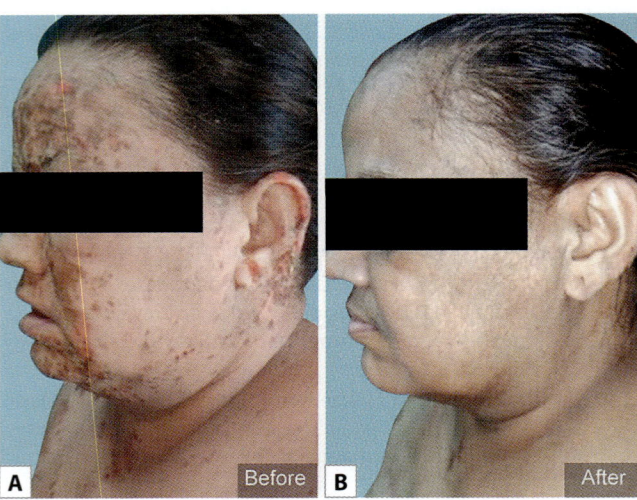

FIGS. 2A AND B: Crusted erosive lesions on face and neck in a patient with drug-associated bullous pemphigoid (DABP).

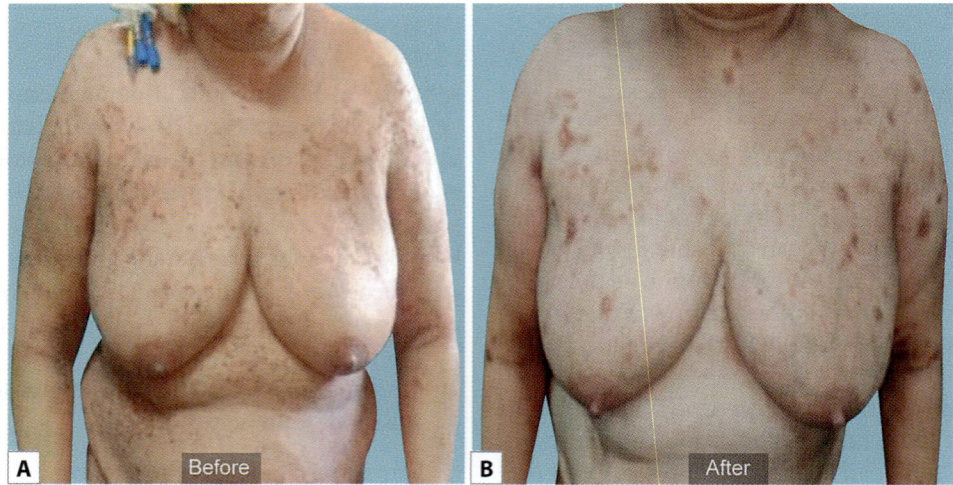

FIGS. 3A AND B: Crusted erosive lesions with bullae on chest and arms in a patient with drug-associated bullous pemphigoid (DABP).

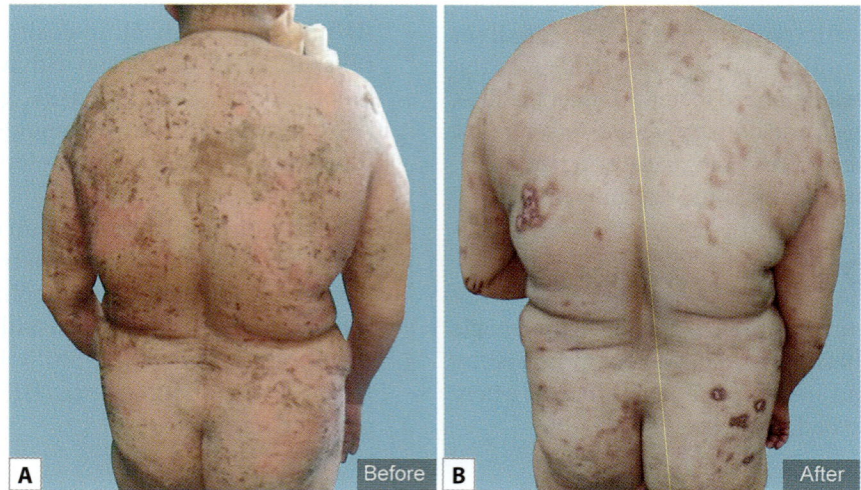

FIGS. 4A AND B: Multiple erosions with bullae on back and buttock in a patient with drug-associated bullous pemphigoid (DABP).

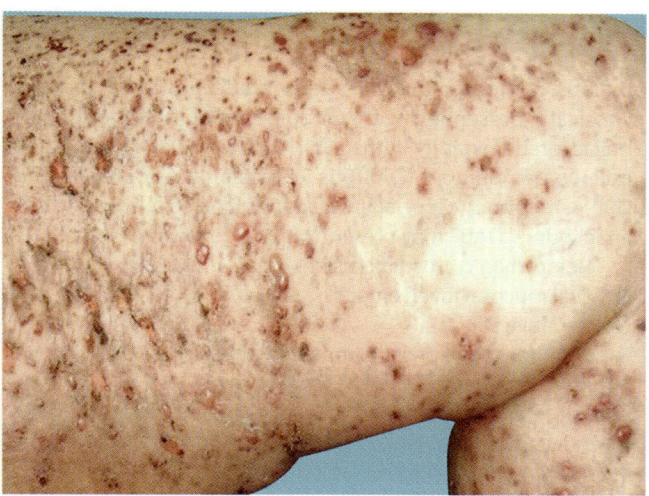

FIG. 5: Tense hemorrhagic bullae on thigh in a patient with drug-associated bullous pemphigoid (DABP).

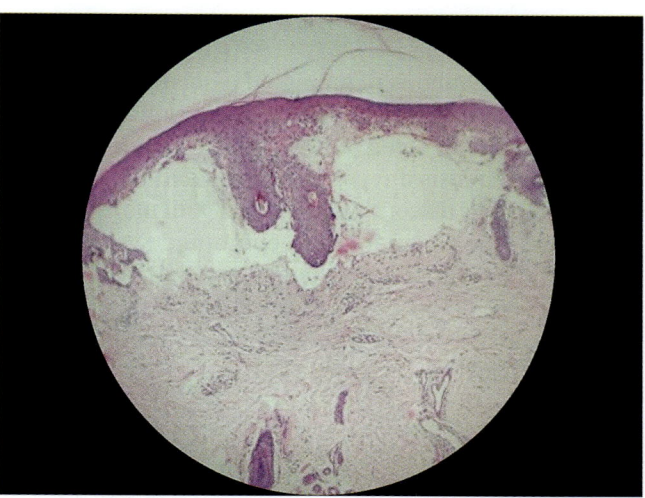

FIG. 7: Histopathological examination (H&E stain) of a patient with drug-associated bullous pemphigoid (DABP).

- Bullous fixed drug eruption
- Idiopathic (autoimmune) BP[1]

MANAGEMENT

Dermatological Management

The patient was hospitalized under dermatology care. All potentially causative medications, including vildagliptin, were discontinued. Initial therapy included intravenous dexamethasone (2 cc once daily), which was gradually tapered and transitioned to oral prednisolone (30 mg daily with milk). Cyclosporine syrup (2 mL once daily) was introduced as an adjunct immunosuppressant. Topical therapy consisted of fusidic acid with betamethasone cream, in addition to regular application of liquid paraffin and white soft paraffin as moisturizers. Wound care was optimized with sterile dressings and supportive nursing measures.[1]

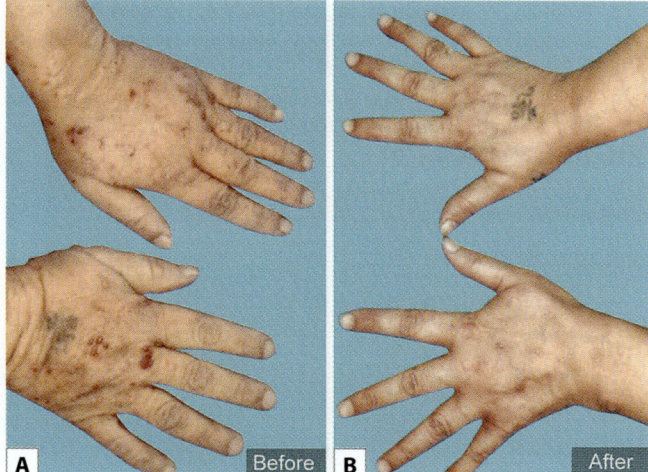

FIGS. 6A AND B: Tense hemorrhagic bullae on dorsa of hands in a patient with drug-associated bullous pemphigoid (DABP).

DIAGNOSIS

Given the clinical presentation and temporal association with vildagliptin initiation, a provisional diagnosis of drug-induced bullous pemphigoid (DIBP) was made.[1] The diagnosis was confirmed as vildagliptin-induced bullous pemphigoid (BP), supported by clinical history, histopathology, and the exclusion of other causes.[1]

DIFFERENTIAL DIAGNOSIS

- Drug-induced linear immunoglobulin A (IgA) dermatosis

Diabetological Management

Diabetes control was maintained with metformin 1,000 mg once daily, following internal medicine consultation. Glycemic status, electrolytes, and systemic parameters were closely monitored. The patient was provided with a comprehensive list of dipeptidyl peptidase 4 (DPP-4) inhibitors and other drugs associated with BP to prevent future recurrences.[1]

With this regimen, the patient's cutaneous lesions showed gradual healing, and both topical and systemic therapies were tapered over 2 months. She was counseled regarding the avoidance of implicated drug classes.[1]

PROGNOSIS

Drug-induced bullous pemphigoid associated with DPP-4 inhibitors, particularly vildagliptin, typically affects younger to middle-aged adults and is characterized by a favorable prognosis if recognized early and the offending drug is promptly discontinued.[1,2] Most patients experience significant improvement with combined systemic and topical immunosuppressive therapy, and the risk of scarring or recurrence is low if re-exposure is avoided. Relapses may occur if the patient is rechallenged with the same or similar agents.[1,2]

Clinical Pearls

Bullous pemphigoid is an autoimmune blistering disease, classically presenting with subepidermal blisters and tense bullae, predominantly in the elderly. However, drug-associated bullous pemphigoid (DABP) is increasingly recognized with DPP-4 inhibitors, especially vildagliptin and to a lesser extent, linagliptin.[1,3] DABP may present with the following:
- Hemorrhagic, crusted erosions
- Oral mucosal involvement
- Negative DIF
- Younger age of onset compared to classical BP
- More localized or atypical distribution

Prompt recognition and withdrawal of the offending drug are essential for optimal outcomes. Notably, vildagliptin carries the highest risk among gliptins for inducing BP.[1,4]

REFERENCES

1. Chouchane K, Di Zenzo G, Pitocco D, Calabrese L, De Simone C. Bullous pemphigoid in diabetic patients treated by gliptins: the other side of the coin. J Transl Med. 2021;19(1):520.
2. González Arnáiz E, Olmos Nieva C, Ariadel Cobo D, Alejo Ramos M, Ballesteros Pomar MD. A clinical case of bullous pemphigoid induced by vildagliptin. Endocrinol Diabetes Nutr (Engl Ed). 2020;67(9):613-4.
3. Pradhan SN, Mitkong M, Belgaumkar V A, Gosavi A P, Bhatt N. Unusual Presentations of Bullous Pemphigoid in Young Patients: A Case Series. J Skin Stem Cell. 2022;9(3):e131978.
4. Moro F, Fania L, Sinagra JLM, Salemme A, Di Zenzo G. Bullous Pemphigoid: Trigger and Predisposing Factors. Biomolecules. 2020;10(10):1432.

Index

Page numbers followed by *f* refer to figure.

A

Abscess 142*f*
  cutaneous 101
  formation 107*f*
  recurrent 141
  scrotal 103
Acanthosis 64*f*
  nigricans 4, 11, 12, 12*f*, 15, 59, 61, 61*f*-65*f*, 65, 148
    drug-induced 66
    malignancy-associated 66
Acne conglobata 142
Acral melanoma 167
Acrochordons 7, 59
  multiple 65
Acyclovir 112
Adalimumab 143
Addison disease 64
Advanced glycation end products 5, 6, 37, 43
Allergic contact
  dermatitis 74, 182
  vaginitis 90
Alopecia areata 14, 144, 144*f*
Altered keratinocyte functions 7*f*
Alternative classification systems 14
Amlodipine 132
Amoxicillin-clavulanic acid 96
Amputated great toe 164*f*
Amputation 164*f*, 167
  urgent referral for 173
Androgenetic alopecia 145
Anhidrosis 14
Ankle-brachial index 166
Annular elastolytic giant cell granuloma 124
Anorexia nervosa 34
Antecubital fossae 64*f*
Antibiotic 170
  therapy 110
Antifibrotic agent 119
Antinuclear antibody 139, 144
Antiplatelet therapy 168
Antiseptic washes 43
Antithyroid peroxidase 144
Apremilast 58
Arterial embolism 170
Aspartate transaminase 34
Aspirin 168
Atorvastatin 65, 111
Atrophic vaginitis 90
Atrophy
  central 24*f*
  drug-related 177
  postsurgical 178
  steroid-induced 177
Autoimmune pigmentary changes 139
Autoimmune skin disorders 12
Azathioprine 188
Azelnidipine 73

B

Bacterial folliculitis, secondary 43
Bacteroides 104
Balanitis xerotica obliterans 88
Balanoposthitis 88*f*
  candidal 88, 91
Betamethasone 191
Bilirubin, total 34
Blood
  glucose, fasting 31, 79, 111, 144
  urea nitrogen 159
Blue toe syndrome 173
Body mass index 40, 118, 156, 159
Buccal mucosa, bilateral 188*f*
Bullosis diabeticorum 8, 13, 28, 30
Bullous drug eruptions 30, 191
Bullous pemphigoid 15, 25, 31, 135, 188, 192
  drugs-associated 190*f*, 191, 191*f*, 192
  gliptin-induced 187
  vildagliptin-induced 189, 191
Burke scale 63

C

Camouflage cosmetics 140
Candida
  albicans 90
  intertrigo 11, 11*f*, 86
Candidiasis 14, 15, 86, 97
  cutaneous 93
Carbuncle 15, 99, 101, 101*f*, 105, 142
Carcinoma, scrotal 103
Carotenemia 36, 37
Carotenoderma 34, 35
Charcot arthropathy 14
Cheiroarthropathy 12
Cholecystectomy 178*f*
Cholesterol embolism 173
Chronic hyperglycemia 6, 11
  damages peripheral nerves 170
Cilostazol 154
Circulation impairment 8
Clindamycin 96, 104, 143
Collagen
  glycosylation of 41
  modification 6
Columnar cells 5
Complete blood count 31, 38, 74, 147, 163
Connective tissue manifestations 113
Contact dermatitis 111
Corticosteroids 140
  intralesional 143
  topical 43, 145
Corynebacterium minutissimum 97
C-reactive protein 147, 166
Creatinine, serum 73
Critical limb ischemia 170
Crohn's disease, cutaneous 142
Crusted erosive lesions 190*f*
Cutaneous lesions, diagnostic importance of 12
Cyclosporine 191

D

Dapagliflozin 37, 73, 93
Dark brown macules 19*f*
  multiple 147*f*
Depigmented macules 139*f*
Dermatitis herpetiformis 15
Dermatologic therapy 124
Dermatology 112, 133, 160
Dermatophytosis 14, 15
Dermatosis, acquired perforating 42, 44, 48, 49
Dexamethasone 191
Diabetes 69, 104, 95, 139
  care 124
  correlation 49
  epidemiology of 3
  management 179
  mellitus 3, 34, 46, 139, 144, 144*f*, 153
    type 1 3, 5, 7*f*, 166
    type 2 3, 5, 7*f*, 19*f*, 36, 36*f*, 42, 52, 57, 70, 89, 91, 93, 121, 134, 144, 159, 162
  uncontrolled 129
  therapies, cutaneous adverse effects of 187
Diabetic bullae 13, 15
Diabetic cheiroarthropathy 13, 14, 41, 115, 116
Diabetic cutaneous manifestations, classification of 13
Diabetic dermopathy 7, 11, 12*f*, 13, 15, 19, 22, 175
Diabetic finger pebbles 40
Diabetic foot
  abscess 95
  dermatology of 151
  gangrene 169
  screening 31
  ulcers 14, 154, 159, 160, 162, 163, 165, 165, 167
Diabetic hand syndrome 12, 115
Diabetic management 66
Diabetic microangiopathy, setting of 11
Diabetic neuropathy 15
Diabetic rubeosis faciei 38
Diabetic scleroderma 118
Diabetic toe gangrene 166
Diabetic truncal neuropathy 132
Digital necrosis 169
Dipeptidyl-peptidase 4 130
Diphenylcyclopropenone 145
Disseminated granuloma annulare 125
Distal onycholysis 79*f*, 83*f*
Distal subungual onychomycosis 80
Draining sinuses 142*f*
Drugs
  administration 143
  eruptions 14
Dry gangrene 163, 166, 168, 166*f*, 169*f*, 173
  development of 166
  extensive 172
  prognosis of 168
Dupuytren's contracture 116
Dyshidrotic eczema 74
Dyslipidemia 73, 111, 159

E

Ecchymosis 111*f*
Eczema, subacute 73, 74
Edema, neuropathic 14
Elastosis perforans serpiginosa 42
Electrocardiogram 163
Electrolytes 163
Endocrine disorders 66
Endocrine syndromes 15
Epidermal barrier
  regulation of 5*f*
  structure of 5*f*
Epidermal hyperplasia 63
Epidermal nevus 64
Epidermis 7
  structure of normal 5
Epidermoid cysts 142
Epidermolysis bullosa acquisita 25, 135
Erosions, multiple 190*f*
Eruptive xanthomas 12, 13, 13*f*, 15, 129, 130
Erythema 38*f*, 88*f*, 95*f*, 101*f*
  annulare centrifugum 82, 123
  mild 73*f*, 91*f*, 97*f*
  multiforme 124
Erythematous halo 129, 129*f*
Erythematous patches 93*f*
Erythematous plaque 86*f*, 127*f*, 183*f*
Erythrasma 15, 96, 97
Erythrocyte sedimentation rate 115, 163
Extensor limbs 44*f*

F

Facial
  acanthosis nigricans 59, 60
  damage, topical steroid-induced 39
  erythema 39
  redness 38*f*
Felon 95
Fibrotic scarring 142*f*
Finger pebbles 40
Fingernails, yellowish discoloration of 79*f*
Fissures 14, 74*f*, 91*f*
Fixed drug eruption 148
Flaccid bullae 28*f*
Folliculitis 43
  decalvans 43
  perforating 42*f*
Foot
  care education 173
  examination 155, 162
  protection 168
  ulcer, nonhealing 153
Foul smelling discharge 141
Fournier's gangrene 5, 9, 14, 103
Fungal opportunists 14
Furuncles, multiple 99*f*, 99*f*
Furunculosis 15, 99, 101
Fusidic acid 96, 112

G

Gangrene 163
  dry 163, 166, 168, 166*f*, 169*f*, 172*f*, 173
  wet 167, 173
Generalized granuloma annulare 127
Genital hygiene, poor 88
Glans
  eczema of 88
  mild erythema of 91*f*
Gliclazide 94
Glimepiride 37, 73, 111, 115, 132, 134
Glucagon-like peptide-1 140
Glucose transporter 7
Glycemic control 69, 112, 123, 130, 145, 168, 173
Glycemic management, degree of 157
Glycemic parameters 172
Glycemic profile 19, 31
Glycemic status 159
Graft-versus-host disease 68
Granulation tissue 153*f*
Granules 5
Granuloma
  annulare 15, 26, 82, 121-123, 130
  postinjection 178
Gravitational eczema 70
Great toe nail 95*f*

H

Hair
  follicle, staphylococcal infection of 99
  loss associations 144
Heel ulceration 169
Hematomas, abdominal wall 133
Hemochromatosis 64
Hemodialysis 46

Hemoglobin 73, 154, 159, 163
    glycated 31, 34, 38, 40, 73, 111, 115, 142, 144, 147, 159, 188
Hepatitis B virus 188
Herpes zoster 112
    hemorrhagic 111
Herpetic whitlow 95
Hidradenitis suppurativa 13, 103, 141, 143
High glucose environment 9
Histoid leprosy 130
Hormonal therapy 143
Human immunodeficiency virus 188
Huntley's papules 40, 41
Hurley staging system 141
Hyperbaric oxygen therapy 157
Hyperglycemia 6, 13
    chronic 6, 11
    steroid-induced 69
Hyperinsulinemia 7
Hyperkeratosis, subungual 79f
Hyperlipidemia 37
Hyperpigmentation 52f
    mild 141f
    perifocal 52f
    peripheral 21f
Hypertension 73
Hypertriglyceridemia, severe 12
Hypothenar areas 38
Hypothyroidism 34, 68, 116

I

Idiopathic guttate hypomelanosis 140
Immune
    dysfunction 11
    dysregulation 8
Immunosuppressive therapy 188
Indian epidemiology of cutaneous involvement in diabetes 4
Infections 8
    bacterial 4, 9, 11
    cutaneous 11, 77
    dermatophyte 79
    fungal 4, 9, 11, 79
    secondary 95, 163
    severe 9
    viral 11
    yeast 86
Inflamed nodules 141f, 142f
Inflammation, chronic 74
Inflammatory markers 154, 172
Ingrown toenail 95
Insulin
    fasting 59
    injection site reactions 177
    pump adhesive 182

    resistance 7, 11
    site changes 14
Intensive insulin therapy 170
Intertrigo 97
Intralesional triamcinolone acetonide 145
Inverse psoriasis 97
Ischemic necrosis 167
Itch, generalized 70
Itraconazole pulse regimen 80

J

Jaundice 36

K

Kaposi's sarcoma 15
Keratinocyte 5, 6
    growth factor 7
Keratolytics 60
    topical 43
Keratosis pilaris 41
Ketoconazole 87
Kidney disease, chronic 46
Klebsiella 104
Knuckle pads, early 41
Koebner phenomenon 139, 140
Kyrle's disease 42, 46

L

Leprous trophic ulcer 170
Lesions
    annular 124f
    magnified view of 71f
    metabolic-related 13
    pigmented 14
    typical 142
    umbilicated 52f
Levothyroxine 121
Lichen
    amyloidosis 130
    nitidus 41, 68, 122
    planus 15, 20, 68, 68f, 74
        annular 123
        pigmentosus 148
    sclerosus 88, 140, 177
    simplex chronicus 58, 68
Lichenification 57f
Lichenoid drug eruption 68
Limb ischemia, acute 167
Limited joint mobility 12, 41
Lipid
    lowering therapy 130
    parameters 37
    profile 34, 172
        assessment 37

Lipoatrophy 177, 178f
    subcutaneous insulin-induced localized 177
Lipodystrophy
    partial 178
    syndromes 178
Lipohypertrophy 14, 177, 180
Liquid paraffin emollient, liberal use of 71
Liraglutide 140
Liver
    disease, chronic 34
    function
        panels 147
        tests 31, 84, 134, 163
Low-density lipoprotein 74
Lower limbs, bilateral 46f
Lupus
    panniculitis 177
    vulgaris 25
Lycopenemia 36
Lymphadenopathy 91f

M

Macroangiopathy 8, 15
Macrovascular damage 170
Maggot infestation 162
    secondary 163
Melanocytes, stimulation of 63
Metabolic derangements, correction of 133
Metabolic profile 40
Metabolic syndrome 60, 73
Metformin 37, 60, 65, 111, 115, 122, 130, 132, 134, 156, 157, 191
Methotrexate 58, 119
Metronidazole 104
Microalbuminuria, screening for 39
Microangiopathy 7, 11, 13, 15, 74, 167
Microbiology 109
Microvascular damage 170
Microvascular thrombosis 104
Minoxidil, topical 145
Mitogen-activated protein kinases, activation of 6
Molluscum contagiosum 130
Mometasone 74
    furoate 71, 140
Monoclonal gammopathy 119, 130
Morphea 177
Motor neuropathy 8
Mucormycosis 173
    cutaneous 170
Multidisciplinary management 170
Multiple hyperpigmented macules 134f

Multiple inflammatory nodular lesions 142f
Mupirocin 96
Mycobacterium
   infection, atypical 160
      cutaneous nontuberculous 106
   skin infections 9

N

Nail
   care 80
   dystrophy 83f
   microscopy 74
Narrowband ultraviolet B 140
Nasal bridge 134f
Necrobiosis lipoidica 13, 24, 25
   diabeticorum 15
Necrobiotic xanthogranuloma 130
Necrosis, central 99f
Necrotic tissue, debridement of 170
Necrotizing fasciitis 14, 103, 163, 173
Negative pressure wound therapy 160, 170
Neoplastic mimics 178
Nephrotic syndrome 34
Nerve dysfunction 8
Neurology 133
Neuropathy 8, 11, 74, 167
   autonomic 8
   foot screening 19
   management 160
   peripheral 9
Neutrophil dysfunction 8
Nodules, erythematous 107f
Norwegian scabies 74
Numerous erythematous plaques 57f
Nutritional care 145
Nystatin 87

O

Obesity 159
Onychomycosis 79, 80, 83, 83f, 163
   lateral subungual 80
Ophthalmic evaluation 19
Opportunistic infections 9
Optimize glycemic control 20, 85
Osteomyelitis 157, 159, 160

P

Pain
   abdominal 133
   management 112
Painless blister 30f
Palm, involvement of 73f

Palmar
   cord thickening 116
   erythema 38, 39
Palmoplantar keratoderma 74
Papillomatosis 7, 63
Papular mucinosis 41
Papular urticaria 122
Papules 141f
   annular 81f, 124f
   arcuate 126f, 125f
   Huntley's 40, 41
   multiple annular 123f
   multiple umbilicated 42f
   pedunculated 65f
   skin-colored 40
   umbilicated 44f, 48f, 52f
   yellow 12
   yellow-red 129f
Papulonodular reddish-brown lesions 46f
Paracetamol 112
Paraproteinemia 130
Paronychia 96
   acute 95, 95f
   chronic 95
Pasini atrophoderma 177
Patch
   hyperpigmented 97f, 134
   testing 74
Peripheral arterial disease 167, 173
   lesions 14
Peripheral embolic infarction 167
Peripheral satellite pustules 86f
Phagocyte dysfunction 8
Phimosis 88, 88f
Phlebotomy 135
Photo-induced facial changes 39
Photosensitivity 121
Phototherapy 58, 119, 179
Phycomycosis 15
Pierini atrophoderma 177
Pigmentation, bilateral yellow-orange 34f
Pigmented purpuric dermatoses 148
Piperacillin-tazobactam 104
Pityriasis
   alba 140
   rubra pilaris 58
   versicolor 97
Plaques 123f, 124f
   hyperpigmented 65f
   urticarial 188f
Plasma glucose, fasting 34
Platelet-derived growth factor 157
Polymicrobial invasion 170
Polymorphic light eruption 122

Porokeratosis 124
Porphyria cutanea tarda 134
Postinflammatory hyperpigmentation 20, 64, 69, 140, 147, 148, 153f, 184
Postprandial blood sugar 188
Potassium hydroxide 74
Prayer sign 12
Prednisolone 188
Pressure ulcers 14
Proximal interphalangeal joints 115f
Prurigo nodularis 68
Pruritic perforating dermatosis 52
Pruritus 15, 70
Pseudohernia, abdominal 132
Pseudoporphyria 135
Psoriasis 15, 68, 74, 88
Pulses, peripheral 153, 156
Punch biopsy 48
Punched-out ulcers 156f
Purpura annularis telangiectodes 20
Purpura fulminans 111
Purulent discharge 99f, 103f
Pus discharge 101f
Pyoderma 15
   gangrenosum 25, 170

R

Random blood glucose 38, 103, 129, 159, 162
Raynaud's phenomenon 116
Reactive oxygen species 7
Reactive perforating collagenosis 42, 48-50
Refractory disease 143
Renal failure, chronic 44
Renal function
   panels 147
   tests 31
Renal parameters 19, 172
Renoprotection 173
Retinoids, topical 43, 60
Revascularization 167
Rheumatoid arthritis 116
Rhinocerebral mucormycosis 9
Rosacea 39
Rosuvastatin 73
Rough skin 6
Rubeosis faciei 38, 38f, 39

S

Salicylic acid 43
Sarcoidosis, cutaneous 26, 124
Scabies 74
Scaly plaques 74f

Scaly skin 11
Scleredema 14, 119
   diabeticorum 13, 118
Scleroderma 15, 116
Scrofuloderma 142
Scrotal ulcer, traumatic 103
Seborrheic dermatitis 58
Sensory neuropathy 8
Serum ferritin 134, 144
Serum glutamic pyruvic transaminase 73
Sexually transmitted infections 88
Shallow transverse fissures 71*f*
Shin spots 19
Silver-based dressings 160
Silvery-white scaling 57*f*
Sinus tract 105*f*
   formation 141
Skin 8
   biopsy 24, 31, 50, 74, 119, 129, 188
   changes, pathogenesis of 5
   conditions 55, 137
   dry 4, 6, 11, 70
   erythematous 31*f*
   infections
      bacterial 14, 95
      viral 111
   necrosis 103*f*
   necrotizing 108
   perfusion, reduced 7
   persistent pruritic dryness of 70
   waxy 12
      thickening of 115*f*
Smoking cessation 168, 173
Sodium 163
   cromolyn 179
   glucose co-transporter 2 74
Soft palate 188*f*
Soft tissue infections 108
Squamous cell carcinoma 25
Staphylococcal infections 9, 99
Stasis dermatitis 20, 26
Statin 168
Stiff skin syndrome 115
Stratum
   corneum 37
      barrier 6
   granulosum 5
   lucidum 5
   spinosum 5
Streptococcus 104
Subacute cutaneous lupus erythematosus 82
Subcutaneous insulin injection sites 180*f*

Subepidermal blisters 192
Subungual debris 83
Superficial fissuring 73*f*
Swollen lateral nail fold 95*f*
Swollen mass 105*f*
Syphilis, secondary 145
Systemic antifungal therapy 80, 84
Systemic lupus erythematosus 135

T

Tacrolimus 74, 179
T-cell lymphoma 58
Telmisartan 73
Telogen effluvium 145
Tenosynovitis 116
Tense bullae 188*f*, 191*f*
   multiple 31*f*, 187*f*
Terbinafine 84
Thyroid
   dysfunction 130
   monitoring 69
   stimulating hormone 69, 115, 129, 139
Tinea 79
   corporis 26, 58
      extensive 81
   cruris 97
   manuum 74
   pedis 14
   versicolor 140
Tissue biopsy 173
Topical therapy 26, 80
Total leukocyte count 163
Tranilast 119
Transepidermal water loss 5, 6
Trichomoniasis 90
Trichoscopy 144
Trichotillomania 145
Triglyceride 74
   serum 129
Trophic ulcer, nonhealing 156
Tropical ulcer 163
Tubercular epididymo-orchitis 103
Tumor necrosis factor alpha 179

U

Ulcer 24*f*, 89*f*
   chronic venous 154
   extensive 153*f*
   multiple punched-out 109*f*
Urinalysis 38, 163
Urinary albumin-to-creatinine ratio 71
Urinary porphyrin profile 134

Urine
   analysis 31
   output 163
   routine 93

V

Vaginal discharge 89*f*
Vaginitis, inflammatory 90
Vaginosis, bacterial 90
Varicella zoster virus 112
Vascular disease, peripheral 160
Vascular endothelial growth factor 6, 7
Vascular studies 172
Vascular surgery management 154
Vasculitis 173
Very-low-density lipoproteins 130
Vesicles, hemorrhagic 111*f*
Vildagliptin 191, 192
   initiation 189, 191
Viral markers 111, 188
Vitamin
   B12 139
   D3 level 144
Vitiligo 14, 15, 139, 140
Vulvar edema, mild 89*f*
Vulvovaginitis, candidal 89, 90

W

Warts, flat 41
Weight reduction 64
Wickham's striae 68*f*, 69
Wood's lamp examination 134, 139
Wound 162*f*
   care 102, 104, 109, 157, 167
   evaluation 159
   follow-up 160
   gangrenous base of 162*f*
   surgery management 160
   swab 163
   traumatic 163
Wrists, flexural surfaces of 68*f*

X

Xanthelasma 15
Xanthogranuloma, juvenile 130
Xanthomatosis 15
Xerosis 4, 6, 11, 70, 70*f*, 74

Z

Ziehl–Neelsen stain 25
Zoon's balanitis 88